Innovative Injectable Techniques in Minimally Invasive Aesthetics

Won Lee
Editor

Innovative Injectable Techniques in Minimally Invasive Aesthetics

Biostimulators, Botulinum Toxin, and Hyaluronic Acid Fillers

Springer

Editor
Won Lee
Yonsei E1 Plastic Surgery Clinic
Anyang, Kyonggi-do, Korea (Republic of)

ISBN 978-981-95-2160-9 ISBN 978-981-95-2161-6 (eBook)
https://doi.org/10.1007/978-981-95-2161-6

This Springer imprint is published by the registered company Springer Nature Singapore Pte Ltd.
The registered company address is: 152 Beach Road, #21-01/04 Gateway East, Singapore 189721, Singapore

Contents

1 **Basic Anatomy for Injectables** 1
Seong Hwan Kim and Won Lee

2 **Target-Specific Sandwich Technique (TSST)** 13
Lim Tingsong and Won Lee

3 **Injectable Biostimulators in Regenerative Aesthetics: Mechanisms, Clinical Applications, and Synergistic Approaches** 25
How Kang Nien, Rungsima Wanitphakdeedecha, and Won Lee

4 **Infraorbital Filler Injection: Advanced Techniques, Adverse Effects and Their Management** 41
Sabrina Shah-Desai and Won Lee

5 **Lower Face Contouring and Rejuvenation with HA Fillers** 61
Juyoung Go and Won Lee

6 **Delayed Inflammatory Reaction Induced by Hyaluronic Acid Filler** 83
Won Lee

7 **Perioral Rejuvenation with Variable Injectables** 93
Kyu Hwa Jung and Won Lee

8 **New Techniques for Ultrasound-Guided Hyaluronic Acid Filler Injection** 107
Benjamin Ascher, Audrey Melin, and Won Lee

9 **Artificial Intelligence and Injectables in Cosmetic Dermatology** 119
Diala Haykal and Won Lee

10 **Superficial Injections to Enhance the Infraorbital Area: When Deep and When Superficial** 139
Marina Landau and Won Lee

11 **Facial Overfilled Syndrome (FOS): Pathophysiology, Diagnosis, and Management** 147
Lim Tingsong and Won Lee

12 Injectables for Hair Loss Treatment 153
Jino Kim and Won Lee

13 Advanced Techniques in Botulinum Toxin Injection 171
Jeongmok Cho and Won Lee

14 Needleless Injection 189
Changwoon Yun and Won Lee

Editors and Authors

About the Editor

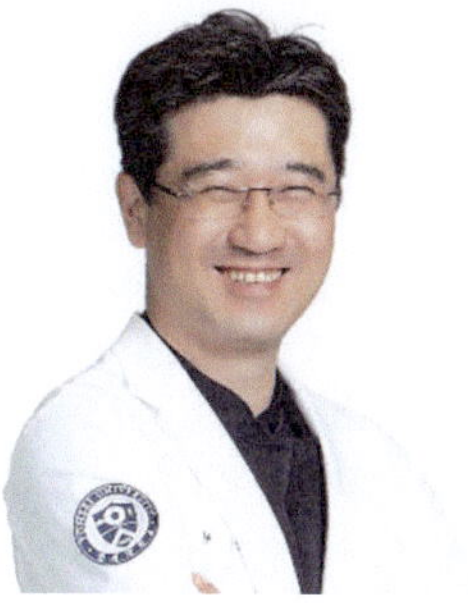

Won Lee is a plastic surgeon. He received his MD from Yonsei University Medical College and PhD from the College of Medicine, Dongguk University, Seoul, South Korea. Currently, he is the Director of Yonsei E1 Plastic Surgery Clinic, Anyang. He is the member of the Korean Society of Plastic and Reconstructive Surgeons, and he is the president of Minimal Invasive Plastic Surgery association from 2022 to 2025. He wrote has published book such as *Filler Complications*, Springer 2019; *Safe Filler Injection Techniques*, Springer 2022; *Minimally Invasive Aesthetic Surgery Techniques*, Springer 2022; *Advances in Hyaluronic Acid Filler Injections*, Springer 2024; and *Lifting Techniques in Plastic Surgery*, Springer 2025. He has published 73 articles about plastic surgery fields until 2025, and he received the "best paper award" from Plastic and Reconstructive Surgery at 2021.

About the Authors

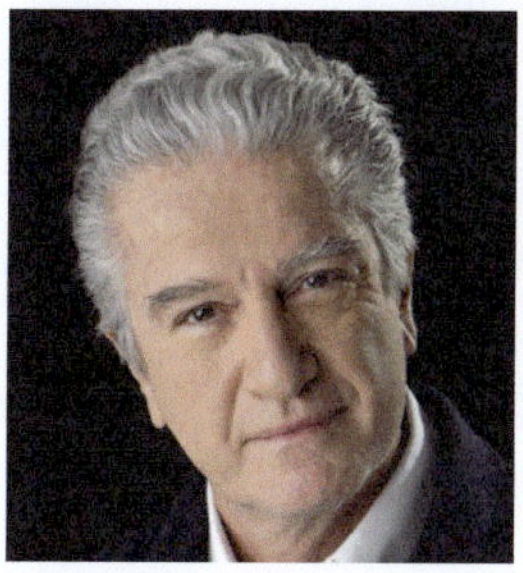

Benjamin Ascher, MD is a board-certified Plastic Surgeon, member of the French, American, and International Societies of Plastic, Reconstructive and Aesthetic Surgery (SOFCPRE, SOFCEP, ASPS, ISAPS).

He is Past Chief Resident, Assistant des Hôpitaux de Paris, and Chairman and Head of the "Clinique of Aesthetic Surgery IENA" in Paris, France.

He is the Founder and President of the I.M.C.A.S company, world leader in medical conferences (Paris, Bangkok, Bali, Cancun, Cartagena, Mumbai,

Goa, Shanghai), dealing with the interface between Plastic Surgery, Cosmetic Dermatology, and Aesthetic Medicine.

The ThinkIn company: leader with VIP Hands on Classes dedicated to Anatomy, Minimal Invasive Live Treatments, Injection and threads Simulator, and Ultrasonography for Injections.

Editor of IMCAS Academy, e-learning digital platform connected with one of the most important networking of the profession.

He is a Member of the International Editorial Board of the *Aesthetic Surgery Journal* (ASJ), Section Editor of the *Aesthetic Plastic Surgery Journal* (APSJ), and Member of the Editorial Board for *Journal of Cosmetic and Laser Therapy*, as well as author of 200 original articles and books published in referenced journals, and review articles.

He works extensively in research and clinical studies-related aesthetic surgical and medical procedures (toxins, fillers, anatomy, ultrasonography, regenerative medicine, lasers and energy-based devices for skin tightening and lipolysis, threads, fat grafting, facelift, and eyelids surgery).

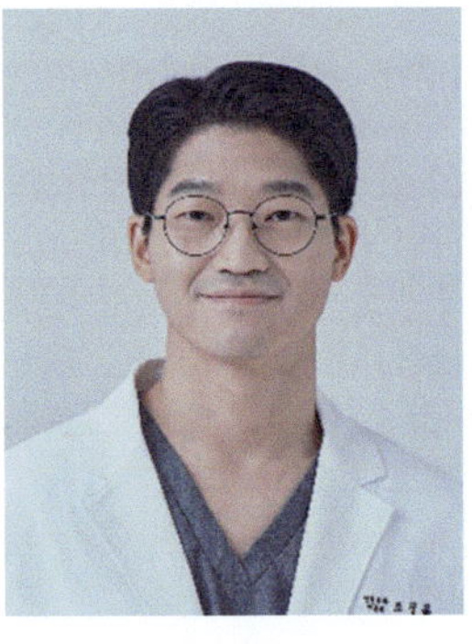

Jeongmok Cho based in Seoul, South Korea, is a globally recognized expert in minimally invasive cosmetic surgery, breast aesthetic surgery, and anti-aging facial surgery. He has made remarkable achievements in the field of plastic surgery with various international lectures and publications. His work focuses on advancing innovative techniques in facial rejuvenation and breast surgery. His clinic has become a sought-after destination for patients from across Asia, including China, Japan, and Taiwan, who seek cutting-edge cosmetic procedures. Besides, he has played an important role in training physicians from these regions, providing hands-on education in advanced surgical techniques. His international collaborations with top institutions and researchers position him at the forefront of minimally invasive nonsurgical treatments in aesthetic medicine.

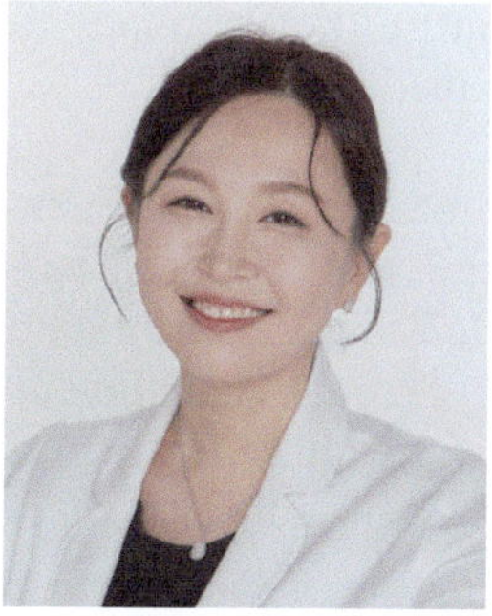

Juyoung Go, MD, PhD, is a board-certified plastic surgeon and the director of Atelier Plastic Surgery Clinic in Seoul, South Korea. She specializes in breast surgery and minimally invasive plastic surgery, combining clinical expertise with academic research. She is a Clinical Professor at Sungkyunkwan University School of Medicine and a consultant for the Bio-Med Connect Center (BMCC) at Samsung Medical Center. She has authored numerous peer-reviewed articles and is an active member of national and international professional societies. Frequently invited to speak at global conferences, she is dedicated to refining surgical techniques and improving patient care. Her contributions continue to advance the field of plastic surgery, benefiting both medical professionals and patients worldwide.

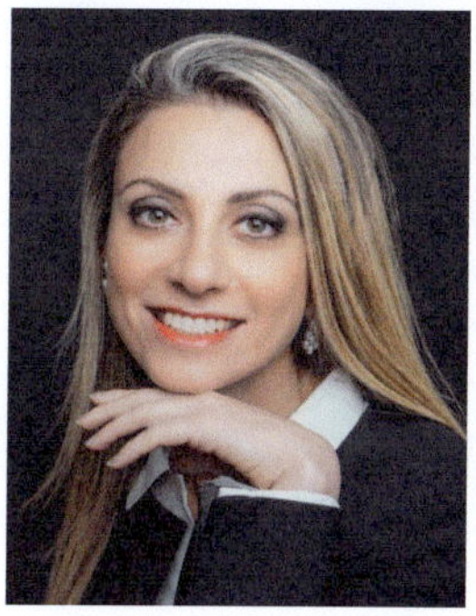

Diala Haykal based in Paris, is a globally recognized expert in aesthetic medicine, lasers, and AI in healthcare, pioneering advancements in precision diagnostics and outcome prediction. She has authored numerous international publications on AI-driven dermatology, skin rejuvenation, and regenerative medicine, shaping the future of personalized skincare. As an editor for esteemed journals, including Springer, *Journal of Cosmetic Dermatology*, and Frontiers, she plays a critical role in advancing scientific discourse in aesthetics and dermatology. With a strong presence in global congresses, she shares her expertise with medical professionals and industry leaders worldwide. Her international collaborations with top institutions and researchers position her at the forefront of integrating AI into aesthetic and laser medicine.

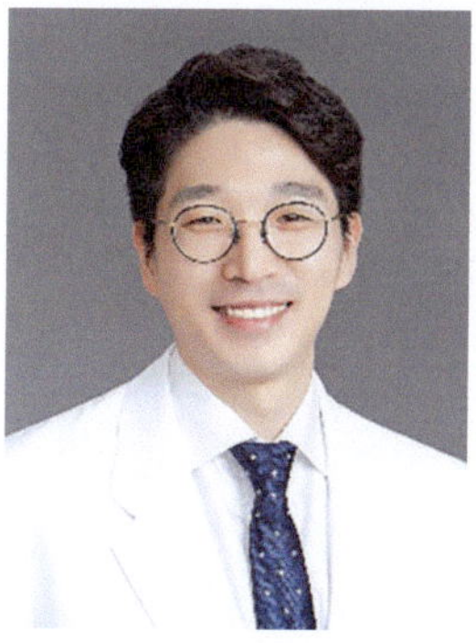

Kyu Hwa Jung is a plastic surgeon specializing in antiaging procedures, including thread lifting, facelift surgery, and injectables. He actively shares his expertise at international conferences and contributes to the development of new medical products. He has published several papers and two books on lifting procedures, recently released in both local and global editions.

Beyond his clinical practice, he has hosted live surgery sessions for international doctors, providing a training in advanced techniques. At overseas conferences, he has delivered thought-provoking presentations, encouraging a new perspective on antiaging. By integrating innovative approaches with practical surgical expertise, he continues to shape the future of aesthetic medicine.

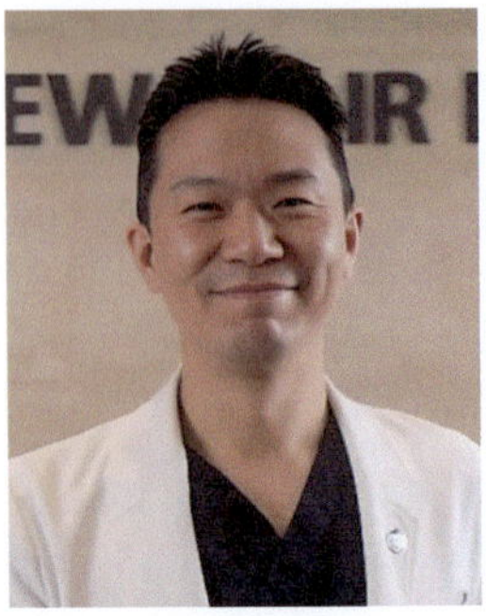

Jino Kim is the Director of New Hair Plastic Surgery Clinic, based in Seoul, and a globally recognized expert in the fields of hair transplantation and hair loss treatment. Through continuous research, development, and the introduction of innovative treatments, he has been leading advancements in this field.

He graduated from Yonsei University College of Medicine and completed his plastic surgery residency at Severance Hospital. He contributes to the advancement of hair transplantation and hair loss treatment by delivering dozens of academic presentations each year. His research is presented at various domestic and international conferences and societies, and he shares his expertise through publications such as Hairology, Hair Restoration, and Hair Transplant 360.

Additionally, he collaborates with multiple pharmaceutical and medical device companies to develop new hair loss treatments and hair transplantation technologies. As a Key Opinion Leader (KOL) for these companies, he provides expert insights into product development and clinical applications, driving the adoption of innovative treatment methods.

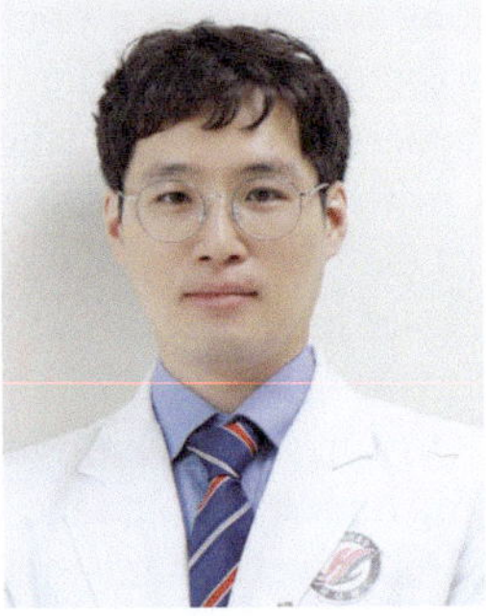

Seong Hwan Kim, MD, PhD is a board-certified plastic surgeon and a Professor at Hallym University Kangnam Sacred Heart Hospital, Seoul. He is a globally recognized expert in plastic and reconstructive surgery, aesthetic medicine, lasers, and AI in healthcare, pioneering advancements in precise diagnostics and outcome prediction.

He has authored numerous international publications on plastic and reconstructive Surgery, AI-driven dermatology, skin rejuvenation, and regenerative medicine, shaping the future of personalized aesthetic and reconstructive treatments.

As an editor of esteemed journals, he plays a critical role in advancing scientific discourse in aesthetic and reconstructive plastic surgery. With a strong presence in global congresses, he shares his expertise with medical professionals and industry leaders worldwide. His international collaborations with top institutions and researchers position him at the forefront of integrating surgical and minimally invasive surgical treatments in aesthetic and reconstructive medicine.

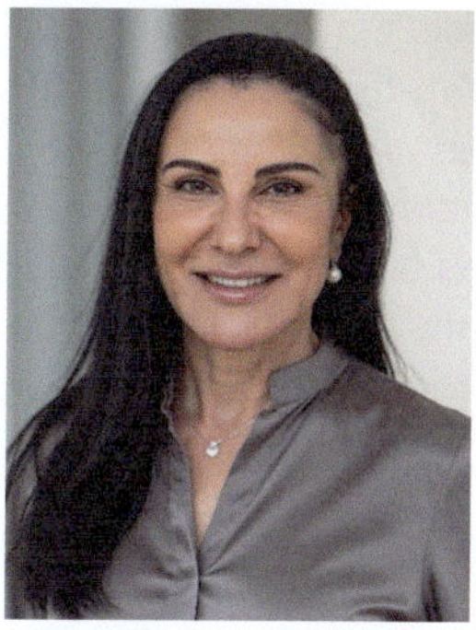

Marina Landau accomplished her dermatology training in the Department of Dermatology in Tel Aviv Medical Center, followed by fellowships in dermatopathology with Dr. Bernard Ackerman in NYU, New York, USA, and Clinical Pharmacology in Sunnybrook Hospital, Toronto, and Pediatric Dermatology, Sick Children Hospital, Toronto, Canada.

She is a founding president of the International Peeling Society.

In addition, she is past President of the Israel Society for Dermatologic Surgery, International Fellow of the American Academy of Dermatology (IFAAD), and a member of the Regional Meetings Committee of the International Society of Dermatology (ISD).

For the last 30 years, she has dedicated to medical and cosmetic dermatology by implementing the most advanced techniques for skin correction and enhancement in her practice.

She is the author of more than 110 scientific articles and a coauthor of chapters in seven textbooks in dermatology and cosmetic dermatology.

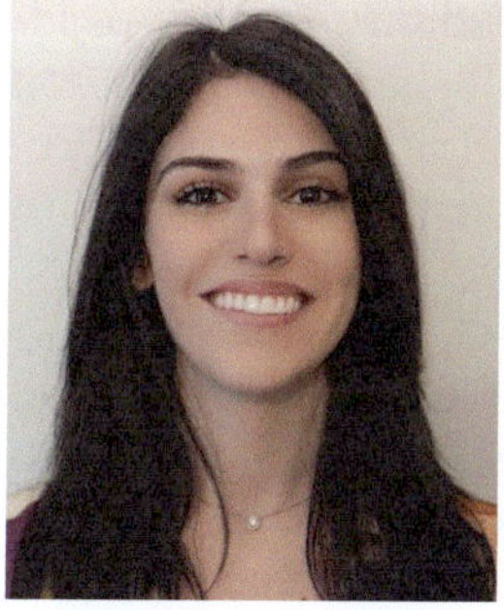

Audrey Melin is a dermatologist with a background in immunology (M2 Immunology, Université Paris-Saclay, INSERM U981) and expertise in aesthetic dermatology and inflammatory skin diseases. Former Chief Resident at CHU Henri Mondor, France, she now practices in both hospital and private practice, focusing on injectables, laser treatments, and dermatological procedures.

She is actively involved in medical training and teaches ultrasound-guided aesthetic injections to enhance precision and safety. She has also contributed to international publications and congresses (SFD, SFME, IMCAS).

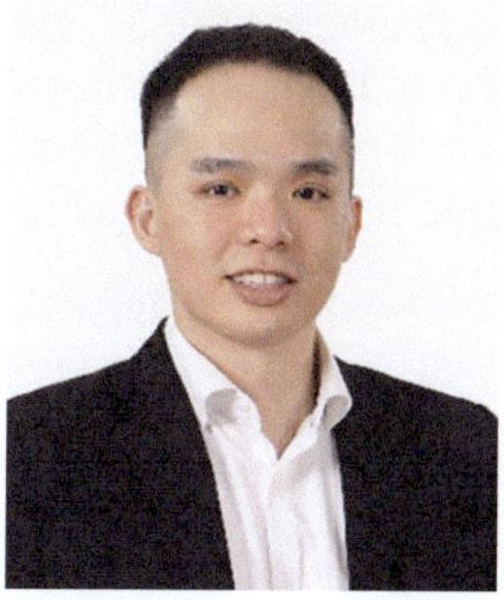

How Kang Nien based in Malaysia, is a consultant dermatologist and dermatologic surgeon renowned for his expertise in aesthetic dermatology and laser surgery. He serves as the Head of Dermatology at Universiti Putra Malaysia and is the Co-founder of Central Dermatology Specialist Clinic. He is a prolific researcher, with a strong publication record in acne, atopic dermatitis, and cosmetic dermatology. He has led and contributed to numerous clinical studies and translational research projects focused on skin rejuvenation, biostimulation, and dermocosmetic formulation. His work has been published in top-tier journals including *Frontiers in Pharmacology*, *Journal of Cosmetic Dermatology*, and *Clinical, Cosmetic and Investigational Dermatology*. A frequent speaker at international dermatology and aesthetic medicine congresses, he bridges clinical practice and research innovation through global collaborations. He is actively involved in guideline development and credentialing committees for dermatology and aesthetic medicine in Malaysia.

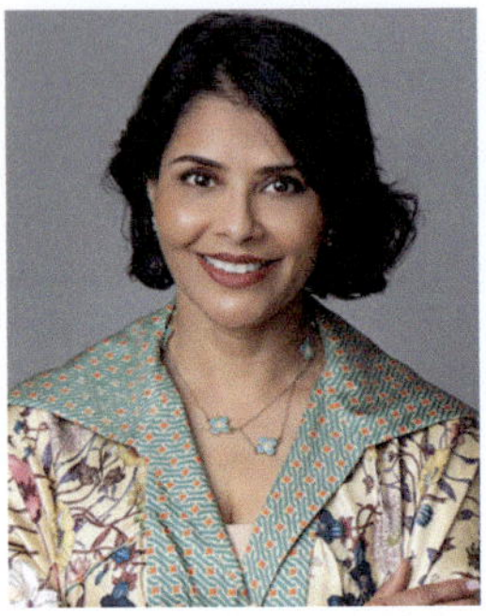

Sabrina Shah-Desai based in London, is a globally recognized expert in Oculoplastic Surgery, aesthetic medicine, and energy-based treatments pioneering advancements in precision diagnostics and outcome prediction. She has authored numerous international publications on Oculoplastic surgery and regenerative medicine, shaping the future of personalized aesthetic treatments. As a global educator and KOL for the aesthetic industry, she plays a critical role in advancing scientific discourse in aesthetics and surgery. With a strong presence in global congresses, she shares her expertise with medical professionals and industry leaders worldwide. Her international collaborations with top institutions and researchers position her at the forefront of integrating surgical and minimally invasive nonsurgical treatments in aesthetic medicine.

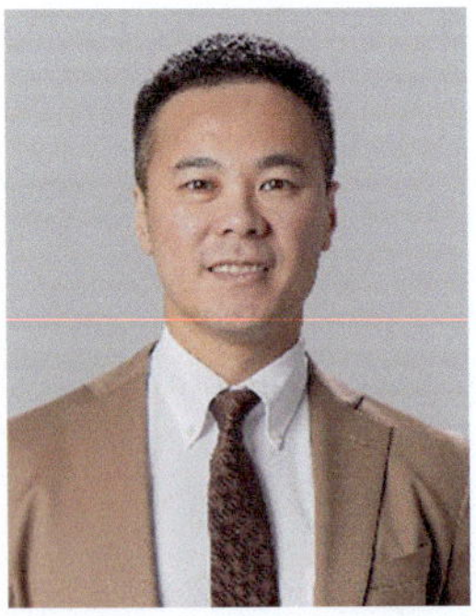

Lim Tingsong as a Letter of Credentialing and Privileging (LCP) holder for Aesthetic Practices in Malaysia, has been actively involved in academic research and training on Asian facial and body aesthetics, clinical application of fillers' rheology, facial overfilled syndrome, pigmentary disorders, energy-based devices, and regenerative medicine.

Graduated from Tohoku University School of Medicine under the Monbusho Scholarship, he is a frequent speaker regionally and internationally. He is currently a Global Key Opinion Leader for injectables, energy-based devices, and noninvasive body contouring. He sat on multiple international advisory board meetings.

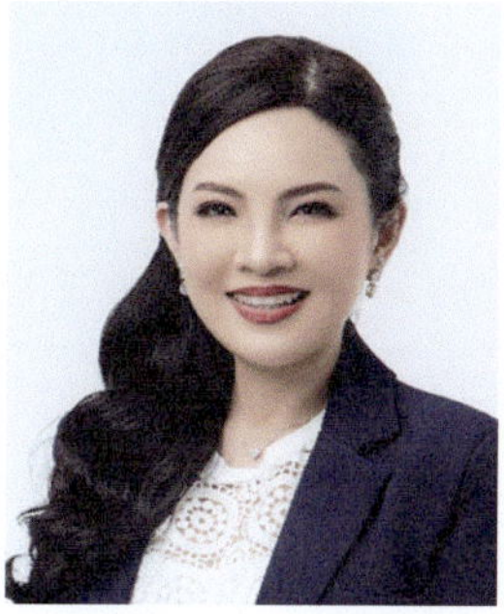

Rungsima Wanitphakdeedecha is a dermatologist and dermatologic surgeon in Bangkok, Thailand. She completed her dermatology residency at Faculty of Medicine Siriraj Hospital, Mahidol University, Bangkok, Thailand. She has been serving as a faculty in the Dermatosurgery Unit, Department of Dermatology, Faculty of Medicine Siriraj Hospital, Mahidol University, since then. She completed her research fellowship training in Procedural Dermatology at the University of Texas-MD Anderson Cancer center, Houston, Texas, USA, and Laser and Cosmetic Surgery at Washington Institute of Dermatologic Laser Surgery, Washington, DC, USA.

Currently, she is appointed as director of Siriraj Skin Laser Center, head of Dermatosurgery Unit, and chairwoman of Department of Dermatology, Faculty of Medicine Siriraj Hospital, Mahidol University, Bangkok, Thailand.

She has lectured nationally and internationally on the topics of dermatologic surgery, laser, injectables, and other cosmetic procedures. She has published many book chapters and manuscripts in peer-reviewed journals.

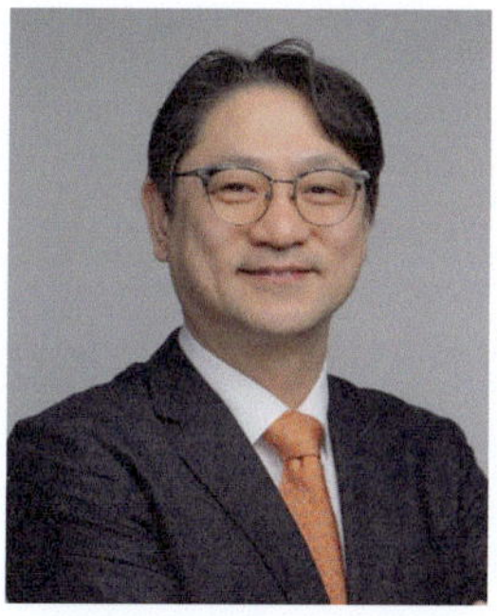

Changwoon Yun is a plastic surgeon based in Seoul, South Korea. He received his MD from Soonchonhyang University Medical College and PhD from the College of Medicine, Soonchonhyang University, Seoul, South Korea. Currently, he is the chief doctor of facial contouring and orthognathic surgery at View Plastic Surgery Clinic, Seoul.

He is the member of the Korean Society of Plastic and Reconstructive Surgeons, and vice president of Minimal Invasive Plastic Surgery association from 2022 to 2025. He has published *Minimally Invasive Aesthetic Surgery Techniques*, Springer 2022. He has published many articles about plastic surgery fields until 2025.

Additionally, he collaborates with multiple pharmaceutical and medical device companies to develop new antiaging treatment technologies. As a Key Opinion Leader (KOL) for these companies, he provides expert technique of thread-lifting field.

Basic Anatomy for Injectables

1

Seong Hwan Kim and Won Lee

1.1 Introduction

A thorough understanding of facial anatomical structures is essential for the safe and effective application of injectables in facial aesthetic procedures. By familiarizing oneself with the anatomical distribution of the face's major blood vessels (arteries and veins), nerves, muscles, fat layers, and retaining ligaments, complications such as vascular occlusion and nerve injury from intravascular injection can be prevented, and optimal aesthetic outcomes can be achieved. In particular, since fillers are used to restore volume and improve contours, it is important to inject them into safe layers considering the neural and vascular structures. This chapter systematically organizes the essential anatomical concepts required for filler and other injectable procedures, aiming to provide evidence-based knowledge for more precise and safer treatments.

S. H. Kim
Hallym University Kangnam Sacred Heart Hospital, Seoul, Republic of Korea

W. Lee (✉)
Yonsei E1 Plastic Surgery Clinic, Anyang, Kyonggi-do, Korea (Republic of)

1.2 Arteries of the Face

Among injectables, fillers are mainly injected into the subcutaneous fat layer, so the possibility of vascular injury is relatively high. Especially when treating areas close to important blood vessels, it is necessary to accurately identify the location and course of vessels passing through the treatment area to avoid complications due to vascular injury. However, there are individual variations in vascular anatomy, and recently, procedures using Doppler ultrasound have been helpful in preventing complications [1–3]. Of the arteries supplying blood to the face, the external carotid artery, which is located on the lateral side of the neck, branches into two major arteries: the external and internal branches (Figs. 1.1 and 1.2). The external branch, which runs outside the skull, includes the facial artery and superficial temporal artery. As the facial and superficial temporal arteries travel, they branch out to supply blood to the lower and midface, the side of the nose, and the temple area [4]. The internal branch, which runs inside the skull, includes the maxillary artery, which branches into the infraorbital artery, buccal artery, and the terminal branch of the inferior alveolar artery (mental artery), supplying blood to the skin and soft tissues of the corresponding facial regions. Additionally, the ophthalmic artery, supraorbital artery, supratrochlear artery, and dorsal nasal artery branch, which arise from the internal carotid artery located on the

W. Lee (ed.), *Innovative Injectable Techniques in Minimally Invasive Aesthetics*,
https://doi.org/10.1007/978-981-95-2161-6_1

inner side of the neck, supply blood to the forehead, glabella, and nose.

(1) Facial Artery

After branching from the external carotid artery, the facial artery runs medially under the mandible, emerges to the surface by winding around the antegonial notch at the anterior border of the masseter muscle, and ascends obliquely toward the medial canthus at the upper inner part of the face [5] (Fig. 1.3). Along its course, the facial artery gives off the horizontal labiomental artery, inferior labial artery, and superior labial artery toward the lips, ascends along the nasolabial fold, then gives off the inferior alar artery and lateral nasal artery toward the nose, and attaches to the border between the nose and cheek, where it

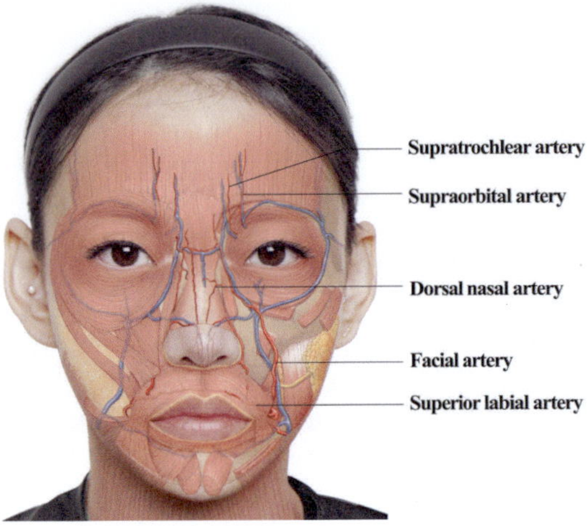

Fig. 1.1 Arteries of the face

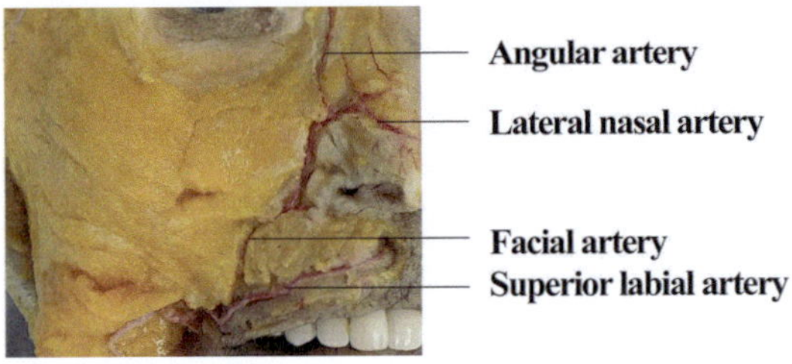

Fig. 1.3 Cadaveric image of facial artery

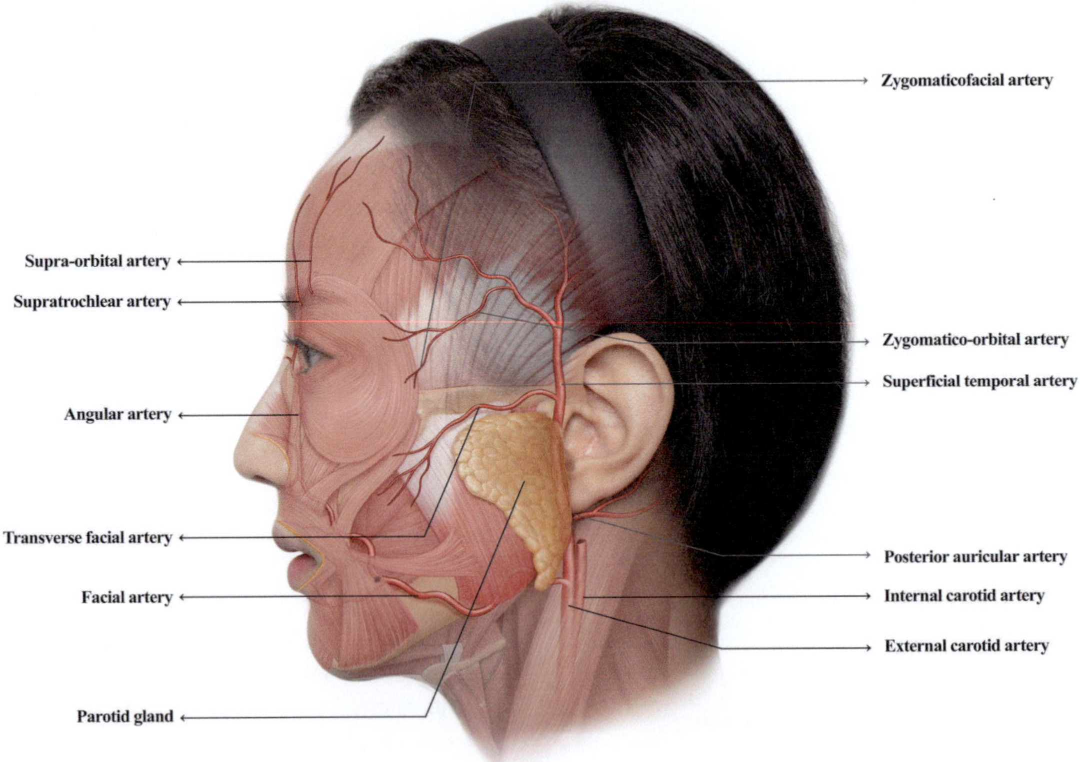

Fig. 1.2 Arteries of the face (lateral)

ascends vertically. The vertically ascending vessel is specifically called the angular artery.

In the glabella and nasal dorsum, branches of the ophthalmic artery, such as the supraorbital artery, supratrochlear artery, and dorsal nasal artery, anastomose with branches of the facial artery.

Another artery branching from the external carotid artery, the superficial temporal artery, ascends toward the temple and divides into anterior (frontal) and posterior (parietal) branches, supplying the temple and lateral forehead. The frontal branch of the superficial temporal artery (anterior temporal), which goes toward the forehead, anastomoses with the supraorbital artery, a branch of the ophthalmic artery.

(2) Supratrochlear Artery

The supratrochlear artery, a branch of the ophthalmic artery, supplies blood to the central forehead and glabella. After exiting the orbit, it runs along the medial side of the supratrochlear nerve on a vertical line drawn from the medial canthus, pierces the orbicularis oculi muscle, and travels on the muscle's surface (Fig. 1.4) [6].

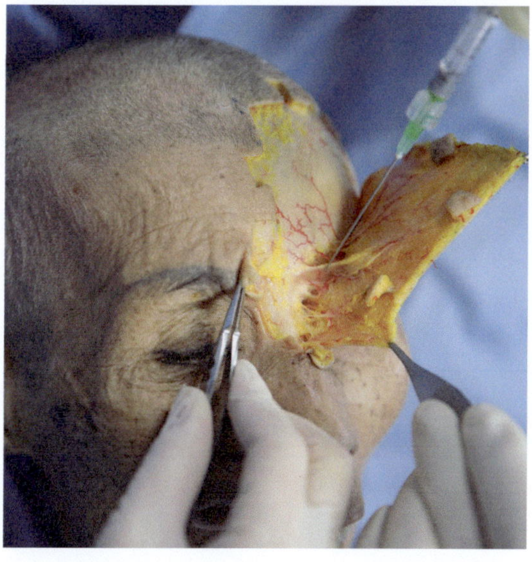

Fig. 1.4 Cadaveric image of supratrochlear artery

(3) Supraorbital Artery

The supraorbital artery exits the orbit through the supraorbital notch or foramen, travels deeply under the orbicularis and frontalis muscles, and at a point about 3 cm lateral to the medial canthus and about 2 cm above the supraorbital rim, pierces the frontalis muscle and anastomoses medially with the supratrochlear artery and laterally with the frontal branch of the superficial temporal artery (Fig. 1.5) [7].

(4) Superficial Temporal Artery

The superficial temporal artery originates from the external carotid artery, passes through the parotid gland, and at a point about 17.7 mm anterior and 37 mm superior to the tragus near the zygomatic arch, divides into anterior and posterior branches and travels in the subcutaneous fat (Figs. 1.6 and 1.7). The anterior branch runs under the superficial temporal fascia toward the anterior forehead, meets the frontalis muscle, connects with branches from the supraorbital artery, and travels over the surface of the frontalis muscle. The zygomaticoorbital artery, a branch of the superficial temporal artery, supplies the orbicularis oculi muscle, usually heads toward the lateral canthus, ascends toward the lateral eyebrow end, and connects with the lacrimal branch and palpebral branches of the ophthalmic artery [8, 9].

(5) Dorsal Nasal Artery

As one of the terminal branches of the ophthalmic artery, the dorsal nasal artery emerges at the medial canthus, passes the medial palpebral ligament, and travels along the dorsum of the nose, supplying blood to the skin, subcutaneous tissue, and cartilage layer of the nasal root and dorsum (Fig. 1.8) [10]. It is connected to the angular artery, and in the event of retrograde flow, a thrombus can enter the ophthalmic artery, potentially causing blindness, or if blood flow is blocked, necrosis of the nasal skin may occur, so caution is required during injectable procedures [11, 12].

(6) Inferior Labial Artery

The inferior labial artery branches from the facial artery near the oral commissure and runs along the vermillion border of the lower lip (Fig. 1.9). It

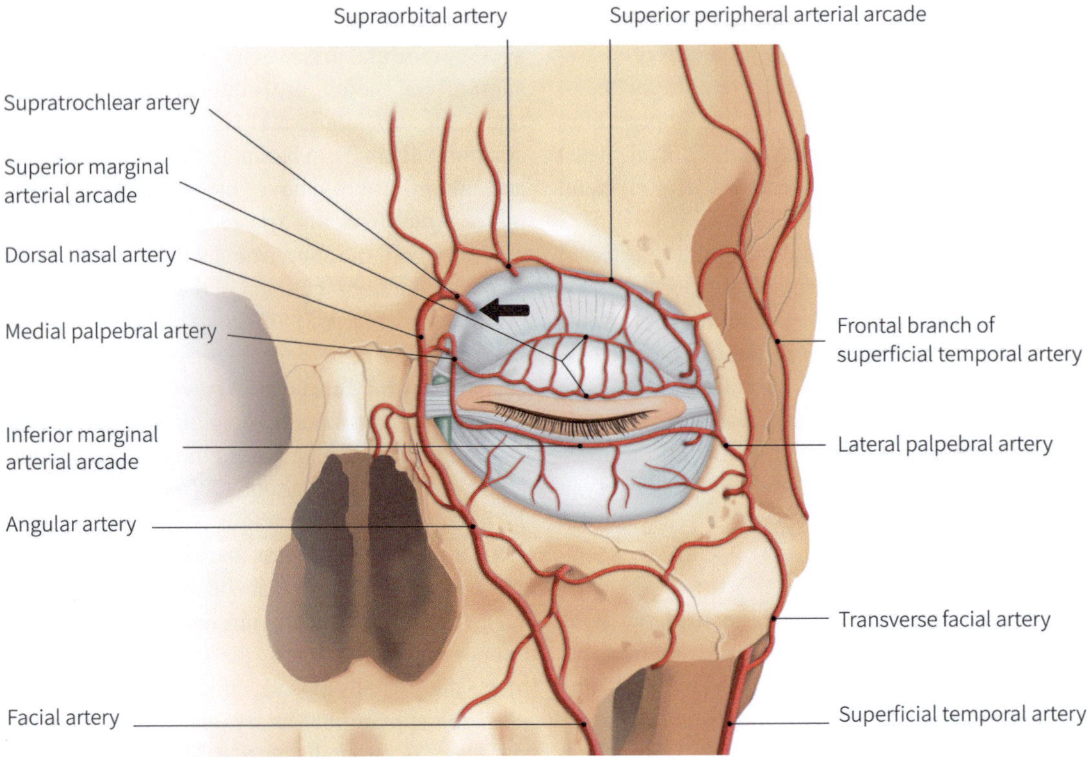

Fig. 1.5 Arteries of the periorbital region

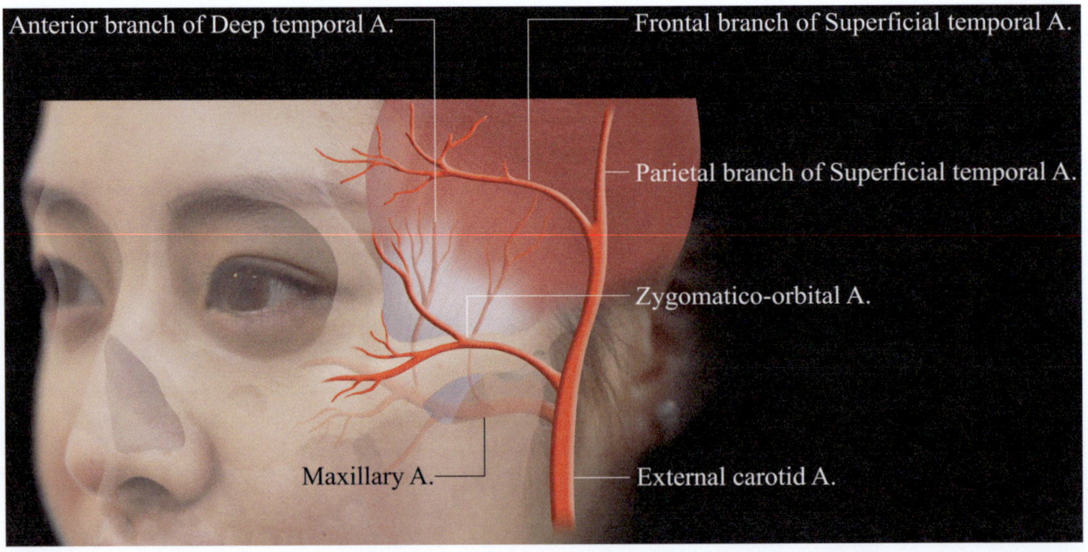

Fig. 1.6 Superficial temporal artery

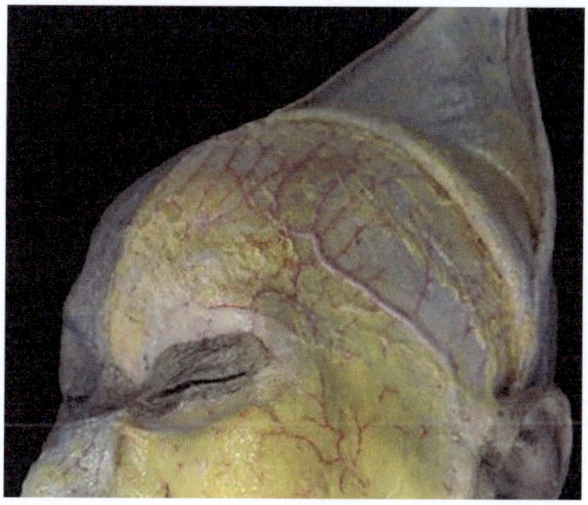

Fig. 1.7 Cadaveric image of STA

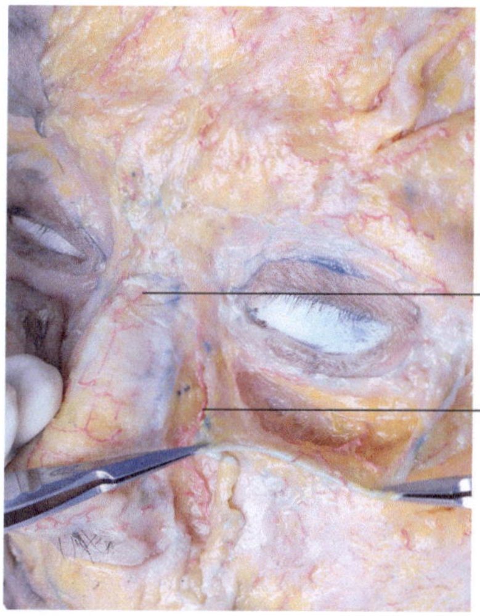

Fig. 1.8 Cadaveric image of dorsal nasal artery

travels deeper than the orbicularis oris muscle, close to the inner wet mucosa of the lip, and as it moves medially from the oral commissure, it becomes more superficial and ascends toward the dry mucosa [13].

(7) Superior Labial Artery

The superior labial artery branches from the facial artery about 1 cm above the oral commissure and runs horizontally, 0.5–1.2 cm above the vermillion border of the upper lip (Fig. 1.10). It is located in a deeper layer than the orbicularis oris muscle, travels close to the wet mucosa of

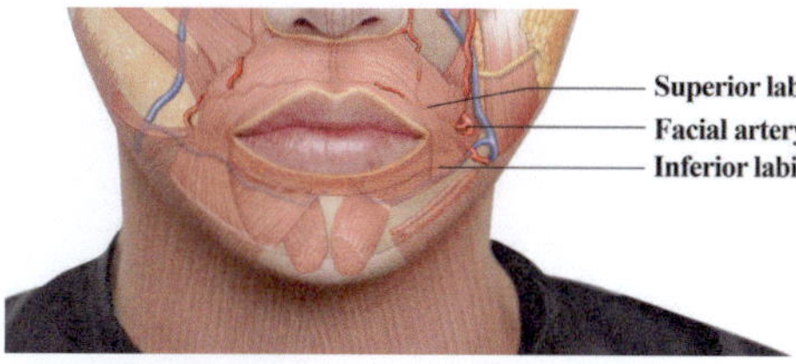

Fig. 1.9 Arteries of the perioral region

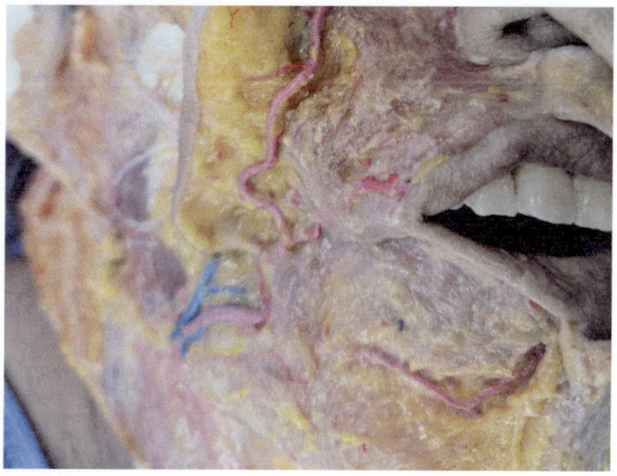

Fig. 1.10 Cadaveric image of perioral area

the lip, and gives off the nasal septal artery near the philtrum. The nasal septal artery has branches that run both superficially and deeply relative to the orbicularis oris muscle, with the superficial branch continuing as the columellar artery [11].

1.3 Veins of the Face

The venous distribution of the face generally resembles that of the arteries, but there are exceptions such as the inferior ophthalmic vein and retromandibular vein. The facial vein is one of the most important veins of the face, running straight about 1.5 cm posterior to the facial artery. The facial vein flows downward and joins the internal jugular vein, but if venous flow is blocked, it can reflux into the cavernous sinus via the superior and inferior ophthalmic veins [14]. Additionally, an intercanthal vein is connecting both angular veins at the medial canthus where the glabella and nasal root meet is reported to exist in about 70% of the population. It crosses

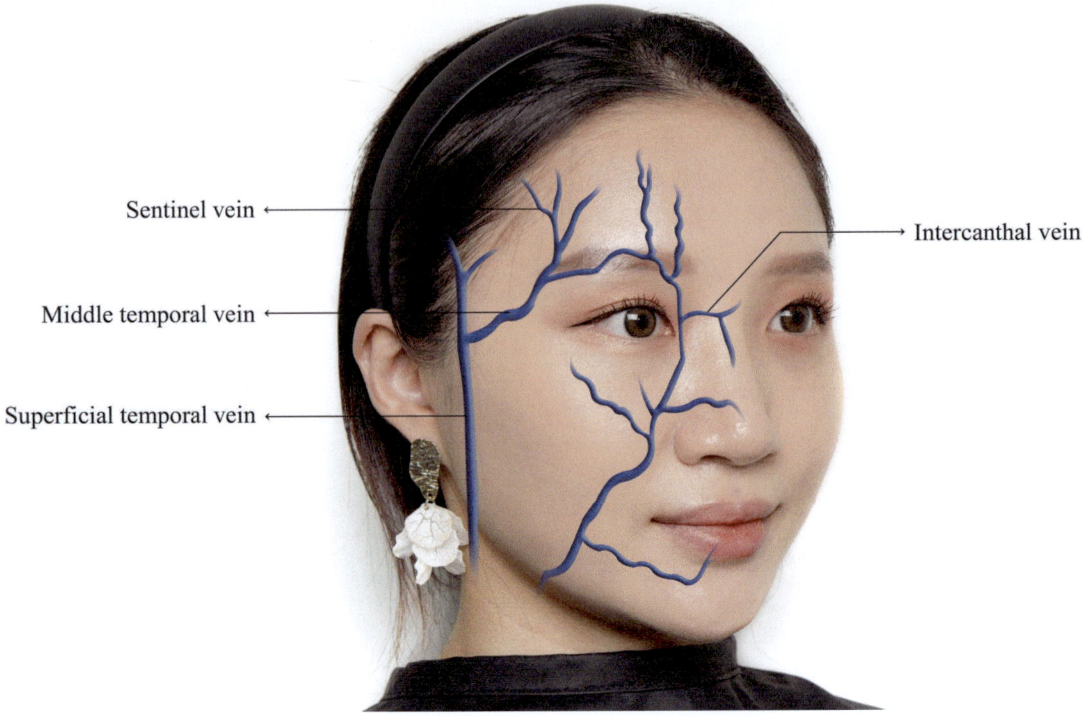

Fig. 1.11 Veins of the face

over the procerus muscle and connects to the cavernous sinus, so care must be taken to avoid injecting into it [15]. In the temporal region, the middle temporal vein is located about 2 cm above the zygomatic arch between the superficial and deep layers of the deep temporal fascia (Fig. 1.11) [16]. Various studies have reported the diameter of the middle temporal vein to range from 0.5 mm to 9.1 mm, and since it continues through the superficial temporal vein, supraorbital vein, and superior ophthalmic vein to the cavernous sinus, it is essential to consider its course when injecting filler into the deep temporal region to ensure safe procedures [17].

1.4 Nerves of the Face

To safely perform injectables and prevent facial nerve injury, or to perform sensory nerve blocks for regional anesthesia, one must accurately understand the location, depth, course, function, and possible symptoms of injury of each nerve in the face (Fig. 1.12).

There are 12 pairs of cranial nerves associated with the face. From the top, these are the following: CN I, olfactory nerve; CN II, optic nerve; CN III, oculomotor nerve; CN IV, trochlear nerve; CN V, trigeminal nerve; CN VI, abducens nerve; CN VII, facial nerve; CN VIII, vestibulocochlear nerve; CN IX, glossopharyngeal nerve; CN X, vagus nerve; CN XI, accessory nerve; and CN XII, hypoglossal nerve [18, 19]. Clinically important cranial nerves are the fifth (trigeminal nerve) and seventh (facial nerve), which pass through the face and neck. Care must be taken as injury during surgery or procedures can result in various neurological symptoms.

(1) Ophthalmic Nerve

The first branch of the trigeminal nerve, responsible for sensation in the forehead, eyes, nasal dorsum, upper eyelid, frontal region, and part of the nasal mucosa. It enters the orbit through the superior orbital fissure, travels laterally in the orbit, and branches into the frontal nerve, nasociliary nerve, and lacrimal nerve. The frontal nerve branches into the supraorbital nerve and

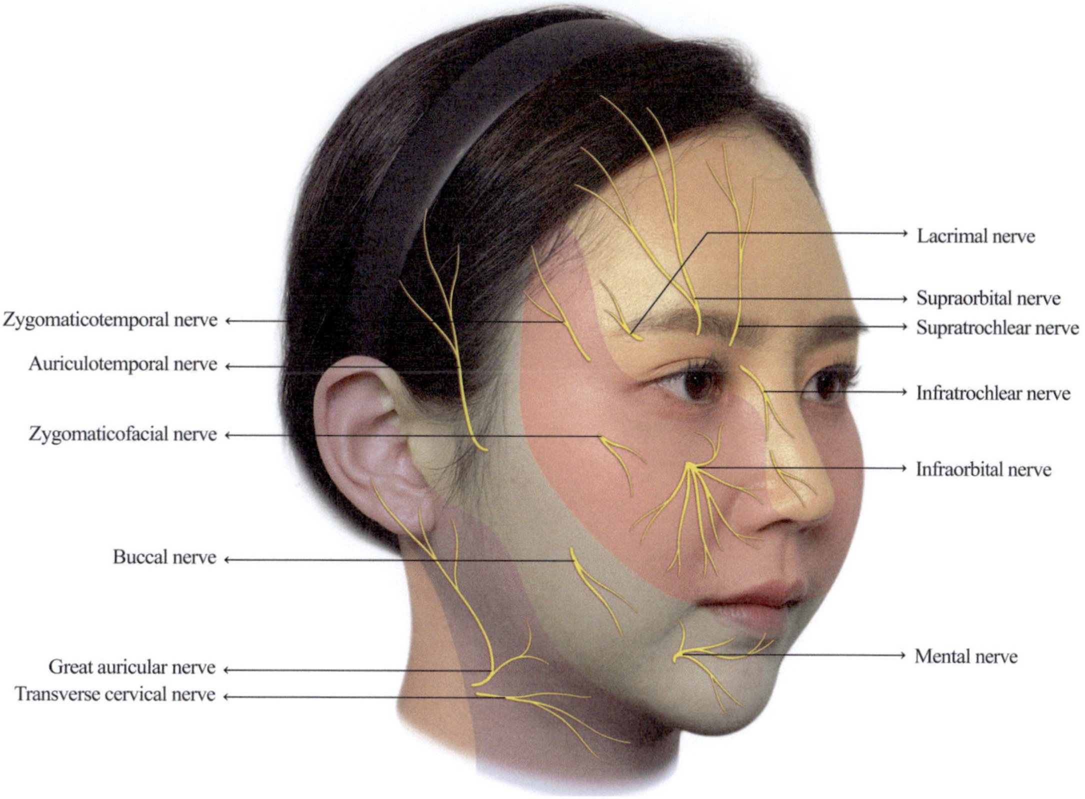

Fig. 1.12 Sensory nerves of the face

supratrochlear nerve via the supraorbital notch, and the nasociliary nerve branches into the infratrochlear nerve and external nasal nerve (anterior ethmoidal nerve) [20].

- Supraorbital nerve: Responsible for sensation in the forehead and anterior scalp
- Supratrochlear nerve: Responsible for sensation in the medial forehead and glabella
- Lacrimal nerve: Sensation of the lateral upper eyelid and lacrimal gland
- Infratrochlear nerve: Sensation of the medial orbit and inner eyelid
- External nasal nerve (anterior ethmoidal nerve): Sensation of the nasal dorsum

(2) Maxillary Nerve

The second branch of the trigeminal nerve, which gives off the zygomatic nerve and ends as the infraorbital nerve exiting the infraorbital foramen. The zygomatic nerve branches into the zygomaticofacial nerve via the zygomaticofacial foramen and the zygomaticotemporal nerve via the zygomaticotemporal foramen, providing sensation to the zygomatic and temporal regions. The infraorbital nerve supplies sensation to the lower eyelid, lateral nose, upper lip, gums, and teeth [21, 22].

(3) Mandibular Nerve

The third branch of the trigeminal nerve, which gives off sensory branches to the mandible and lateral regions and motor branches to the muscles of mastication. The auriculotemporal nerve supplies sensation to the skin around the ear and temporal region; the buccal nerve supplies sensation to the skin and mucosa of the cheek. The inferior alveolar nerve passes through the mental

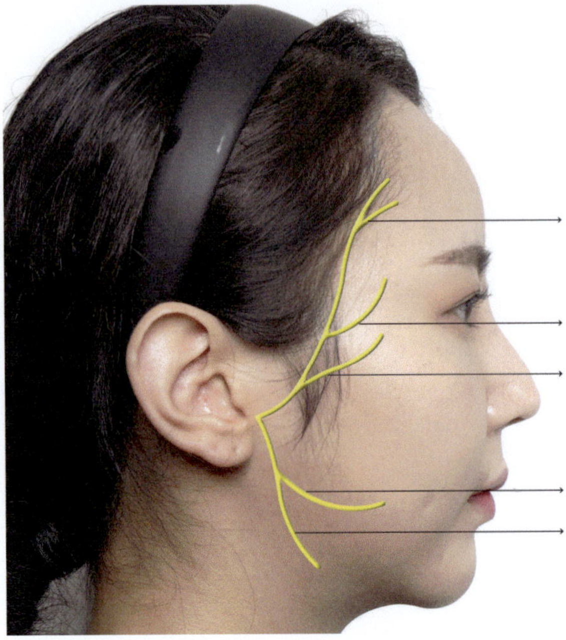

Fig. 1.13 Facial nerve

foramen to become the mental nerve, which supplies sensation to the lower lip and chin skin [23].

(4) Cervical Plexus

Cutaneous branches of the cervical plexus emerge from the middle posterior border of the sternocleidomastoid muscle. The great auricular nerve supplies the skin of the mastoid process, parotid gland, angle, and inferior margin of the mandible. The transverse cervical nerve supplies the skin of the anterior triangle, providing cutaneous sensation [24].

(5) Facial Nerve

The facial nerve passes through the stylomastoid foramen, divides into five branches within the parotid gland, exits the edge of the parotid gland, and runs covered by the SMAS, generally traveling deep to the facial expression muscles (Fig. 1.13) [25]. The temporal branch consists of several branches, exits the parotid gland, crosses the zygomatic arch, and runs anterosuperiorly, innervating the upper parts of the frontalis, corrugator supercilii, and orbicularis oculi muscles [26]. The zygomatic branch innervates the lower part of the orbicularis oculi and the zygomaticus major and minor muscles. The buccal branch runs with the parotid duct and innervates muscles responsible for movement around the lips and nose. The zygomatic and buccal branches anastomose and, as they travel along the lateral aspect of the nose, give off branches to the nasalis, procerus, and corrugator supercilii muscles [27]. The marginal mandibular branch innervates the orbicularis oris, depressor anguli oris, depressor labii inferioris, and mentalis muscles, allowing for pursing of the lips, pulling down the oral commissure and lower lip, and drawing the skin and soft tissue of the chin [28]. The cervical branch innervates the platysma muscle, which tenses and controls the skin of the neck.

1.5 Muscles of the Face

When performing botulinum toxin injections, it is important to know the exact location and depth of the facial muscles for precise treatment. In filler procedures, knowing whether to inject above or below the muscle and considering the effects of muscle movement is necessary, so accurate anatomical knowledge is required (Fig. 1.14).

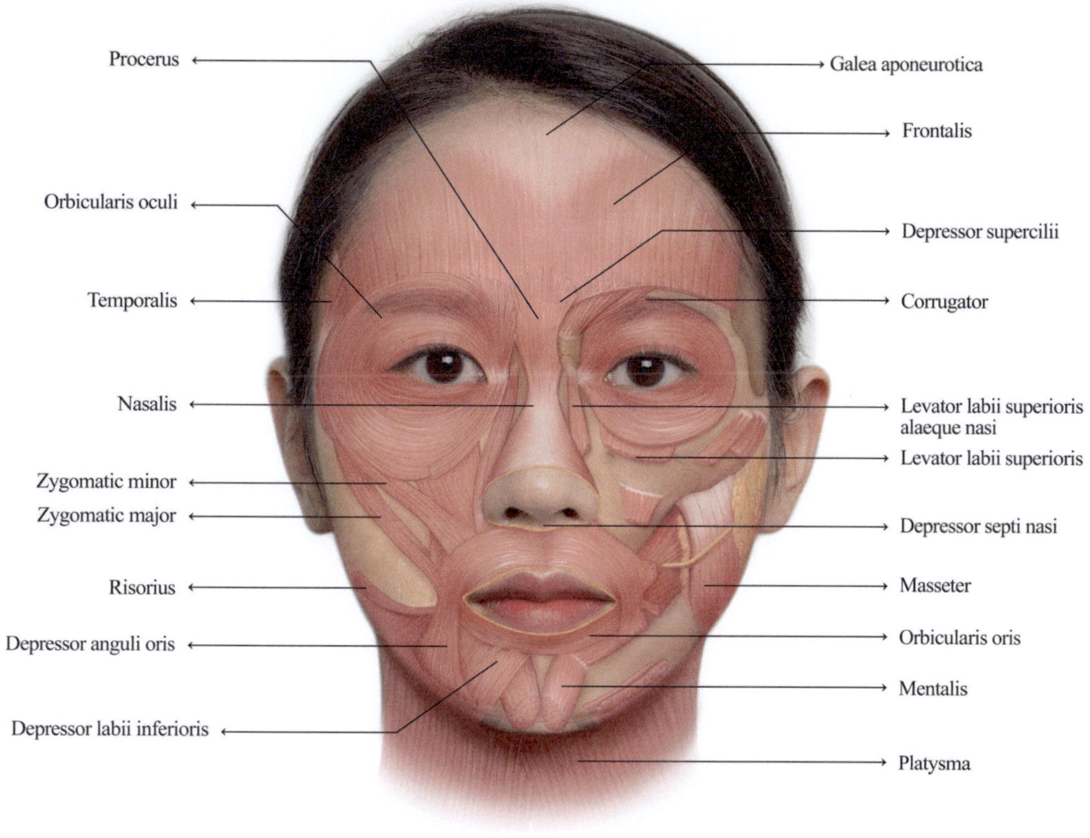

Fig. 1.14 Muscles of the face

1.6 Superficial and Deep Fat Compartments of the Face

The facial fat layer is divided into a superficial fat layer above the SMAS (Fig. 1.15) and a deep fat layer below the SMAS. These fat layers are composed of several compartments, which vary by region. In the midface, both superficial and deep fat layers are clearly distinguished, but in the upper and lower face, the thickness and distribution of the two layers may differ. Therefore, it is important to plan injectable procedures considering the differences in fat layers by region [29]. According to studies, adipocytes in the deep fat compartments are smaller than those in the superficial compartments, and as aging progresses, the volume of deep fat compartments decreases, weakening support and causing skin sagging. The rate of fat absorption also varies by region and over time (Fig. 1.16). These changes, along with sagging of the skin and soft tissues, contribute to the accentuation of existing wrinkles. In particular, as facial volume loss and tissue descent progress, wrinkles become more pronounced in specific areas associated with each fat compartment [30, 31]. Therefore, understanding the anatomical structure of the face and the relationship between fat compartments allows for appropriate volume restoration using injectables, helping to restore skin elasticity and naturally alleviate wrinkles.

Fig. 1.15 Compartments of superficial fat layer

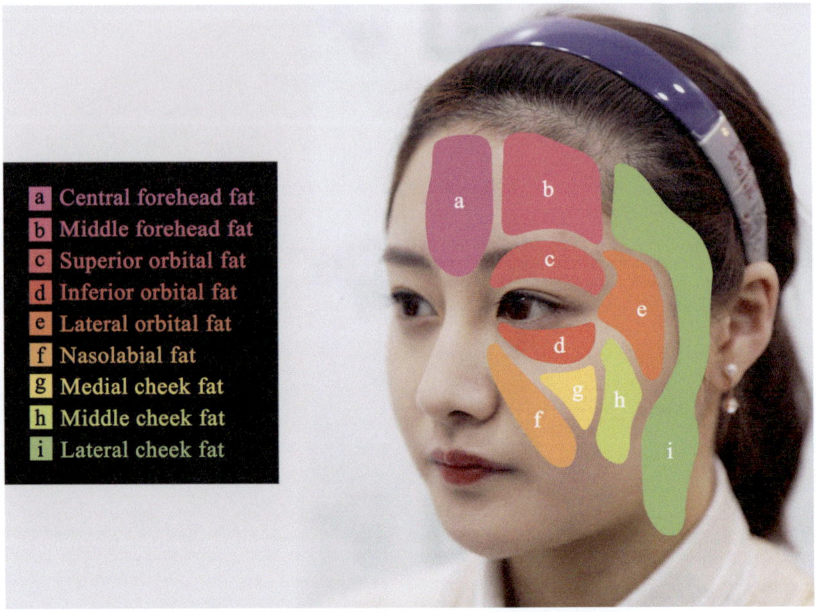
a Central forehead fat
b Middle forehead fat
c Superior orbital fat
d Inferior orbital fat
e Lateral orbital fat
f Nasolabial fat
g Medial cheek fat
h Middle cheek fat
i Lateral cheek fat
a
b
c
d
e
f
g
h
i

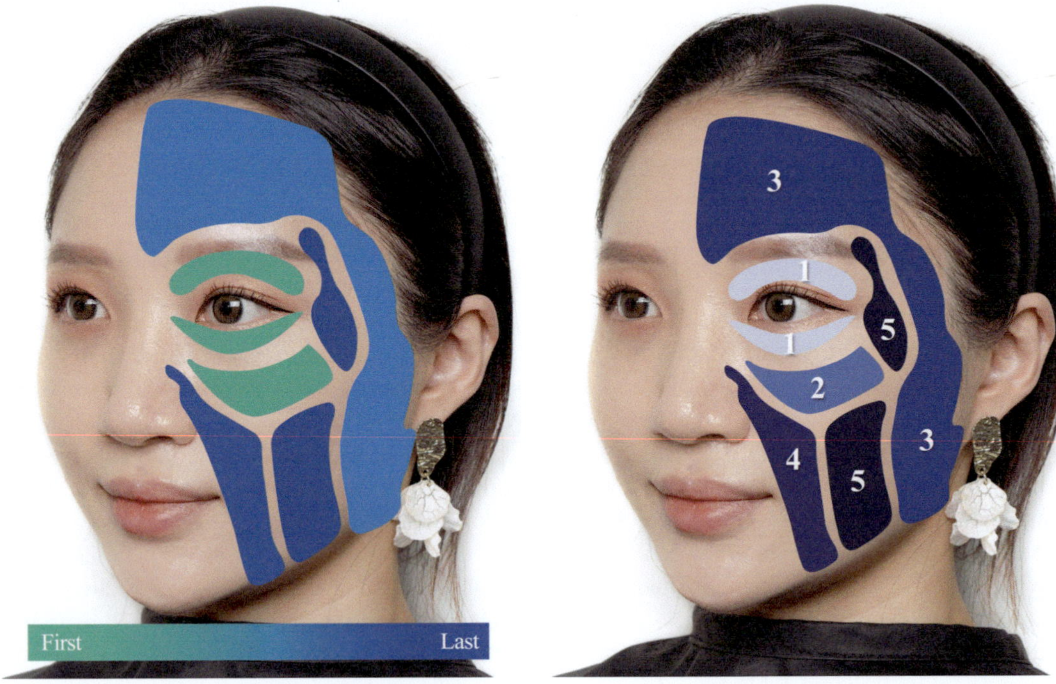
First
Last
3
1
1
5
2
3
4
5

Fig. 1.16 Changes in facial fat absorption over time

1.7 Retaining Ligament of the Face

The face contains various ligamentous structures that connect the skin to the bone or subcutaneous fat layer. Retaining ligaments are strong fibrous structures that extend vertically from the periosteum or deep fascia to the dermis, playing important roles in facial support, expression, and aging. These ligaments are located in specific regions, define different fat compartments, and separate facial spaces. Thus, understanding these anatomical structures is necessary not only for various cosmetic procedures such as injectable treatments but also for surgical approaches (Fig. 1.17). For example, the orbicularis retaining ligament, which maintains the lid-cheek junction, is important for tear trough filler injections, and the zygomatic retaining ligament must be considered in midface lifts and malar augmentation [32].

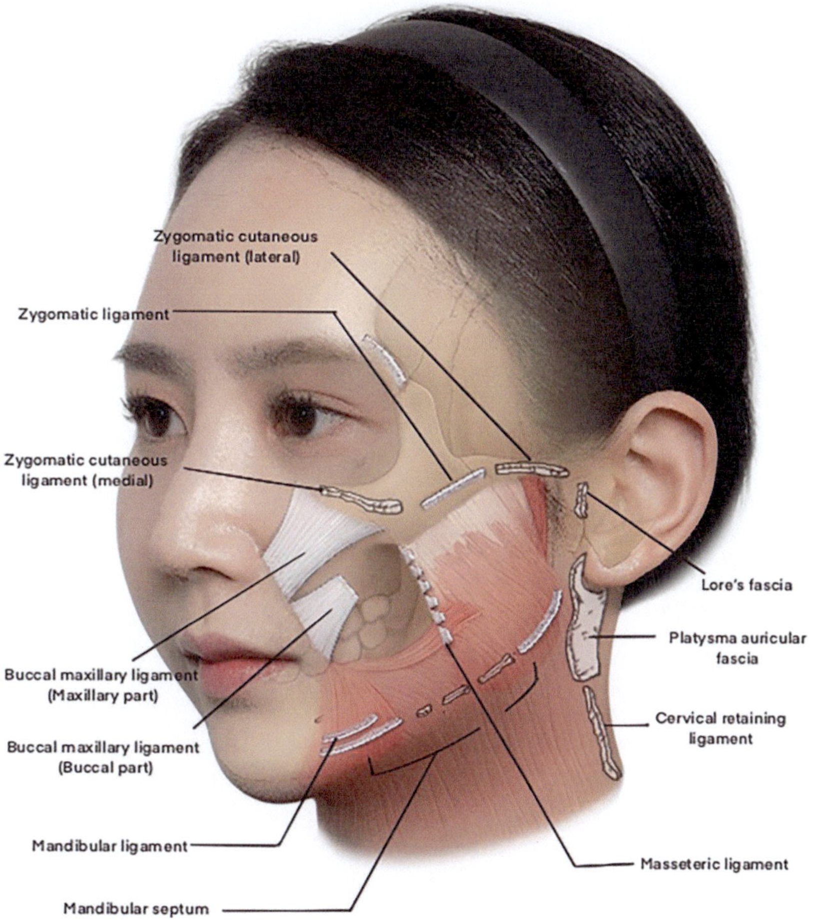

Fig. 1.17 Retaining ligament of the face

References

1. Lee W, et al. A safe Doppler ultrasound-guided method for nasolabial fold correction with hyaluronic acid filler. Aesthet Surg J. 2021;41(6):NP486–92.
2. Rocha PS, Guerra TA, Teixeira DA. Description of a safe doppler ultrasound-guided technique for hyaluronic acid filler in the face – A method to avoid adverse vascular events. J Cosmet Dermatol. 2022;21(7):2783–7.
3. Cotofana S, Schelke LW, Velthuis PJ. Commentary on: Doppler ultrasound-guided filler injections: useful tips to integrate ultrasound in daily practice. Aesthet Surg J. 2023;43(7):784–5.
4. Marur T, Tuna Y, Demirci S. Facial anatomy. Clin Dermatol. 2014;32(1):14–23.
5. Yang HM, et al. New anatomical insights on the course and branching patterns of the facial artery: clinical implications of injectable treatments to the nasolabial fold and nasojugal groove. Plast Reconstr Surg. 2014;133(5):1077–82.
6. Cong LY, et al. Topographic analysis of the supratrochlear artery and the supraorbital artery: implication for improving the safety of forehead augmentation. Plast Reconstr Surg. 2017;139(3):620e–7e.
7. Kim YS, et al. The anatomical origin and course of the angular artery regarding its clinical implications. Dermatol Surg. 2014;40(10):1070–6.
8. Sykes JM, et al. Upper face: clinical anatomy and regional approaches with injectable fillers. Plast Reconstr Surg. 2015;136(5 Suppl):204S–18S.
9. Lee JG, et al. Frontal branch of the superficial temporal artery: anatomical study and clinical implications regarding injectable treatments. Surg Radiol Anat. 2015;37(1):61–8.
10. Choi DY, et al. Topography of the dorsal nasal artery and its clinical implications for augmentation of the dorsum of the nose. J Cosmet Dermatol. 2018;17(4):637–42.
11. Janis JE, et al. The anatomy of the corrugator supercilii muscle: Part II. Supraorbital nerve branching patterns. Plast Reconstr Surg. 2008;121(1):233–40.
12. Saban Y, et al. Nasal arterial vasculature: medical and surgical applications. Arch Facial Plast Surg. 2012;14(6):429–36.
13. Lee SH, Lee M, Kim HJ. Anatomy-based image processing analysis of the running pattern of the perioral artery for minimally invasive surgery. Br J Oral Maxillofac Surg. 2014;52(8):688–92.
14. Scheuer JF 3rd, et al. Facial danger zones: techniques to maximize safety during soft-tissue filler injections. Plast Reconstr Surg. 2017;139(5):1103–8.
15. Lee HJ, et al. Description of a novel anatomic venous structure in the nasoglabellar area. J Craniofac Surg. 2014;25(2):633–5.
16. Jung W, et al. Clinical implications of the middle temporal vein with regard to temporal fossa augmentation. Dermatol Surg. 2014;40(6):618–23.
17. Kapoor KM, et al. A systematic literature review of the middle temporal vein anatomy: 'Venous Danger Zone' in temporal fossa for filler injections. Aesthetic Plast Surg. 2020;44(5):1803–10.
18. SS. Gray's anatomy. 41st ed. Edinburgh: Elsevier; 2016.
19. Moore KL, DA, Agur AM. Clinically oriented anatomy. 8th ed. Philadelphia: Wolters Kluwe; 2018.
20. Gil YC, et al. Three-dimensional topography of the supratrochlear nerve with reference to the lacrimal caruncle, and its danger zone in asians. Dermatol Surg. 2017;43(12):1458–65.
21. Hu KS, et al. Branching patterns of the infraorbital nerve and topography within the infraorbital space. J Craniofac Surg. 2006;17(6):1111–5.
22. Kim HS, et al. Three-dimensional courses of zygomaticofacial and zygomaticotemporal canals using micro-computed tomography in Korean. J Craniofac Surg. 2013;24(5):1565–8.
23. Song WC, et al. Location of the infraorbital and mental foramen with reference to the soft-tissue landmarks. Plast Reconstr Surg. 2007;120(5):1343–7.
24. Brennan PA, et al. Communication between the transverse cervical nerve (C2,3) and marginal mandibular branch of the facial nerve: a cadaveric and clinical study. Br J Oral Maxillofac Surg. 2019;57(3):232–5.
25. Hwang K. Surgical anatomy of the facial nerve relating to facial rejuvenation surgery. J Craniofac Surg. 2014;25(4):1476–81.
26. Agarwal CA, et al. The course of the frontal branch of the facial nerve in relation to fascial planes: an anatomic study. Plast Reconstr Surg. 2010;125(2):532–7.
27. Dorafshar AH, et al. Surface anatomy of the middle division of the facial nerve: Zuker's point. Plast Reconstr Surg. 2013;131(2):253–7.
28. Huettner F, et al. The relationship of the marginal mandibular nerve to the mandibular osseocutaneous ligament and lesser ligaments of the lower face. Aesthet Surg J. 2015;35(2):111–20.
29. Rohrich RJ, Pessa JE. The fat compartments of the face: anatomy and clinical implications for cosmetic surgery. Plast Reconstr Surg. 2007;119(7):2219–27.
30. Gierloff M, et al. Aging changes of the midfacial fat compartments: a computed tomographic study. Plast Reconstr Surg. 2012;129(1):263–73.
31. Rohrich RJ, Pessa JE, Ristow B. The youthful cheek and the deep medial fat compartment. Plast Reconstr Surg. 2008;121(6):2107–12.
32. Mohammed A, Mark AC. Retaining ligaments of the face: review of anatomy and clinical applications. Aesthet Surg J. 2013;33(6):769–82.

2 Target-Specific Sandwich Technique (TSST)

Lim Tingsong and Won Lee

2.1 Introduction

Hyaluronic acid (HA) fillers have long been the gold standard in non-surgical facial rejuvenation, sought after for their ability to restore lost volume, enhance facial contours, and reduce wrinkles. Their popularity has been driven by their biocompatibility, ease of administration, and minimal recovery time. However, a significant shift in patient attitudes is emerging. Once celebrated for their safety and reversibility, HA fillers are now met with growing apprehension due to concerns about overfilling, migration, and long-term inflammatory reactions [1]. The rising fear of an "overfilled" or unnatural appearance—exacerbated by high-profile cases of filler complications—has led many patients to seek alternatives that prioritize subtlety, safety, and longevity.

Traditional multi-point injection techniques, which often rely on large filler volumes, have been increasingly scrutinized for contributing to complications such as asymmetry, excessive swelling, and delayed inflammatory responses [2]. The growing backlash against the overuse of HA fillers highlights the urgent need for refined techniques that minimize risks while achieving natural, long-lasting results.

To address this shift in patient concerns, target-specific sandwich technique (TSST)—a novel approach designed to optimize filler placement while reducing overall product use is much preferable. This technique strategically layers small amounts of HA filler with varying rheological properties at different tissue depths, ensuring structural support without excessive volumization. By adopting this tailored method, we aim to provide a safer, more precise, and patient-conscious approach to facial rejuvenation.

2.2 The Changing Landscape of HA Fillers

Despite the global HA filler market surpassing $5.5 billion in 2022 and projected to grow at 9.3% annually [3], the industry faces a paradox: demand for minimally invasive treatments is rising, but so is patient hesitation. Once viewed as a simple solution for age-related volume loss, HA fillers are now frequently associated with "filler fatigue," a phenomenon where patients feel their facial contours have been subtly distorted over time due to cumulative filler treatments [4]. Social media, which once fueled the filler boom, has now contributed to a widespread critique of

L. Tingsong
Clique Clinic, Kuala Lumpur, Malaysia
e-mail: drlim@cliqueclinic.com

W. Lee (✉)
Yonsei E1 Plastic Surgery Clinic,
Anyang, Kyonggi-do, Korea (Republic of)

W. Lee (ed.), *Innovative Injectable Techniques in Minimally Invasive Aesthetics*,
https://doi.org/10.1007/978-981-95-2161-6_2

the "pillow face" effect and the potential long-term impact of repeated HA injections.

The overfilled look, initially popularized by excessive midface augmentation, is increasingly seen as unnatural, leading patients to question the longevity and aesthetic risks of fillers. Recent cases of chronic swelling, nodule formation, and delayed inflammatory reactions have reinforced these concerns [5], making patients more cautious about treatment choices. Additionally, emerging research suggests that repeated filler injections may contribute to soft tissue malpositioning, particularly in aging faces, further fueling skepticism [6, 7].

In response to these evolving perceptions, the aesthetic industry is shifting toward techniques that use less filler while achieving superior, natural-looking results. The TSST aligns with this trend, offering a refined approach that strategically distributes fillers to enhance structure without excess volume [8].

2.3 Safety Considerations and the Future of HA Fillers

While HA fillers remain a cornerstone of nonsurgical aesthetics, their use requires greater caution and advanced technique refinement. Common risks such as filler migration, vascular occlusion, Tyndall effect, and delayed inflammatory responses have heightened patient concerns, necessitating safer, more conservative application methods [9, 10].

2.4 The Need for a More Targeted Approach

Given the increasing patient demand for natural and undetectable enhancements, it is essential to move away from traditional volumizing techniques that rely on high filler quantities. The TSST was developed to address these concerns, ensuring precise filler placement with minimal product use, ultimately reducing complications and patient anxiety [11, 12].

By focusing on layered filler application at specific anatomical sites, TSST allows for structural support without excessive bulking, addressing the key aesthetic concerns that have fueled filler skepticism. This approach offers a balance between volume restoration and facial harmony, preventing the heavy, overfilled appearance that has led to growing patient distrust in HA fillers.

2.5 Applying Fillers Rheology in TSST

Various HA fillers with distinct rheological properties are available for specific treatment objectives [13]. In TSST, three variants of filler were used and applied specifically in certain areas, chosen for their favorable safety and ability to achieve sustainable aesthetic outcomes:

- Filler with good projection capacity with relative moldability: ideal for deep supraperiosteal injections to restore volume and provide structural support in areas with thin skin, e.g., periorbital area, perioral area, temple, and forehead.
- Filler with good elasticity: High elasticity and resistance to deformation, best suited for shaping and structural enhancement in deeper tissues, e.g., the nose, chin, and mandibular angle.
- Fillers with good tissue integration: High cohesivity with homogenous tissue integration, making it suitable for superficial placement in mobile facial areas such as periorbital and perioral areas, without migration concerns.

2.6 The Target-Specific Sandwich Technique (TSST)

With the patient in an upright position, entry points are disinfected.

Recommendations:

- 25G × 40 or 50 mm cannula for multilayer distribution of fillers.
- 27G × 40 mm needle for direct pre-periosteal implantation.

For safety, a 25G cannula minimizes vascular injury risk while optimizing filler distribution. The midface entry point, designated as the X-point, is positioned between the lateral canthus and the oral commissure. Using the cannula, filler with good projection capacity and moldability is deposited in precise, minute quantities (0.05–0.1 cc) at key anatomical landmarks (Fig. 2.1) [14]:

- V-frame deformity (deep fat pad)
- Lateral orbital floor, along the lateral orbital rim
- Canine fossa, via the superficial nasolabial fat pad (Fig. 2.2)
- Interfascial space at the temple
- Subgaleal space at the forehead

Subsequently, fillers with good tissue integration are applied in the same regions at a more superficial depth (superficial sub-orbicularis oculi fat, SOOF) (Fig. 2.3).

Fillers with good elasticity are injected in small aliquots (0.02 cc) at the T-hollow, mandibular angle, and chin using a 27G sharp needle [15]. 25G × 40 or 50 mm cannula is being used for nose bridge instead (Fig. 2.4).

All the procedures can be performed by one entry point (Figs. 2.5, 2.6, 2.7, 2.8, 2.9, 2.10, 2.11, and 2.12). Additional needle injection can be performed (Figs. 2.13, 2.14, and 2.15).

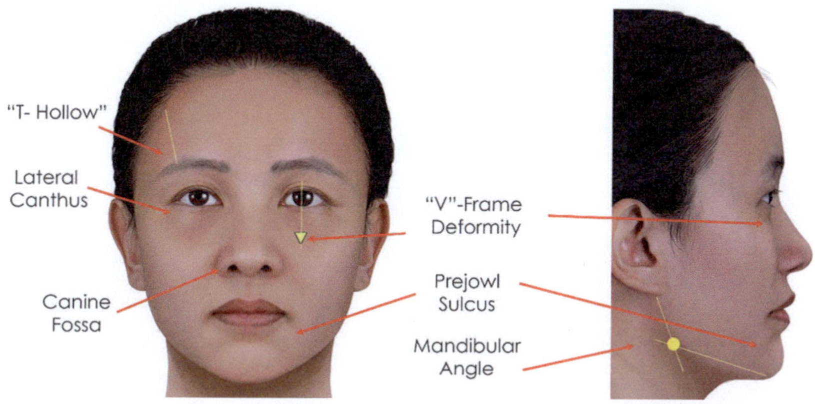

Fig. 2.1 Key anatomical landmark of the face

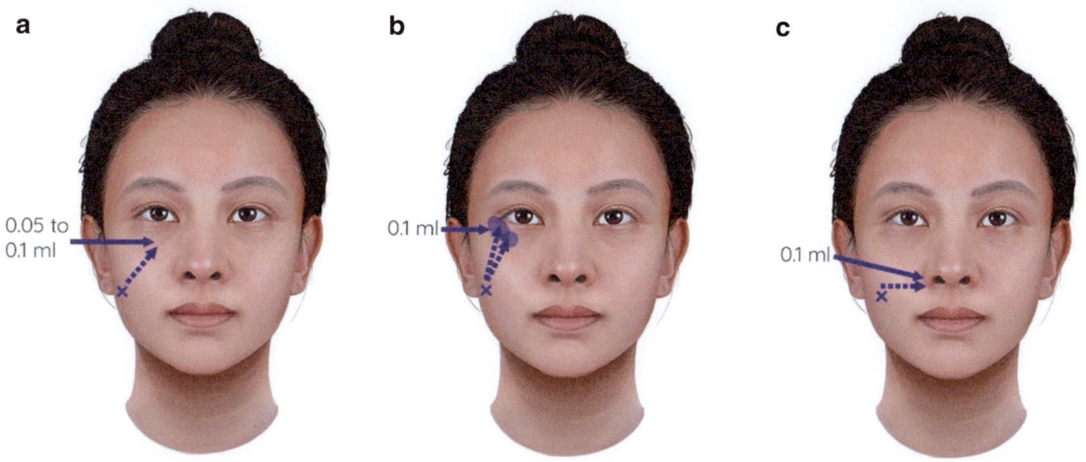

Fig. 2.2 Correction of tear trough deformity and nasolabial fold (**a**) tear trough correction (**b**) lateral canthus (**c**) nasolabial fold of tear trough deformity and nasolabial fold

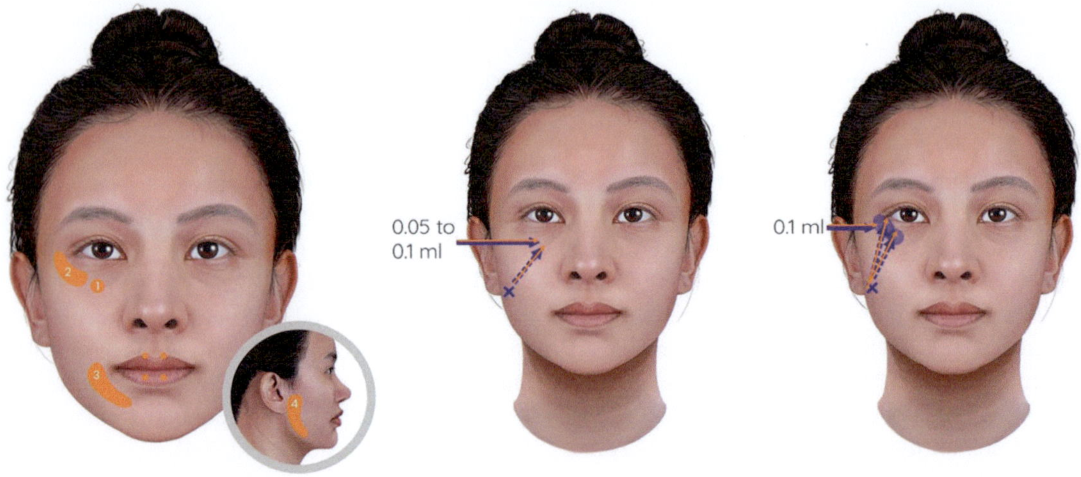

Fig. 2.3 Superficial injection

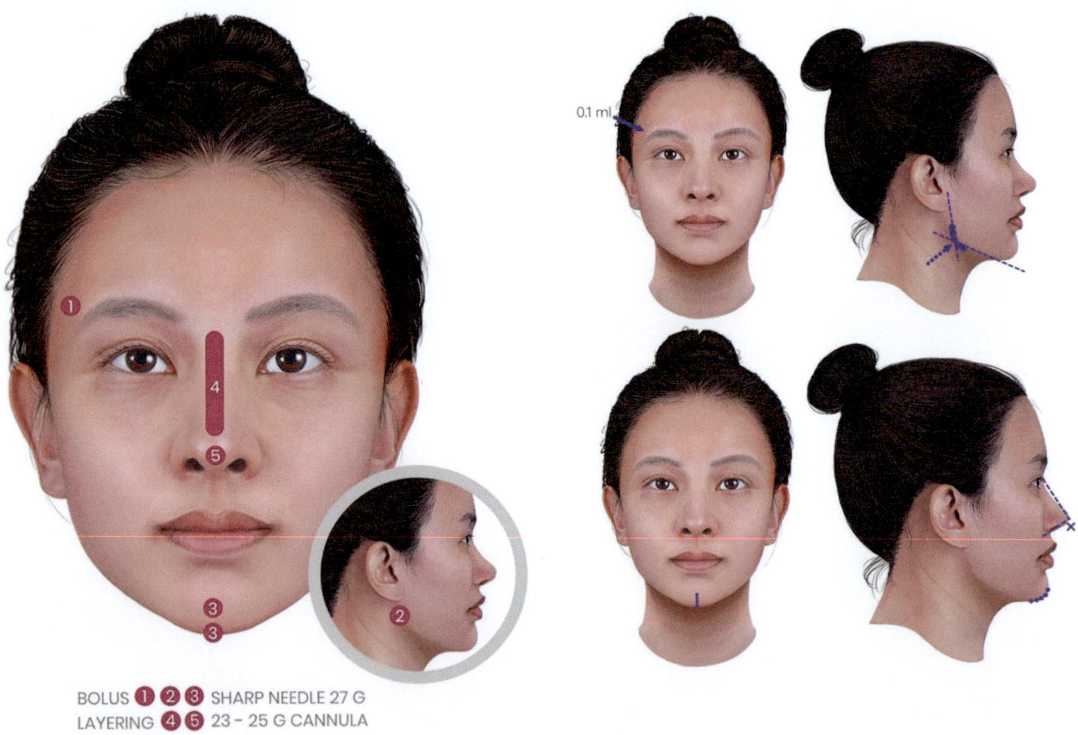

Fig. 2.4 Nose augmentation by cannula

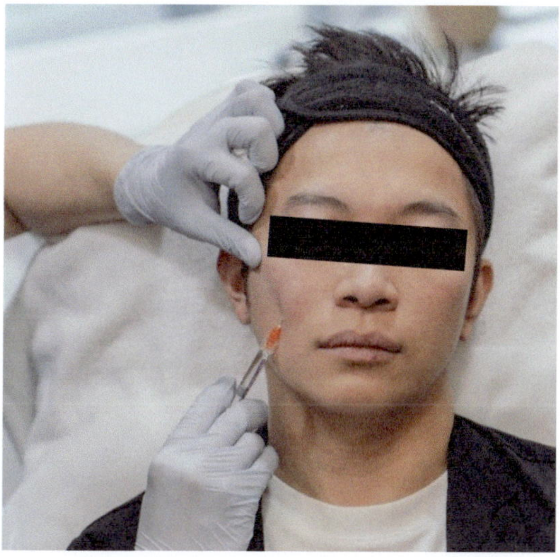

Fig. 2.5 Entry point of the cannula

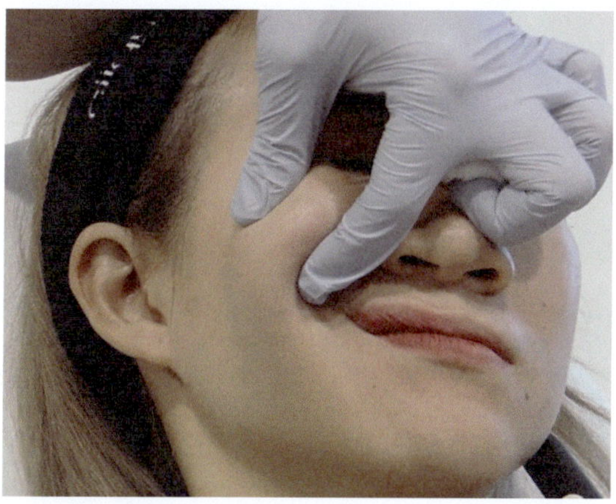

Fig. 2.6 Determining the entry point of the cannula

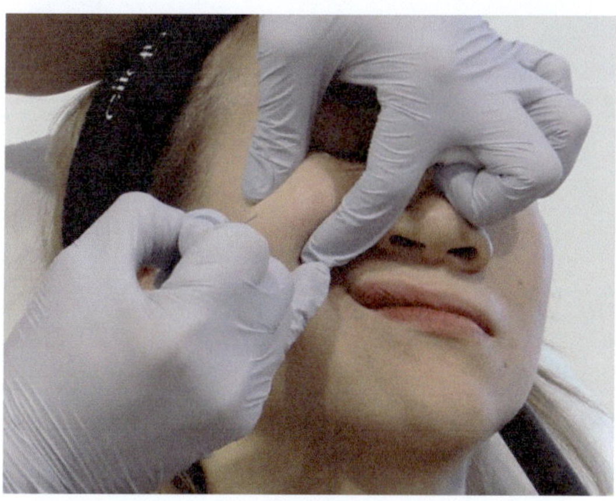

Fig. 2.7 Making insertion point of the cannula

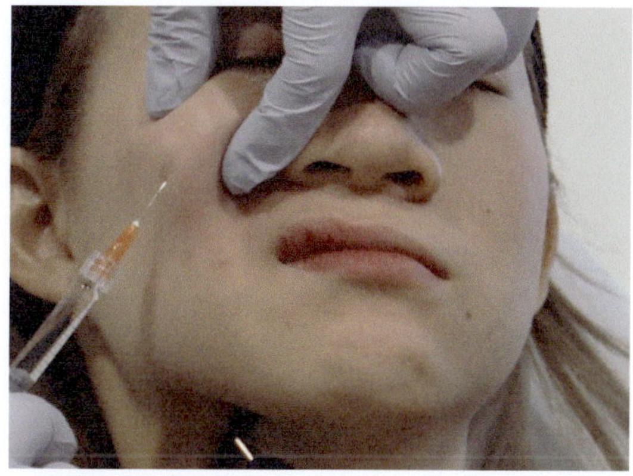

Fig. 2.8 Delivering fillers with good projection capacity and plasticity at the V-frame deformity

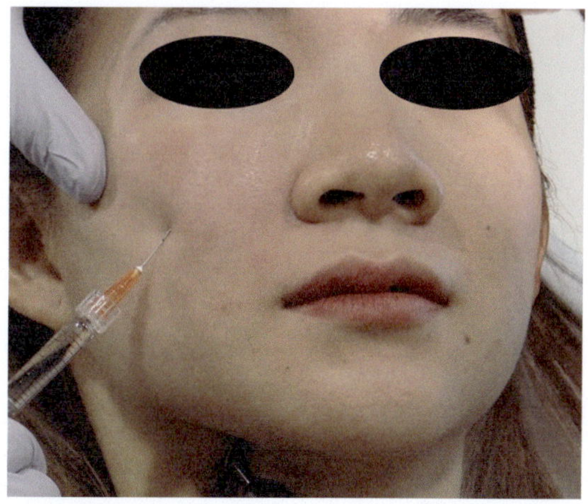

Fig. 2.9 Placing fillers at the V-frame deformity

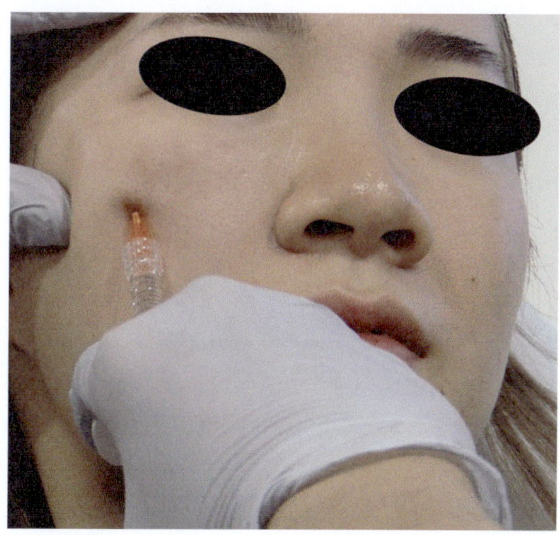

Fig. 2.10 Placing fillers at the lateral canthus

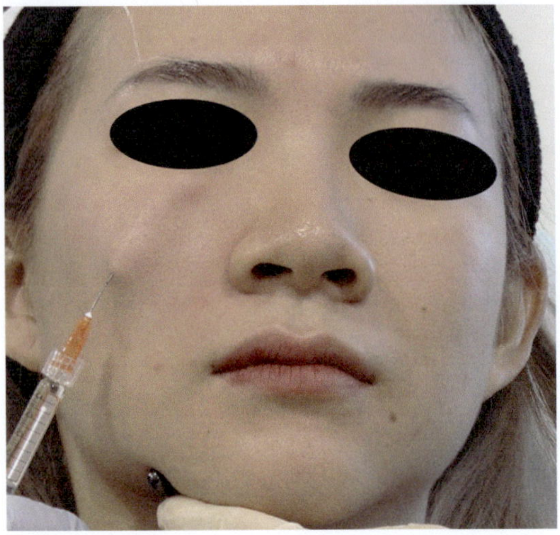

Fig. 2.11 Placing fillers with good tissue integration superficially at the v frame deformity

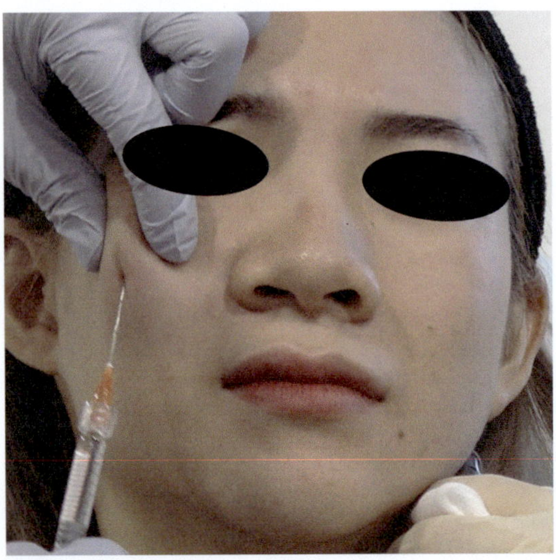

Fig. 2.12 Place fillers laterally at lateral canthus with fillers with good tissue integration

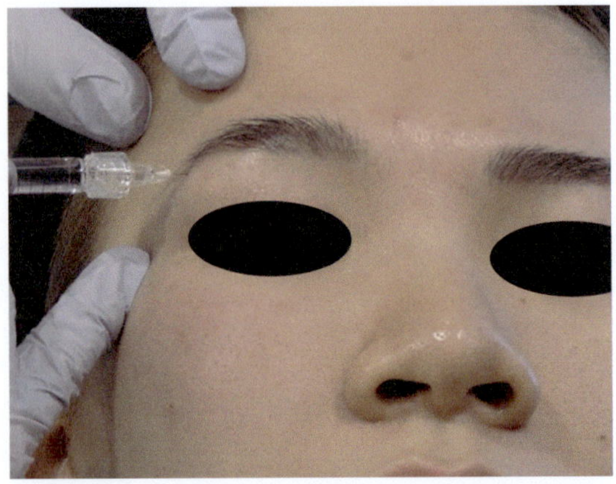

Fig. 2.13 Targeting the T-hollow with fillers with good elasticity using the walk-on-the-bone technique

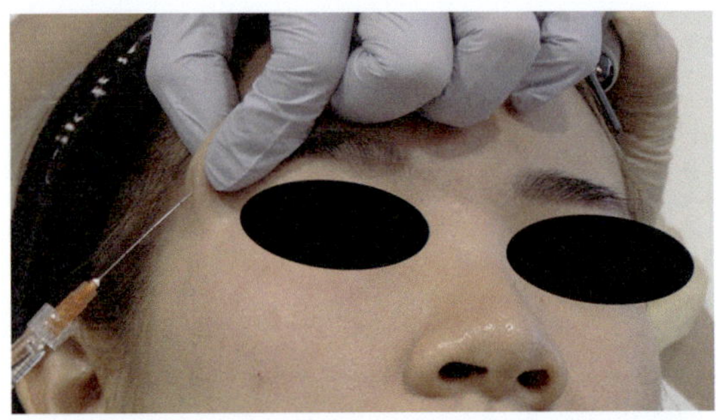

Fig. 2.14 Targeting the temple interfascial space with fillers with good projection capacity and plasticity using cannula

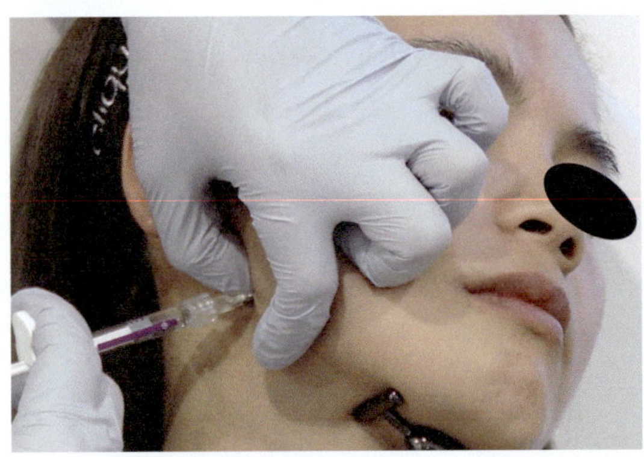

Fig. 2.15 Targeting the mandibular angle using a filler with good elasticity

2.7 Clinical Outcomes and Advantages

TSST reduces the number of injection points while optimizing filler distribution, resulting in the following:

- Reduced risk of vascular complications and product wastage
- Enhanced safety with controlled, low-pressure injections
- A natural, rejuvenated appearance without adding excessive weight to the soft tissue (Figs. 2.16, 2.17, 2.18, 2.19, and 2.20)

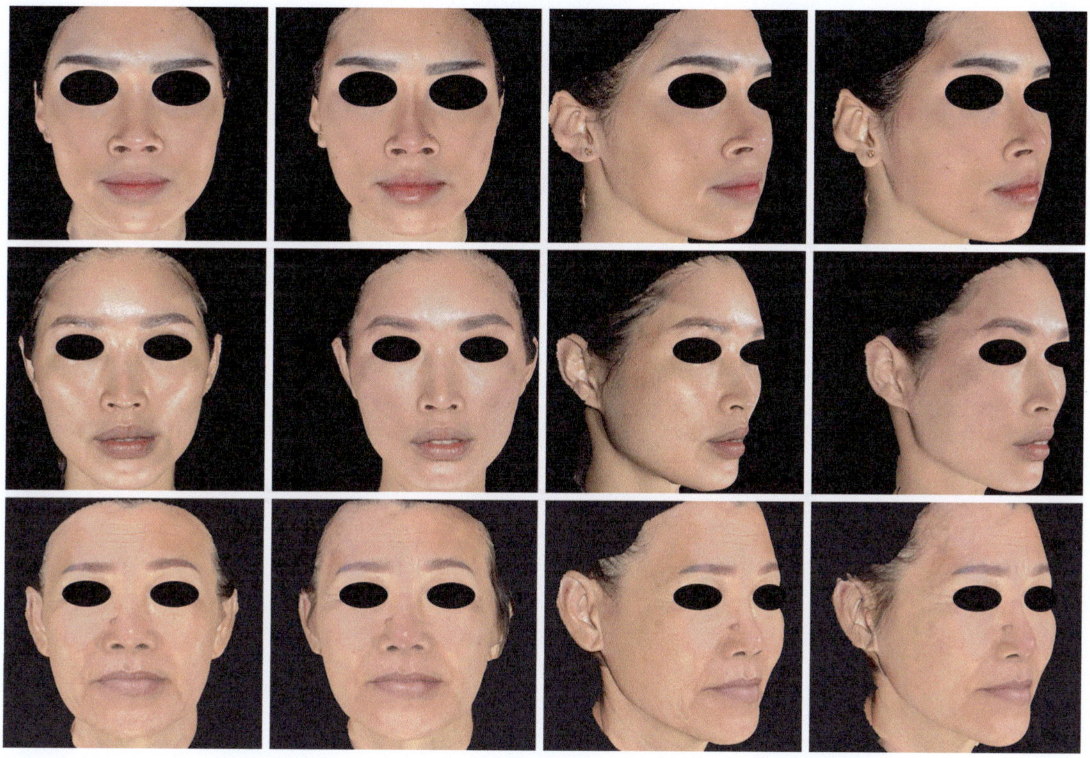

Fig. 2.16 Placing fillers with TSST has shown to maintain the natural features of the three patients

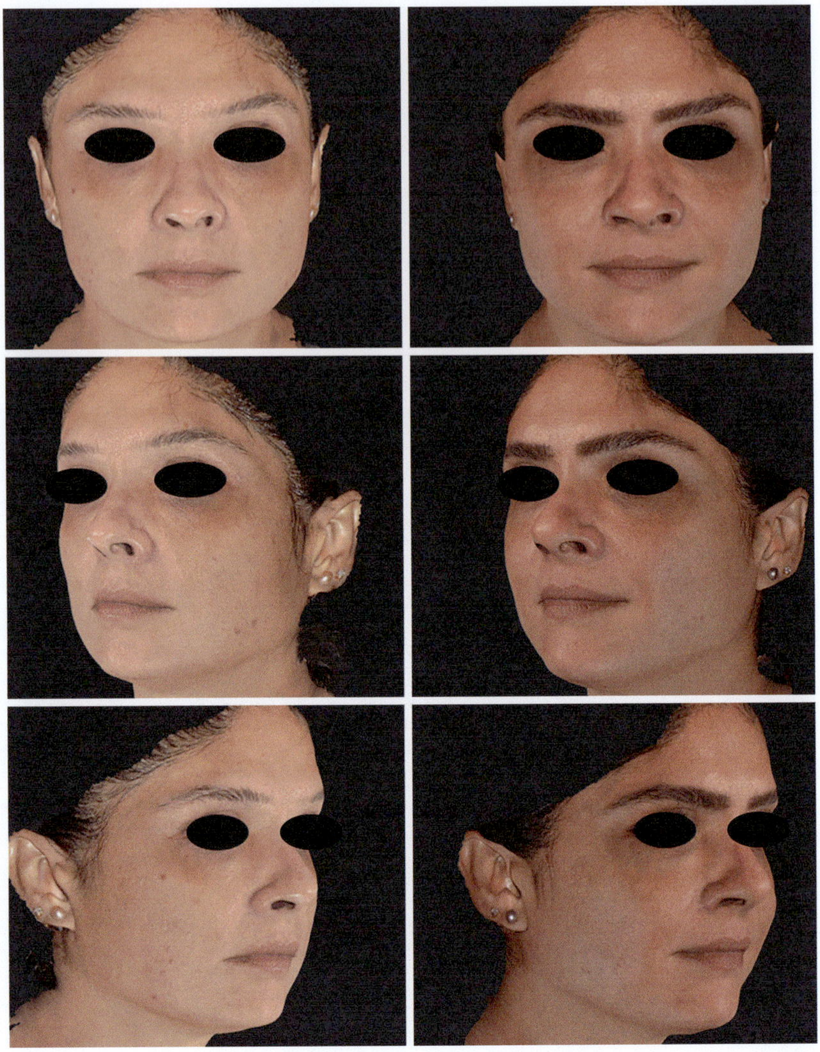

Fig. 2.17 Placing fillers with TSST has shown to maintain the natural features of the patient

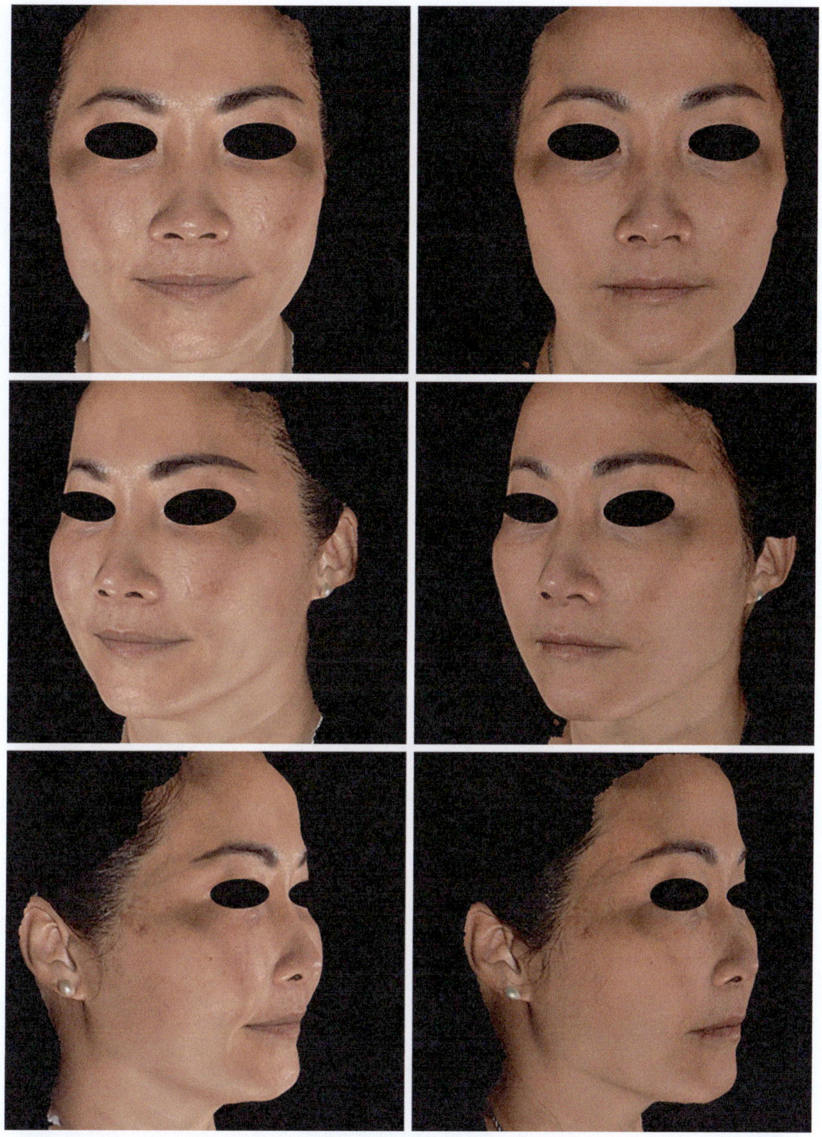

Fig. 2.18 Placing fillers with TSST has shown to maintain the natural features of the patient

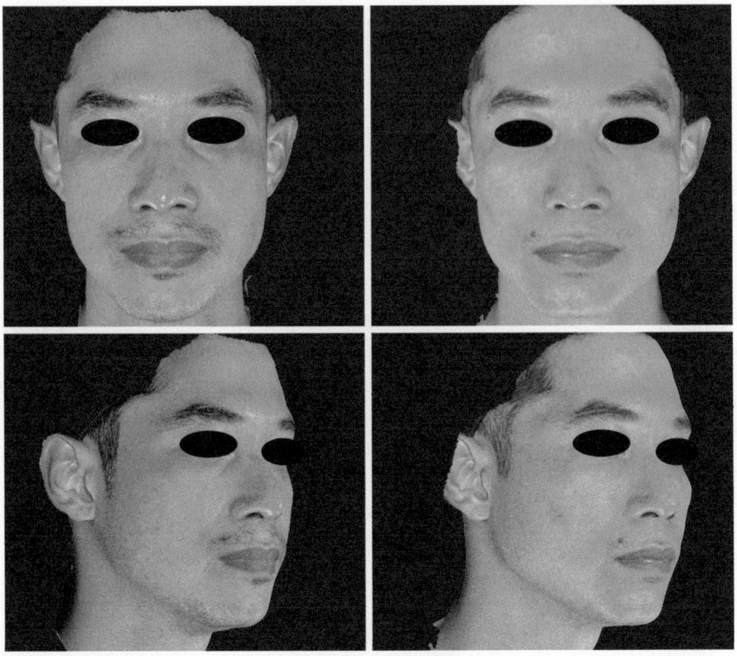

Fig. 2.19 Placing fillers with TSST has shown to maintain the natural features of the patient

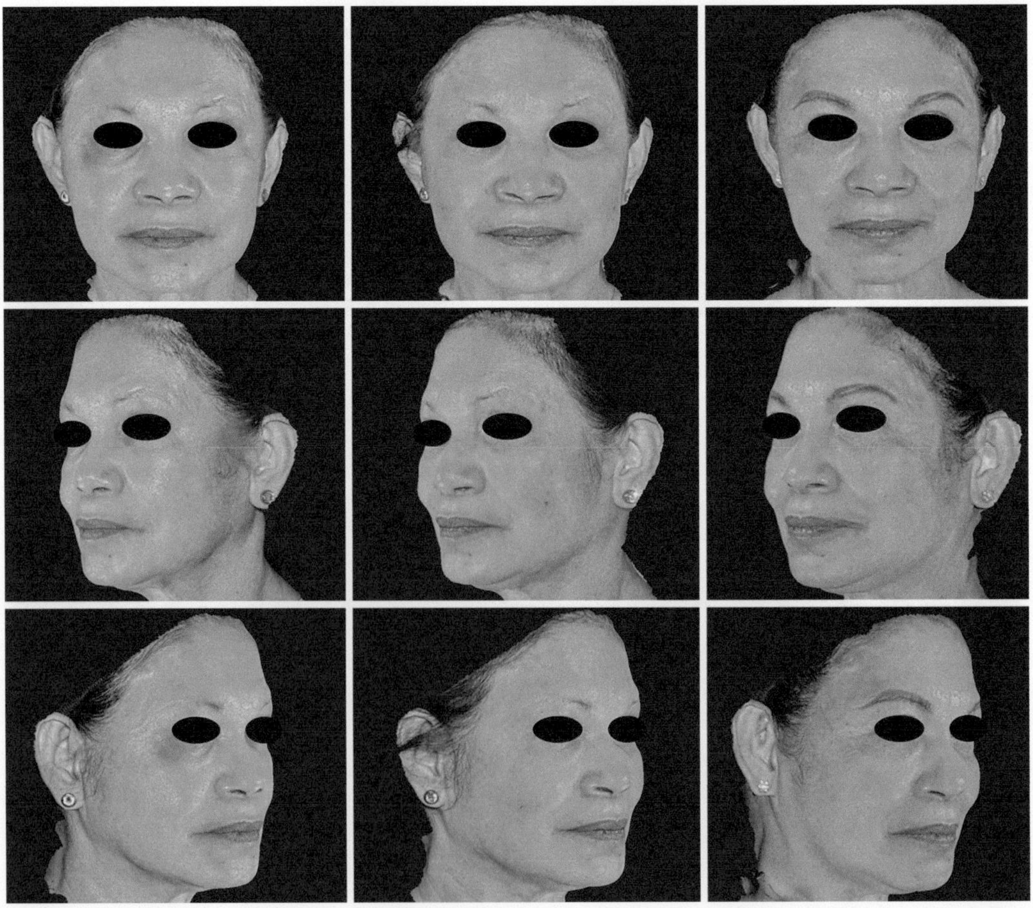

Fig. 2.20 Placing fillers with TSST has shown to maintain the natural features of the patient

2.8 Limitations and Future Considerations

Although TSST is effective in both Asian and Caucasian patients, injection sites must be adapted to accommodate ethnic anatomical differences [16]. Additionally, TSST requires advanced skills in cannula use and facial assessment, which may pose challenges for inexperienced practitioners. Despite these considerations, the technique offers a promising advancement in non-surgical facial rejuvenation, prioritizing safety and efficacy.

2.9 Conclusion

The TSST, by emphasizing precise, layered injections, represents a crucial step in addressing the growing fear surrounding HA fillers. By reducing filler volume and focusing on anatomical precision, this technique offers a more sustainable and patient-reassuring approach to facial rejuvenation.

As patient expectations evolve, aesthetic practitioners must adapt by prioritizing subtlety, safety, and longevity in their techniques. The future of HA fillers lies in minimizing risk while maximizing aesthetic outcomes, ensuring that patients regain confidence in these treatments without fear of unnatural results or long-term complications.

References

1. Edwards PC, Fantasia JE. Review of long-term adverse effects associated with the use of chemically-modified animal and nonanimal source hyaluronic acid dermal fillers. Clin Interv Aging. 2007;2(4):509–19.
2. Beer K, Avelar R. Relationship between delayed reactions to dermal fillers and biofilms: facts and considerations. Dermatologic Surg. 2014;40(11):1288–97.
3. Grand View Research. Hyaluronic acid market size report, 2023.
4. Wu WT, Peng PH, Liew S, et al. Consensus on current injectable treatment strategies in the Asian face. Aesth Plast Surg. 2016;40(2):202–14.
5. Lazzeri D, Agostini T, Figus M, et al. Blindness following cosmetic injections of the face. Plast Reconstr Surg. 2012;129(4):995–1012.
6. Liew S, Wu WT, Chan HH, et al. Consensus on changing trends, attitudes, and concepts of Asian beauty. Aesth Plast Surg. 2016;40(2):193–201.
7. Cotofana S, Schenck TL, Trevidic P, et al. The anatomy of the aging face: a review. Facial Plast Surg. 2016;32(3):253–60.
8. Lim TS, Frank RG. Target-specific sandwich technique: facial rejuvenation leveraging CPM technology. J Cosmet Dermatol. 2021;20(7):2024–30.
9. DeLorenzi C. Complications of injectable fillers, part 2: vascular complications. Aesthet Surg J. 2014;34(4):584–600.
10. Ginat DT, Schatz CJ. Imaging features of midface injectable fillers and associated complications. AJNR Am J Neuroradiol. 2013;34(8):1488–95.
11. Prasetyo AD, Sari MI, Bachtiar YA, et al. Hyaluronic acid fillers with cohesive polydensified matrix for soft-tissue augmentation and rejuvenation: a literature review. Clin Cosmet Investig Dermatol. 2016;9:257–80.
12. Lorenc ZP, Lambros V, Monheit GD, et al. Review of key Belotero Balance safety and efficacy trials. Plast Reconstr Surg. 2013;132(4 Suppl 2):33S–40S.
13. Sundaram H, Fagien S. Cohesive polydensified matrix hyaluronic acid for fine lines. Plast Reconstr Surg. 2015;136(5 Suppl):149S–63S.
14. Raspaldo H, Gassia V, Niforos FR, Michaud T. Global, 3-dimensional approach to natural rejuvenation: part 1–recommendations for volume restoration and the periocular area. J Cosmet Dermatol. 2012;11(4):279–89.
15. Patel U, Fitzgerald R. Facial shaping: beyond lines and folds with fillers. J Drugs Dermatol. 2010;9(8 Suppl ODAC Conf Pt 2):s129–37.
16. Landau M. Universal concepts of beauty and their implications on clinical approach to female cosmetic patient. In: Gender and dermatology. Springer; 2018. p. 255–65.

Injectable Biostimulators in Regenerative Aesthetics: Mechanisms, Clinical Applications, and Synergistic Approaches

3

How Kang Nien, Rungsima Wanitphakdeedecha, and Won Lee

3.1 Introduction

The rising demand for minimally invasive aesthetic procedures has led to significant advancements in soft tissue injectables, with injectable biostimulators gaining attention for their ability to stimulate collagen production and enhance skin structure over time. Offering a longer-lasting solution compared to traditional hyaluronic acid (HA) fillers, biostimulators are increasingly recognized for their role in skin rejuvenation, volume restoration, and overall structural support. Unlike traditional dermal fillers, which provide immediate volumization through gel-like substances, biostimulators work by triggering a controlled inflammatory response that stimulates fibroblast activity and enhances extracellular matrix production. These products are designed for deep tissue integration, leading to gradual aesthetic improvement and long-term remodeling, making them a cornerstone in regenerative aesthetics. Their rising popularity is attributed to their ability to improve skin laxity, texture, and structure while providing more natural-looking results with reduced maintenance compared to conventional fillers. Studies have shown that biostimulators not only enhance skin thickness, elasticity, and hydration but also contribute to facial contouring and structural support. As the global aesthetic market evolves and regenerative medicine gains momentum, the interest in biostimulators continues to grow, reinforcing their role as a key player in non-surgical aesthetic treatments.

This book chapter will explore the mechanism of action of biostimulators, detailing their role in collagen production and tissue remodeling. It will compare different biostimulators, highlighting their composition, longevity, and indications. The chapter will also cover dilution methods, application across various body areas, and management of potential complications such as nodules and delayed inflammatory reactions. Additionally, it will discuss the synergistic use of biostimulators with energy-based devices like HIFU, RF, and lasers to optimize outcomes.

H. K. Nien
Universiti Putra, Serdang, Selangor, Malaysia
e-mail: hkangnien@upm.edu.my

R. Wanitphakdeedecha
Siriraj Skin Laser Center, Bangkok, Thailand

W. Lee (✉)
Yonsei E1 Plastic Surgery Clinic,
Anyang, Kyonggi-do, Korea (Republic of)

3.2 Mechanism of Action of Biostimulators: An Overview

When a biostimulator is injected, it creates a controlled "injury" that engages the immune system and resident skin cells. Macrophages are among the first responders. They recognize the foreign material and orchestrate the healing response.

W. Lee (ed.), *Innovative Injectable Techniques in Minimally Invasive Aesthetics*,
https://doi.org/10.1007/978-981-95-2161-6_3

The biomaterial's presence polarizes macrophages into activation states that influence outcomes. M1 macrophages (classically activated) initiate inflammation and can secrete signals that recruit fibroblasts and endothelial cells for angiogenesis, while M2 macrophages (alternatively activated) secrete anti-inflammatory cytokines and growth factors (like TGF-β, IL-10) that promote tissue repair and collagen synthesis [1]. In the context of biostimulatory fillers, the goal is a balanced, regenerative inflammation: enough immune activity to induce collagen, but not so much as to cause fibrosis or scarring. The injected scaffold material can modulate this balance. For instance, CaHA has been shown to induce predominantly an M2-type response with minimal pro-inflammatory cell recruitment [1]. This favorable immune profile means that as CaHA particles are phagocytosed and cleared by macrophages, the macrophages release wound-healing signals that drive collagen deposition rather than chronic inflammation [1].

Fibroblasts are the key effector cells that actually produce new collagen and other ECM components. They are activated both by direct interaction with the scaffold and by cytokines from macrophages. Fibroblasts infiltrate the area and attach to or surround the biostimulator material. In some cases, the material provides mechanical cues, for example, spherical CaHA microparticles create local stretch/tension that directly stimulates fibroblasts via mechanotransduction [1]. This leads to secretion of collagen, elastin, and glycosaminoglycans in the surrounding tissue. In other cases (e.g., poly-L-lactic acid), the stimulation is more immune-mediated: the material alone does not directly cause fibroblasts to produce collagen until macrophages and giant cells release growth factors like TGF-β [1, 2]. Once activated, fibroblasts increase production of collagens (types I and III), as well as elastin and hyaluronic acid/proteoglycans, thereby rebuilding a healthy dermal matrix. Notably, studies have demonstrated increases in fibroblast numbers and activity in skin treated with biostimulatory fillers. Indeed, histological analyses in animal models show higher counts of fibroblasts and robust collagen fiber formation in tissue treated with CaHA or PCL compared to untreated controls [3]. Similarly, in vitro experiments indicate that fibroblast proliferation and collagen gene expression rise when co-cultured with these scaffold materials, especially in the presence of macrophages [1, 4]. Over time, some fibroblasts differentiate into α-SMA expressing myofibroblasts, which can contract and remodel the newly formed tissue, helping integrate the collagen scaffold into the surrounding skin [4]. This orchestrated interaction between macrophages and fibroblasts, with the biostimulator as the catalyst, underlies the neocollagenesis and tissue remodeling seen with these treatments.

Importantly, the quality of the ECM produced is improved, not just the quantity. Biostimulators can restore a more youthful architecture to the dermis. For instance, CaHA has been shown to improve collagen fiber organization and thickness, yielding aligned, mechanically robust fibers [1]. The new collagen III acts as a template that stabilizes and enhances the alignment of collagen I, resulting in a stronger, well-structured dermis [1]. In addition to collagen, regenerative fillers increase elastin (improving elasticity) and proteoglycans/hyaluronic acid (improving hydration and turgor) in the skin [1]. They also stimulate angiogenesis (growth of new capillaries) in the treated area, likely through macrophage and fibroblast release of VEGF and other factors [1, 5]. This richer blood supply nourishes the new tissue. Overall, the interaction of biostimulators with fibroblasts and immune cells leads to the synthesis of a full spectrum of dermal matrix components, remodeling aged or damaged tissue into a healthier state.

3.3 Comparative Biostimulatory Effects of Different Materials

Biostimulator products in aesthetics come in various compositions, each with unique properties that influence their collagen-stimulating behavior. Key examples include poly lactic acid (including poly-L-lactic acid and poly-D-L-lactic acid), calcium hydroxylapatite (CaHA), polycaprolactone (PCL), polydioxanone (PDO), and polynucleotides (PN). All serve as resorbable regenerative scaffolds, but they differ in how they interact with tissue, the intensity/duration of collagen stimulation, and their degradation profiles [6]. Below are some differences in biostimulatory mechanisms among these materials:

3.3.1 Poly-Lactic Acid Family: Poly-L-Lactic Acid (PLLA) and Poly-D-L-Lactic Acid (PDLLA)

Poly-lactic acid (PLA) biostimulators induces neocollagenesis through a controlled foreign-body reaction. Two stereochemical forms are used in aesthetics: poly-L-lactic acid (PLLA), a semi-crystalline polymer of L-lactide, and poly-D-L-lactic acid (PDLLA) a racemic (50:50) copolymer of D- and L-lactide that is fully amorphous. Both materials share a common mechanism of stimulating fibroblasts via macrophage-mediated pathways, but they differ in microstructure and biological response. PLLA's irregular particles tend to provoke a stronger initial M1 response (classically activated, pro-inflammatory macrophage), upregulating IL-6 secretion [4]. In contrast, the smoother PDLLA microspheres may elicit a milder initial inflammatory response. Indeed studies had found that PDLLA preferentially skew macrophages toward the M2 phenotypes, which is the alternatively activated, pro-healing type [7, 8]. This difference in macrophage skew leads to a difference in the cytokine milieu.

PLLA has been shown to upregulate Th2/M2 cytokines IL-4 and IL-13 in treated skin, which drive macrophages toward M2 polarization [4]. PLLA-activated macrophages secrete abundant TGF-β1 (transforming growth factor beta), a key fibrogenic cytokine, to stimulate fibroblast collagen production [4]. However, PLLA may also transiently elevate pro-inflammatory mediators. In a preclinical study, PLLA stimulation caused significant increases in four M1-associated cytokines (e.g. IL-6, TNF-α) and two M2-associated cytokines, reflecting an initial mixed response [4]. By contrast, PDLLA induces a more clearly anti-inflammatory cytokine profile. PDLLA-treated macrophages release high levels of IL-10, a potent anti-inflammatory cytokine, along with TGF-β [7, 8]. IL-10 secretion is a hallmark of M2 polarization and helps dampen TNF-α and NF-κB-mediated inflammation [7, 8]. Indeed, PDLLA has been shown to enhance NRF2 in macrophages, a transcription factor that inhibits NF-κB and oxidative stress, thereby reducing M1 cytokines (like TNF-α) while boosting IL-10 [7, 8]. The clinical improvement of the patient receiving PLLA is shown in Fig. 3.1.

Both PLLA and PDLLA are able to induce an transition from initial type III to predominant type I collagen, providing long-lasting structural support. However, the exact timing of the type I/III switching may vary. In human biopsy studies, PLLA caused a significant increase in type I collagen by 3–6 months, with only a slight, non-significant rise in type III [9]. By approximately 4 months post-injection, new type III collagen becomes detectable in the treated tissue, but it is soon followed and overtaken by robust type I deposition [10]. On the other hand, histology from animal studies confirms that collagen fibers appear within weeks of PDLLA placement: total collagen is evident by week 4, and by 8–12 weeks, abundant type I collagen is present between and even inside the PDLLA microspheres [11].

In conclusion, both PLLA and PDLLA share a common regenerative outcome, with slight difference in macrophage activation and scaffold structure. PLLA leans on a slower more inflammatory start that transition to remodeling, whereas PDLLLA takes a faster, more M2-friendly track. Ultimately both creates collagen-rich tissue with minimal residual implant, improved vascularity, and restoration of dermal thickness. However, PLLA offers a longer track record of efficacy and durability in inducing neocollagenesis [10].

3.3.2 Calcium Hydroxylapatite (CaHA)

Calcium hydroxylapatite is an inorganic bioceramic composed of calcium phosphate particles

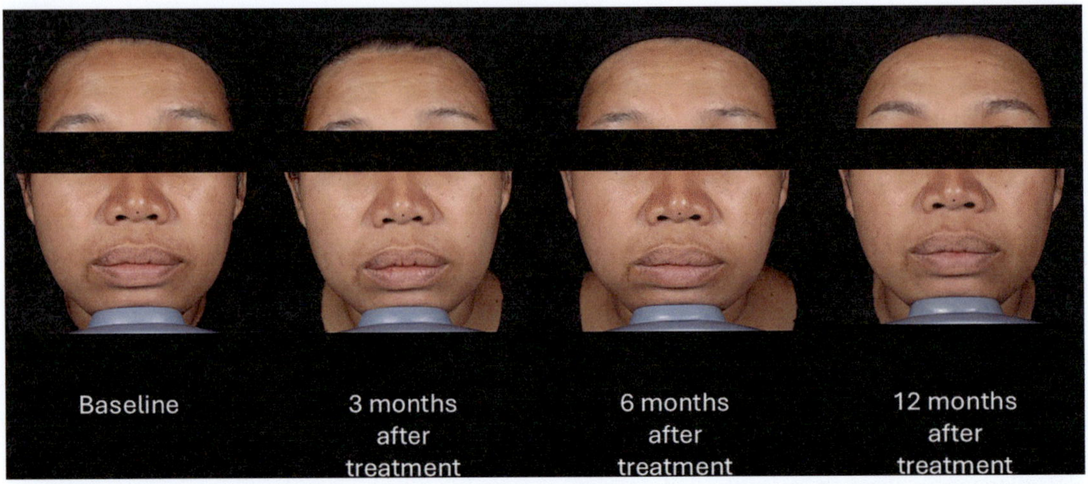

Fig. 3.1 A 45-year-old female patient receiving a single treatment session of poly-L-lactic acid (PLLA) injection. The images depict the progression from baseline to 3 months, 6 months, and 12 months post-treatment. Over time, notable improvements are observed, including enhanced skin brightness, smoother texture, and a reduction in visible pores

(~25–45 μm) suspended in a carboxymethylcellulose gel. CaHA provides an immediate filling effect from the gel carrier and a longer-term scaffold effect from the microspheres. Its mechanism is twofold, namely, direct fibroblast stimulation and gentle immune modulation. The smooth CaHA spheres create a supportive matrix in which fibroblasts can attach and proliferate, and they also exert mechanical tension on surrounding cells. This mechanotransduction quickly triggers fibroblasts to produce new collagen [1]. CaHA also induces neocollagenesis in vivo with minimal inflammation: within 1 month of injection, there is often collagen deposition around the microspheres with only scant inflammatory cells present [1]. As the gel carrier is absorbed over a few weeks, space is created for cellular ingrowth, such as fibroblasts and capillaries, between the CaHA particles [1]. Macrophages do participate in clearing CaHA eventually, but CaHA's immunological footprint is mild. It tends to avoid strong adaptive immune activation; studies note that CaHA causes little to no chronic inflammation or T-cell infiltration [1]. Instead, macrophages interacting with CaHA lean toward an M2 phenotype that facilitates regenerative healing [1]. The result is robust collagen type I and III production, along with increased elastin and proteoglycans in the area [1]. A hallmark of CaHA's collagen stimulation is the presence of type III collagen early on, which gradually matures to type I [1]. This is analogous to natural wound healing and yields a well-organized collagen matrix. CaHA's biostimulatory effect has been demonstrated in both animals and humans: canine studies showed a steady increase in collagen content from 4 weeks through 78 weeks after CaHA injection, corresponding to the particles gradually resorbing and being replaced by collagen fibers [1]. Clinically, CaHA improves skin firmness and elasticity; histologically it has been shown to increase dermal collagen fiber density and thickness for up to a year or more [1]. In summary, CaHA acts as a regenerative scaffold that "tricks" the tissue into rebuilding itself: it provides immediate structure and over time is replaced by the body's own collagen with minimal long-term inflammation [1].

3.3.3 Polycaprolactone (PCL)

Polycaprolactone is a synthetic aliphatic polyester that, like PLLA, comes as biodegradable microspheres (e.g. in Ellansé). PCL has the

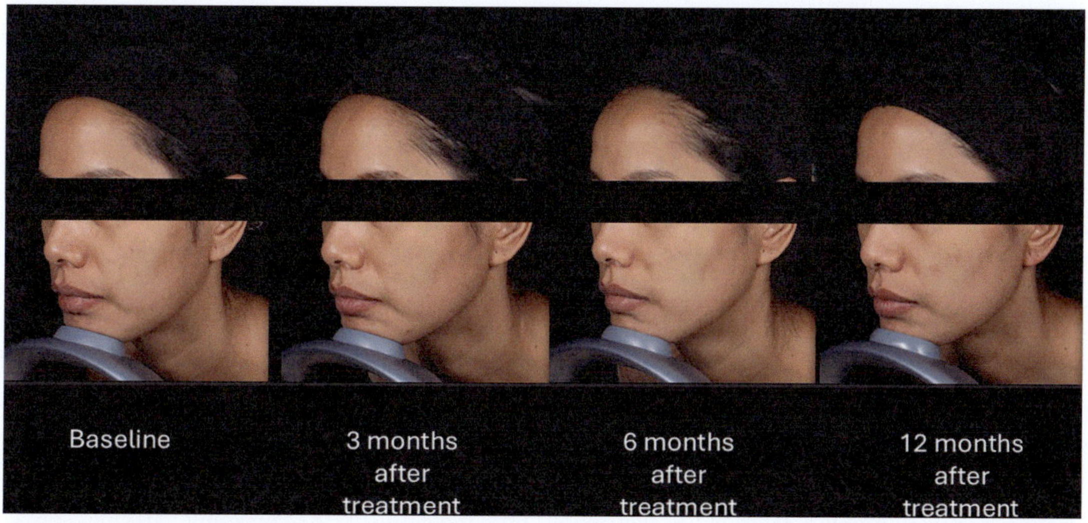

Fig. 3.2 A 40-year-old female patient undergoing three treatment sessions of polycaprolactone (PCL) injections, administered at 1-month intervals. The images illustrate the progression from baseline to 3 months, 6 months, and 12 months post-treatment. Over time, noticeable enhancements are observed, including increased skin brightness, smoother texture, and overall improvement in skin quality

longest persistence of the common biostimulatory fillers, owing to very slow hydrolysis of its polymer chains [6]. Mechanistically, PCL's stimulation of collagen is often compared to PLLA's, since both are foreign-body type stimulators. Injection of PCL microspheres triggers a localized foreign body reaction where macrophages and giant cells surround the particles, releasing growth factors that induce fibroblast activity. The key difference is kinetics: PCL breaks down over 2–4 years, depending on formulation, providing a prolonged stimulus. In vivo studies have shown that PCL and CaHA are equally effective in boosting collagen in the mid-term. For example, a head-to-head rat study demonstrated that at 2 and 4 months post-injection, both PCL and CaHA had significantly increased dermal collagen content (with higher collagen I and III levels) relative to controls and with no difference between the two fillers in total collagen yield [3]. However, PCL tended to sustain fibroblast activation longer—by 4 months, the PCL-treated skin had a higher number of fibroblasts than CaHA-treated skin, suggesting a more prolonged biostimulatory phase [3]. This aligns with PCL's slower resorption; the microspheres remain to stimulate tissue remodeling for an extended period. Clinically, PCL fillers achieve results that can last around 3 years or more, with gradual collagen accumulation maintaining volume and skin quality. The immune response to PCL is generally moderate: like PLLA, it can incite a foreign-body reaction, but the slower degradation may spread out the inflammatory stimulus, potentially reducing the intensity of any one inflammatory burst. Some literature indicates that PCL particles being smooth and uniform might lead to a more controlled macrophage response (less spiky than PLLA particles) [1]. Overall, PCL combines a PLLA-like mechanism of collagen induction with a CaHA-like longevity (yielding a durable scaffold). Its biostimulatory profile is characterized by steady, long-term collagenogenesis with a good safety profile when properly injected (low incidence of granulomas reported, likely due to its sustained, gentle stimulation). The clinical improvement of the patient receiving PCL treatment is shown in Fig. 3.2.

3.3.4 Polydioxanone (PDO)

PDO is a biodegradable polymer conventionally used in PDO threads for tissue lifting and collagen stimulation. PDO has been recently formulated as a powdered microsphere for collagen stimulation. Combining with carboxymethylcellulose as a carrier, it is marketed as a "liquid PDO threads," with 200 mg vial essentially similar to approximately 1400 PDO monofilament. Similar to many other biostimulators, PDO trigger a mild foreign body inflammatory response that ultimately stimulate fibroblast to produce collagen [12]. Macrophages drawn to the PDO particles are pivotal "middleman" in biostimulation. However, its role on M1 and M2 macrophage is not well described. In vitro direct contact of PDO with fibroblast alone also does not significantly increase collagen production [2], indicating that in vivo immune/fibroblast interplay is that who drives neocollagenesis.

Though PDO threads and PDO powder rely on the same material and basic mechanism, but their tissue interaction differ. Threads are larger implant that cause collagen to form along the thread's length, often creating a fibrous "sheath" around the thread [2]. Thread can provide an immediate mechanical lift in addition to delayed collagen deposition. In contrast, PDO powder provides pure biostimulatory effect, with collagen gradually improving skin firmness and texture overtime [13]. Indeed, one animal study comparing injectable PLLA vs. PDO found that both induced a similar amount of collagen by 12 weeks, with both showing a higher proportion of type III collagen in the early phase of healing [12]. Interestingly, PDO particles caused slightly less intense granulomatous inflammation than PLLA in that model, suggesting PDO might be a gentler stimulator when used as an implant material [2]. As PDO powder has a higher surface-area-to-volume ratio, it is postulated that it allows faster hydrolysis.

3.3.5 Polynucleotides (PN)

Unlike the above structural fillers, polynucleotides are biochemical biostimulators. They are fragments of nucleic acids (DNA/RNA polymers, often derived from salmon DNA or synthesized) used in injectable skin treatments (sometimes called PDRN for polydeoxyribonucleotide). Polynucleotides do not provide significant volume or a physical scaffold for cells; instead, they work by engaging cell receptors and improving the tissue environment. One primary mechanism is through activation of adenosine A2A receptors on immune cells and fibroblasts [5]. When PN fragments bind these receptors, cAMP/PKA signaling is triggered, leading to increased production of growth factors such as VEGF and other regenerative signals [5]. This results in enhanced angiogenesis and has an anti-inflammatory effect, as A2A activation shifts macrophages toward a healing phenotype [5]. In parallel, polynucleotides can enter the "salvage pathway" of nucleotide metabolism [5], whereby enzymes break them down into nucleosides and bases that can be reused by cells for DNA/RNA synthesis. In tissues with high turnover or damage, this supply of nucleotides supports cell proliferation and repair. Research shows PN injections stimulate fibroblast growth and activity, leading to increased synthesis of collagen and hyaluronic acid in the dermis [5]. Unlike the other materials, PN does not invoke a foreign body reaction; rather, it creates a bioactive milieu that encourages cells to regenerate. It may also form a transient gel-like matrix upon injection that slightly hydrates and volumizes the tissue and could serve as a temporary scaffold at the microscopic level. PN treatments are known for improving skin quality, which correlates with the increased collagen/elastin content and improved ECM organization observed in studies. Another interesting aspect is that polynucleotides have been reported to scavenge free radicals and protect cells from UV-induced damage, further aiding tissue repair. Notably, these effects have been noted in dermatologic studies of PDRN [5]. The biostimulatory effect of PN is subtle and gradual; typically a series of injections over weeks is done. Since PN are water-soluble and metabolized quickly, their direct action is short, but they set in motion regenerative pathways that outlast their presence. There is usually minimal inflammation. Overall, polynucleotide injectables function as cellular stimulants and regenerative signals rather than physical fillers, directly targeting fibroblasts and macrophages to induce collagen remodeling in an especially biocompatible, gentle manner.

3.4 Preparation for Different Biostimulators

Injectable biostimulators such as PLLA, PDLLA, CaHA, PCL, PDO, and PN are collagen-stimulating fillers supplied as either lyophilized powders or suspensions. These products often require proper dilution (reconstitution with a diluent) before injection. Dilution technique is critical because it influences product handling, safety, and clinical outcomes. Table below listed the manufacturer recommended dilution protocols for injectables biostimulators. However, hybrid biostimulators such as PDLLA/HA are not listed (Table 3.1).

Table 3.1 Manufacturer-recommended dilution protocols for injectable biostimulators

Biostimulator (brand)	Composition (active + excipient)	Forms (molecular size)	Reconstitution method (manufacturer instruction)	Diluents used	Mixing technique
PLLA (Sculptra®, Galderma)	150 mg PLLA; 90 mg CMC; 127.5 mg mannitol	Lyophilized powder (40–63 µm)	According to product information leaflet. Option 1: Add 5 mL SWFI per vial (previous recommendation) Option 2: 8 mL SWFI +1 mL lidocaine for immediate injection (total 9 mL per vial)	SWFI, optional 1–2 mL of 2% lidocaine	Sit for hydrate for at least 2 h to up to 72 h (if refrigerated)
PDLLA (Aesthefill®, REGEN Biotech)	154 mg PDLLA +46 mg CMC	Lyophilized powder (30–70 µm, porous spherical structure)	Depending on treatment indication. In general 7–8 mL (superficial fine lines) of SWFI per vial [14–16]	SWFI, optional 1–2 mL of 1% lidocaine [16] DO NOT use NSS to avoid slow mixing[a]	Standing time in 10–30 min, agitate manually before injection further dilution with NSS is possible with back and forth method [14, 16]
Hybrid PDLLA (Juvelook, VAIM Global)	42.5 mg PDLLA +7.5 mg non-crossed-linked hyaluronic acid	Lyophilized powder (10–40 µm, porous spherical structure)	8 ml of SWFI or NSS other protocols had been described[a]	SWFI or NSS. 1 ml of lidocaine 2% can be added	Vortex for 30 min before injecting Unused preparation can be stored in refrigerator up to 72 h

(continued)

Table 3.1 (continued)

Biostimulator (brand)	Composition (active + excipient)	Forms (molecular size)	Reconstitution method (manufacturer instruction)	Diluents used	Mixing technique
Hybrid PDLLA (Lenisna, VAIM Global)	170 mg PDLLA +30 mg non-crossed-linked hyaluronic acid	Lyophilized powder (40–80 μm, porous spherical structure)	Face: 16mls of SWFI or NSS Body: 20mls of SWFI or NSS other protocols had been described[a]	SWFI or NSS 1 ml of lidocaine can be added	Add 5 ml of SWFI +1 ml of lidocaine (6 ml of SWFI if no lidocaine added) followed by vortex for 30 min Solution is then withdrawn and 10 ml of SWFI will be added in a 20 ml syringe. Mixture is then transferred back and forth between two connected 20 ml syringes for four times
CaHA (Radiesse®, Merz)	30% Calcium hydroxyapatite +70% aqueous gel of glycerin + sodium CMC + SWFI) ± 0.3% lidocaine premixed	Smooth, cohesive off white gel (25–45 μm)	No reconstitution required if meant for contouring. 1:2–4 ml dilution with NSS has been described.	0.9% Normal Saline (NSS), lidocaine	Using two interconnected tube, desired volume of NSS is aspirated, and mixture is then transferred back and forth between two connected 20 ml syringes for 20 times
PCL (Ellansé®, Sinclair)	30% PCL microspheres +70% excipients (CMC)	Pre-filled syringe, smooth white suspension gel (25–50 μm)	No reconstitution needed (pre-filled syringes); optional 0.1–0.3 mL of 2% lidocaine per 1 mL filler to improve injection comfort	Lidocaine (1–2%), if needed	
PCL (Gouri®, Dexlevo)	21% (210 mg/ml) PCL fully solubilized in proprietary solvent system	Pre-filled syringe, milky solution (fully solubilized with no microparticles)	No reconstitution needed	–	–

(continued)

Table 3.1 (continued)

Biostimulator (brand)	Composition (active + excipient)	Forms (molecular size)	Reconstitution method (manufacturer instruction)	Diluents used	Mixing technique
PN (Poly-nucleotides)—Rejuran®, Plinest	10–20 mg/mL polynucleotide + excipients		Ready-to-use; no dilution required, but optional ~0.1 mL lidocaine for pain reduction	No dilution required; optional lidocaine	

SWFI sterile water for injection

[a]PDO powder (Ultracol 100 & 200, Ultra V) is commercially available and marketed with the claim that each vial is equivalent to 1400 PDO threads in biostimulatory effect. However, standardized dilution methods and injection techniques are not widely documented online. To date, only minimal clinical study has evaluated PDO powder for volumizing the nasolabial folds, but the reconstitution and mixing protocol was not clearly detailed in the publication [13, 17]

3.5 Common Indication for Biostimulators

Biostimulators are commonly used for the treatment of aging and sagging skin, subcutaneous tissue restructuring, and atrophic scars. It is also utilized to prevent sagging and aging, as well as for subcutaneous or deep replacement of facial folds. Non-facial indications extend to areas such as the neck, décolletage, arms, thighs, abdomen, buttocks, hands, knees, and the genital/peri-genital region. However, not all biostimulators are suitable for every treatment area, as their mechanism of action, particle size, viscosity, and collagen-stimulating effects vary. Some carry higher risks of nodule formation, vascular complications, or poor integration in delicate areas like the forehead, periorbital, and perioral regions. Below is a summary on whether each product is recommended, cautiously used, or contraindicated in specific treatment zones (Table 3.2).

Key Considerations

- Not all biostimulators are suitable for every area.
  - PLLA, PDLLA, CaHA, and PCL are deep injectables.
  - PDO and PN are superficial injectables.
- High-risk areas (not recommended):
  - Forehead and periorbital: Risk of vascular occlusion and nodules.
  - Lips: Risk of visible lumps and poor tissue integration.
- Best for skin rejuvenation (superficial placement, no volume effect):
  - PDO and PN → Ideal for fine wrinkles, hydration, elasticity improvement.
- Best for deep volume and structural support:
  - PLLA, PDLLA, PCL, CaHA → Best for jawline, cheeks, chin, temples (Table 3.3)

Table 3.2 Biostimulator suitable by area

Biostimulator	Forehead	Temple	Midface (cheek, malar, submalar)	Nasolabial folds	Perioral region (lips, marionette lines)	Jawline and chin	Neck and décolletage	Hands	Body (arms, abdomen, knees, buttocks, thighs)
PLLA (Sculptra) [18, 19]	Not recommended	Safe	Safe	Safe	Not recommended	Safe	Caution	Safe	Safe
PDLLA (Aesthefill)	Not recommended	Safe	Safe	Safe	Caution[a,b]	Safe	Inadequate recommendation		
CaHA (Radiesse) [20, 21]	Not recommended	Safe	Safe	Safe	Not recommended	Safe	Safe	Safe	Safe
PCL (Ellansé) [22]	Safe	Safe	Safe	Safe	Safe	Safe	Inadequate recommendation		
PDO (Ultracol 100, Ultracol 200)	Inadequate recommendation								
PN (Rejuran, Plinest, Newest) [23]	Intradermal for skin quality improvement and rejuvenation. Also suitable for crow feet reduction		Safe (intradermal injection)	Safe (intradermal injection)	Intradermal for skin quality improvement and rejuvenation.		Inadequate recommendation		

Table 3.3 Injection protocols by treatment area [16, 18, 19, 21, 23]

Area	Injection techniques	Injection planes	Immediate care	Aftercare	Follow-up
Forehead	Linear threading Cross-hatching, fanning with 22–25G cannula Serial puncture, depot, microdroplet technique with 27G—30G needle	Supraperiosteal (preferred), subdermal	Immediate massage is recommended to spread product evenly. Certain products may be required consistent massage for the subsequent few days (manufacturer guidelines should be referred) Ice packs if swelling	Keep face clean, avoid make up, avoid excessive facial movement, pressure, alcohol, smoking, excessive heat and radiation exposure (sun and sauna), swimming, bathing	Based on the severity of the condition Mild and preventive cases: one session may suffice Moderate cases: may require 2–3 sessions Severe cases: may need three or more sessions Can combine with other treatment modalities Minimum interval between sessions: 30 days
Temple		Deep supraperiosteal, interfascia plane, or subdermal			
Midface (cheeks, malar, submalar)		Subdermal, supraperiosteal			
Nasolabial folds		Supraperiosteal upper one third with subdermis over lower two-thirds			
Perioral region (lips, marionette lines)		Subdermal			
Jawline an Chin		Supraperiosteal, subdermal			
Neck and décolletage		Superficial subdermal			
Hands		Dorsal superficial lamina or dorsal intermediate lamina was described			
Body (arms, abdomen, knees, buttocks, thighs)		Deep dermis, subcutaneous			

3.6 Contraindication for Biostimulators

Below are common contraindications that should be taken into account before injection.

Absolute contraindication	Active inflammatory or infectious processes at the application site Active collagen disorders Presence of permanent fillers in the same location and plane Ongoing pregnancy Active herpes infections near the treatment area
Relative contraindication	Other active inflammatory processes Autoimmune diseases (including collagen disorders in remission) Blood dyscrasia and anticoagulation Liver dysfunctions Different types of permanent fillers in other locations or planes Lactation The use of anti-inflammatory or immunosuppressive drugs Recent surgical intervention at treatment site (within the last 2 months) Other significant disruptions in homeostasis Uncontrolled diabetes and metabolic syndrome

3.7 Complications Related to Biostimulators

Mild adverse events such as pain, swelling, and bruising at the treatment site are common and should be anticipated. The incidence of nodule formation ranges from 0.4% to 6.9%, with a lower likelihood observed when higher reconstitution volumes are used [24–26]. Nodules are more frequently reported in dynamic facial areas, which are therefore recommended to be avoided when possible [21]. Persistent palpable subcutaneous papules or nodules at injection sites are characteristic of intermediate-onset (months) and late-onset (>2 years) adverse reactions [27].

Intermediate-onset papules are typically small (1–3 mm), gradually develop over several months post-injection, remain stable in size, and generally resolve spontaneously within 3 months [1, 8]. Late-onset papules and nodules, on the other hand, present abruptly, may be associated with tissue edema and often exhibit periodic flare-ups followed by partial regression, persisting for several years [27].

Early-onset nodules can be managed with vigorous massage and intralesional normal saline injections. Late-onset nodules should be approached by first ruling out infection and inflammation. Antibiotic is necessary if infection and biofilms are suspected [28]. Refractory non-infected nodules can be approached using intralesional corticosteroid, intralesional 5-fluorouracil injections, and systemic corticosteroids. Other adjuvant therapeutic approaches that were described include fractional CO_2 laser therapy, radiofrequency, and extraction using micro-liposuction cannula with negative pressure. Ultimately refractory cases should be surgically excised [28, 29].

Severe adverse events, including embolization leading to blindness or skin necrosis, have been reported [30, 31], with the highest incidence occurring following dorsal nasal injections [30, 31]. Several consensus guidelines have been established for the management of vascular compromise associated with hyaluronic acid-based fillers [32, 33]. However, standardized treatment protocols for managing intravascular complications following biostimulator injections remain limited. To date, CaHA is the only biostimulator with a published consensus on intravascular complication management [34].

Intravascular complications involving CaHA requires early recognition, aspiration (if feasible), and vasodilatory measures such as warm compresses, massage, and systemic vasodilators (sildenafil, tadalafil) [34]. Antiplatelet therapy (aspirin, 500–625 mg loading dose, followed by maintenance at 75–100 mg for 3–5 days) and systemic anticoagulation (low molecular weight heparin) are recommended in cases of early ischemia [34]. Adjunctive therapies such as hyperbaric oxygen therapy (HBOT), platelet-rich plasma (PRP), and low-level laser therapy (LLLT) may aid in tissue recovery [34]. For ocular complications, immediate referral, ocular massage, acetazolamide, and beta-blocker eye drops should be initiated to reduce intraocular pressure [34]. Hyaluronidase is still recommended to be commenced in accordance to DeLorenzi protocol [33, 34], even if it is a non HA based filler. Hyaluronidase may help in view of its edema reduction, anti-inflammation, and capillary permeability effects. This protocol should be repeated every 2 h (for 3–4 h) if no improvement is observed [34].

Emerging in vivo studies on PCL demonstrate a high risk of persistent intravascular thrombosis, distinct from CaHA and hyaluronic acid fillers, as PCL microspheres do not degrade enzymatically and trigger prolonged inflammatory reactions. Preclinical animal models demonstrate that a 100 U intravascular heparin injection administered adjacent to necrotic tissue induced by 120 μL of filler injected at 40 μL/min, in combination with 200 μL of nitroglycerin applied directly over the affected area, effectively reduces thrombosis and enhances tissue perfusion by 80% on day 7 post-procedure. This finding suggest the use of vasodilators and anticoagulants in the treatment of PCL related intravascular complications. However, the optimal type, dosage, and way of commencement will require further study [35].

Management for intravascular associated with other biostimulators, such as PLLA, PDLLA, PDO, and PN, are limited. It is encouraged that it should be approached according to the CaHA and HA protocol, including commencing of the hyaluronidase [32–34]. Nevertheless, prevention is better than cure. High-risk area should be avoided if possible and slow injection, with cannula approach is encouraged if needed to proceed.

3.8 Advances in Biostimulators

The evolution of biostimulatory fillers has led to the development of hybrid injectable systems, combining collagen-stimulating polymers with immediate volumizing agents. Traditional biostimulators mentioned previously are known for their gradual tissue remodeling but offer minimal immediate volumization, which may not satisfy patients seeking instant results. To address this limitation, new-generation formulations incorporate non-cross-linked hyaluronic acid or other hydrophilic carriers, enhancing immediate hydration and soft tissue augmentation while maintaining long-term regenerative effects. Among these advancements, PDLLA/HA and CaHA/HA hybrid fillers have gained prominence, offering a balance of structural support, collagen induction, and hydration.

Hybrid formulations such as Juvelook and Lenisna integrate PDLLA microspheres with non-cross-linked hyaluronic acid (HA) to improve injectability, tissue integration, and immediate volumization. Juvelook contains 42.5 mg of PDLLA and 7.5 mg of HA (particle size 10–40 μm), while Lenisna features 170 mg of PDLLA and 30 mg of HA (particle size 40–80 μm) [36]. Due to its smaller particle size, Juvelook is suitable for superficial intradermal applications, including periorbital rejuvenation, atrophic scar treatment, and facial fine-line correction [36]. It can be delivered via autosensing mesotherapy injectors, microjet systems, sharp needles, or superficial cannula injections into the deep dermal layer [36, 37]. Clinical studies have demonstrated improvements in skin elasticity, hydration, and texture, particularly in the tear trough region and periorbital area. However, misuse of higher-particle PDLLA formulations in delicate areas has been associated with complications, including nodule formation and posterior ischemic optic neuropathy, underscoring the need for careful product selection and precise injection techniques [29, 38].

Calcium hydroxylapatite (CaHA) is widely recognized for its dual functionality as a volumizer and collagen stimulator. The introduction of CaHA/HA hybrid fillers, such as HArmonyCa™, further refines its application by combining CaHA microspheres (55.7%, 25–45 μm) with hyaluronic acid (HA, 20 mg/mL) [39]. This formulation enables immediate volumization via HA while maintaining CaHA's long-term collagen-stimulating effects. Unlike traditional CaHA fillers, which are suspended in carboxymethylcellulose (CMC) gel, HArmonyCa's HA carrier enhances hydration and biocompatibility [40]. Clinically, this hybrid filler has demonstrated significant improvements in skin viscoelasticity, dermal thickness, and facial contouring [41]. The recommended injection technique involves retrograde linear threading using a 23G cannula, primarily in areas requiring structural support, such as the mandibular border, preauricular region, and deep dermis [39]. HArmonyCa™ is also being explored for post-acne scar treatment, solar elastosis correction, and midface volume restoration, highlighting its potential beyond volumization [39–42]. Due to its biostimulatory properties, HArmonyCa™ serves as a longer-lasting alternative to traditional HA fillers while avoiding excessive inflammation often associated with PLLA or PDLLA.

These hybrid fillers exemplify the next phase of regenerative aesthetics, offering enhanced longevity, structural support, and tissue hydration. However, understanding the molecular properties, injection techniques, and clinical indications of each formulation remains critical to optimizing outcomes while minimizing complications.

Synergy with Energy-Based Devices

The combination of biostimulators with energy-based devices (EBDs) has gained increasing attention for enhancing collagen remodeling, optimizing skin quality, and improving treatment longevity. Biostimulators stimulate neocollagenesis and extracellular matrix (ECM) remodeling, while energy-based devices, such as monopolar radiofrequency (RF), microfocused ultrasound (MFU-V), ablative and non-ablative lasers, and microneedling radiofrequency (MNRF), induce controlled thermal injury, triggering wound healing pathways that further enhance tissue regeneration.

Clinical studies suggest that MFU-V and monopolar RF can enhance the collagen-stimulating effects of biostimulators by increasing heat-induced fibroblast activation and promoting deeper dermal remodeling [43, 44]. Additionally, ablative fractional CO_2 lasers and microneedling RF can improve biostimulator integration by increasing transdermal permeability and stimulating collagen renewal at multiple depths [45–47]. The combination approach may also accelerate biostimulator degradation in cases of complication management, as seen with CO_2 laser-assisted resolution of nodules from PDLLA and PLLA injections [29]. However, the sequence and interval between treatments must be carefully planned to prevent overstimulation of the inflammatory response, which could lead to excessive fibrosis or prolonged erythema. Consensus recommendations on combination therapy remain limited, necessitating further clinical studies to establish best practices for timing, energy parameters, and biostimulator selection in combination regimens.

3.9 Summary

Injectable biostimulators represent a paradigm shift in aesthetic medicine, offering progressive tissue remodeling, long-lasting collagen induction, and a more natural approach to facial and body rejuvenation. Unlike traditional fillers, biostimulators stimulate fibroblast proliferation, enhance extracellular matrix synthesis, and integrate into the dermal structure over time. The choice of biostimulator depends on biodegradability, particle size, and inflammatory profile, with options ranging from PLLA, PDLLA, CaHA, PCL, PDO, and PN. Each has unique indications, injection techniques, and safety considerations, particularly in high-risk anatomical areas such as the forehead, periorbital region, and lips, where vascular compromise and nodule formation are concerns.

New-generation hybrid fillers, such as PDLLA/HA (Juvelook, Lenisna) and CaHA/HA (HArmonyCa), have been introduced to bridge the gap between immediate volumization and long-term biostimulation. Their combination of hyaluronic acid for hydration and biostimulatory microspheres for neocollagenesis offers a synergistic approach to facial rejuvenation, reducing downtime and improving skin elasticity. Advances in combination therapy with energy-based devices further optimize results, but standardized protocols for sequencing and safety remain under investigation.

3.10 Conclusion

The future of injectable biostimulators lies in personalized treatment protocols, optimizing product selection, dilution techniques, and combination approaches to achieve predictable, natural, and long-lasting results. The development of hybrid formulations and improved application techniques has expanded treatment possibilities, allowing practitioners to tailor regenerative therapies to different facial and body areas while minimizing risks.

However, challenges remain in terms of complication management, particularly in vascular occlusion and nodule formation. While hyaluronidase has been explored for non-HA fillers, newer approaches, such as heparin and nitroglycerin for PCL-induced thrombosis, are being investigated. Future research should focus on refining treatment algorithms, establishing guidelines for combination therapies with EBDs, and identifying patient-specific factors that influence long-term outcomes. As regenerative aesthetics continue to evolve, biostimulators will remain at the forefront of non-surgical tissue restoration, paving the way for enhanced safety, efficacy, and patient satisfaction.

References

1. Aguilera SB, McCarthy A, Khalifian S, Lorenc ZP, Goldie K, Chernoff WG. The role of calcium hydroxylapatite (Radiesse) as a regenerative aesthetic treatment: a narrative review. Aesthet Surg J. 2023;43(10):1063–90.
2. Ermino José Souza JRAB, Tambeli CH, Parada CA, de La Torre G, Canales MB, de Souza C, Gobbi RC, de Oliveira CMR-B. Polydioxanone powder induces collagen synthesis in fibroblast culture? A pilot study. Aesthet Med. 2023;9:e2023007.
3. Yanatma I, Sarac G, Gul M, Gul S, Kapicioglu Y. Comparison of polycaprolactone and calcium hydroxylapatite dermal fillers in a rat model. Dermatol Ther. 2021;34(1):e14716.
4. Oh S, Lee JH, Kim HM, et al. Poly-L-lactic acid fillers improved dermal collagen synthesis by modulating M2 macrophage polarization in aged animal skin. Cells. 2023;12(9):1320.
5. Lee KWA, Chan KWL, Lee A, et al. Polynucleotides in aesthetic medicine: a review of current practices and perceived effectiveness. Int J Mol Sci. 2024;25(15):8224.
6. Christen MO. Collagen stimulators in body applications: a review focused on poly-L-lactic acid (PLLA). Clin Cosmet Investig Dermatol. 2022;15:997–1019.
7. Oh S, Seo SB, Kim G, et al. Poly-D,L-lactic acid filler increases extracellular matrix by modulating macrophages and adipose-derived stem cells in aged animal skin. Antioxidants. 2023;12(6):1204.
8. Lee KWA, Chan LKW, Lee AWK, Lee CH, Wong STH, Yi KH. Poly-d,l-lactic acid (PDLLA) application in dermatology: a literature review. Polymers (Basel). 2024;16(18):2583.
9. Goldberg D, Guana A, Volk A, Daro-Kaftan E. Single-arm study for the characterization of human tissue response to injectable poly-L-lactic acid. Dermatologic Surg. 2013;39(6):915–22.
10. Ao YJ, Yi Y, Wu GH. Application of PLLA (Poly-L-Lactic acid) for rejuvenation and reproduction of facial cutaneous tissue in aesthetics: a review. Medicine. 2024;103(11):e37506.
11. Lin JY, Fu JP, Hsu NJ, Lin CY. Early-stage volume effect difference between injectable poly-l-lactic acid and injectable poly-d,l-lactic acid. J Cosmet Dermatol. 2023;22(5):1702–3.
12. Bernardo RTR, Oliveira RCG, Freitas KMS, Albergaria-Barbosa JR, Rizzatti-Barbosa CM. Effect of poly-L-lactic acid and polydioxanone biostimulators on type I and III collagen biosynthesis. Skin Res Technol. 2024;30(4):e13681.
13. Trinh T-TT, Chien PN, Le LTT, et al. An assessment of the effectiveness and safety of ULTRACOL100 as a device for restoring skin in the nasolabial fold region. Cosmetics. 2023;11(1):4.
14. Chen S-Y, Lin J-Y, Lin C-Y. The back-and-forth method: a quick and simple technique for reconstitution of injectable poly-D,L-lactic acid. Arch Aesthetic Plast Surg. 2020;26(2):79–83.
15. Lin JY, Lin CY. Adjusting thickness before injection: a new trend for preparing collagen-stimulating fillers. Plast Reconstr Surg Glob Open. 2021;9(6):e3653.
16. Magacho-Vieira FN, Vieira AO, Soares A Jr, et al. Consensus recommendations for the reconstitution and aesthetic use of poly-D,L-lactic acid microspheres. Clin Cosmet Investig Dermatol. 2024;17:2755–65.
17. Giang NN, Kim HJ, Chien PN, et al. An evaluation of the effectiveness of 'ULTRACOL 200′ in enhancing nasolabial fold wrinkles through cutaneous repair. Skin Res Technol. 2024;30(4):e13679.
18. Haddad A, Avelar L, Fabi SG, et al. Injectable Poly-L-lactic acid for body aesthetic treatments: an international consensus on evidence assessment and practical recommendations. Aesthetic Plast Surg. 2024;49:1507–17.
19. Avelar L, Ong A, Ong D, et al. Consensus recommendations on the use of injectable poly-l-lactic acid in Asian patients. J Cosmet Dermatol. 2023;22(12):3223–31.
20. Corduff N, Chen JF, Chen YH, et al. Pan-Asian consensus on calcium hydroxyapatite for skin biostimulation, contouring, and combination treatments. J Clin Aesthet Dermatol. 2021;14(8):E76–85.

21. de Almeida AT, Figueredo V, da Cunha ALG, et al. Consensus recommendations for the use of Hyperdiluted calcium hydroxyapatite (Radiesse) as a face and body biostimulatory agent. Plast Reconstr Surg Glob Open. 2019;7(3):e2160.
22. de Melo F, Nicolau P, Piovano L, et al. Recommendations for volume augmentation and rejuvenation of the face and hands with the new generation polycaprolactone-based collagen stimulator (Ellanse((R))). Clin Cosmet Investig Dermatol. 2017;10:431–40.
23. Lampridou S, Bassett S, Cavallini M, Christopoulos G. The effectiveness of polynucleotides in esthetic medicine: a systematic review. J Cosmet Dermatol. 2025;24(2):e16721.
24. Baumann K, Alm J, Norberg M, Ejehorn M. Immediate use after reconstitution of a biostimulatory poly-L-lactic acid injectable implant. J Drugs Dermatol. 2020;19(12):1199–203.
25. Palm M, Mayoral F, Rajani A, et al. Chart review presenting safety of injectable PLLA used with alternative reconstitution volume for facial treatments. J Drugs Dermatol. 2021;20(1):118–22.
26. Duracinsky M, Leclercq P, Herrmann S, et al. Safety of poly-L-lactic acid (New-Fill(R)) in the treatment of facial lipoatrophy: a large observational study among HIV-positive patients. BMC Infect Dis. 2014;14:474.
27. Reszko AE, Sadick NS, Magro CM, Farber J. Late-onset subcutaneous nodules after poly-L-lactic acid injection. Dermatologic Surg. 2009;35(Suppl 1):380–4.
28. Philipp-Dormston WG, Goodman GJ, De Boulle K, et al. Global approaches to the prevention and management of delayed-onset adverse reactions with hyaluronic acid-based fillers. Plast Reconstr Surg Glob Open. 2020;8(4):e2730.
29. Seo SB, Wan J, Yi KH. Energy-based device management of nodular reaction following Poly-D, L-lactic acid injection for tear trough rejuvenation. J Cosmet Dermatol. 2025;24(1):e16575.
30. Povolotskiy R, Oleck NC, Hatzis CM, Paskhover B. Adverse events associated with aesthetic dermal fillers: a 10-year retrospective study of FDA data. Am J Cosmet Surg. 2018;35(3):143–51.
31. Rayess HM, Svider PF, Hanba C, et al. A cross-sectional analysis of adverse events and litigation for injectable fillers. JAMA Facial Plast Surg. 2018;20(3):207–14.
32. Cohen JL, Biesman BS, Dayan SH, et al. Treatment of hyaluronic acid filler-induced impending necrosis with hyaluronidase: consensus recommendations. Aesthet Surg J. 2015;35(7):844–9.
33. DeLorenzi C. New high dose pulsed hyaluronidase protocol for hyaluronic acid filler vascular adverse events. Aesthet Surg J. 2017;37(7):814–25.
34. van Loghem J, Funt D, Pavicic T, et al. Managing intravascular complications following treatment with calcium hydroxylapatite: an expert consensus. J Cosmet Dermatol. 2020;19(11):2845–58.
35. Khan A, Gong L, Wang Y, et al. Combination administration of heparin and nitroglycerin for the treatment of polycaprolactone-induced intravascular embolism: a preclinical investigation. Aesth Plast Surg. 2024;48(17):3195–205.
36. Seo SB, Park H, Jo JY, Ryu HJ. Skin rejuvenation effect of the combined PDLLA and non cross-linked hyaluronic acid: a preliminary study. J Cosmet Dermatol. 2024;23(3):794–802.
37. Oh DY, Seo SB, Jang YJ, Park EJ, Kim KH. Facial skin rejuvenation using poly- dl -lactic acid injected with a laser-generated needle-free microjet injector. Dermatologic Surg. 2024;50(8):739–45.
38. Joo HJ, Kim DH. Posterior ischemic optic neuropathy following skin booster injection. J Neuroophthalmol. 2025;45(1):e60–2.
39. Proietti I, Spagnoli A, Favaroni A, et al. HArmonyCa hybrid filler to restore connective tissue: an Italian real-life retrospective study. J Cosmet Dermatol. 2024;23(12):3883–92.
40. Urdiales-Galvez F, Braz A, Cavallini M. Facial rejuvenation with the new hybrid filler HArmonyCa: clinical and aesthetic outcomes assessed by 2D and 3D photographs, ultrasound, and elastography. J Cosmet Dermatol. 2023;22(8):2186–97.
41. Barone M, De Bernardis R, Persichetti P. Minimally invasive post-acne scars treatment with the hybrid filler HArmonyCa. Aesth Plast Surg. 2024;48:5251.
42. Barone M, Salzillo R, Persichetti P. Minimally invasive facial rejuvenation with the hybrid filler HArmonyCa. Aesth Plast Surg. 2024;48(23):5251–3.
43. Ramirez S, Scherz G, Leprince R. Pilot study: single-depth superficial ultrasound with subdermal injections of diluted calcium hydroxylapatite for improving lower face skin quality. Plast Reconstr Surg Glob Open. 2024;12(10):e6210.
44. Suh DH, Chen LC, Chung HJ, Lee SJ, Kim J. An 18-year comprehensive safety study on microfocused ultrasound and monopolar radiofrequency combined with cosmetic injectables in 1,040 patients. Arch Dermatol Res. 2025;317(1):251.
45. Wu X, Cen Q, Wang X, Xiong P, Wu X, Lin X. Microneedling radiofrequency enhances poly-L-lactic acid penetration that effectively improves facial skin laxity without lipolysis. Plast Reconstr Surg. 2024;154(6):1189–97.
46. Hyeong JH, Jung JW, Seo SB, Kim HS, Kim KH. Intradermal injection of poly-d, l-lactic acid using microneedle fractional radiofrequency for acne scars: an open-label prospective trial. Dermatologic Surg. 2022;48(12):1306–11.
47. Rkein A, Ozog D, Waibel JS. Treatment of atrophic scars with fractionated CO2 laser facilitating delivery of topically applied poly-L-lactic acid. Dermatologic Surg. 2014;40(6):624–31.

Infraorbital Filler Injection: Advanced Techniques, Adverse Effects and Their Management

4

Sabrina Shah-Desai and Won Lee

4.1 Introduction

The infraorbital area plays a crucial role in non-verbal signalling of health and vitality. The periorbital area can impact perceived attractiveness [1] and affect self-confidence, as structural changes can make individuals look sad, tired or unwell. Infraorbital (IO) hyaluronic acid (HA) filler injections have rapidly gained popularity, since they were first used in 2005, due to their minimally invasive nature and immediate results. The "tear trough area" of IO hollows were rated as the second most likely area to be treated in the 30- to 34-year age group and third most likely facial area to be treated and all age groups [2]. However, the complex nature of IO anatomy, its assessment and the rising risk of complications have made practitioners and patients wary of undertaking these treatments.

This chapter reviews the anatomy and assessment underpinning safe injection strategies, potential early and delayed adverse effects of infraorbital filler injections and current evidence-based strategies for their management.

S. Shah-Desai
Perfect Eyes Ltd, London, UK

W. Lee (✉)
Yonsei E1 Plastic Surgery Clinic,
Anyang, Kyonggi-do, Korea (Republic of)

4.2 Oculo-Facial Ageing, Infraorbital (IO) Anatomy and Assessment

IO hollows can be the result of a number of different aetiologies with contributions from deep skeletal, soft tissue and skin changes.

The first step in managing IO ageing concerns is to assess the various aetiologic factors present so that the most appropriate customised therapy can be crafted, as a spectrum of treatment strategies exist. These including non-invasive options such as office-based treatments with soft tissue fillers and energy-based treatment, as well as more invasive surgical interventions.

Understanding and assessing the complex anatomy of the infraorbital region is crucial for safe filler injection and minimizing adverse events.

4.2.1 Eyelid Skin

The eyelid skin is thinnest in the human body [3] and progressively thins and changes texture and elasticity with age. The average skin thickness of the lower eyelid is 0.37 mm to over 2 mm [4]. Eyelid skin ageing is a multifactorial process that is influenced by genetic, environmental and lifestyle factors. Evidence indicates significant variability in ageing patterns between sex- and race-based subgroups. Characteristic ageing

W. Lee (ed.), *Innovative Injectable Techniques in Minimally Invasive Aesthetics*,
https://doi.org/10.1007/978-981-95-2161-6_4

Table 4.1 Assessment of skin ageing changes

Thin skin vs thick skin
Excess skin (mild, moderate, severe)
Elastosis of the skin
Texture of the skin (smooth vs "crepey" texture)
Skin dyschromia/pigmentation (brown, grey-brown, reddish)
Static fine lines and wrinkles vs dynamic wrinkles
Presence of blue veins and telangiectasia

changes in Caucasians include fine rhytid formation in the periorbital regions and skin sagging. In comparison, Asian patients have thick skin and more subcutaneous fat, which often delays the onset of fine lines and rhytids [5] (Table 4.1).

In clinical practice, the assessment for pigmentation and erythema is visual and often subjective and may lead to variability in observations among clinicians. Objective and quantitative techniques are preferred for a precise evaluation of the skin quality and the treatment's efficacy. The author advocates assessing the skin objectively using photography (e.g. the VISIA® skin analysis system is the most frequently used device for full-face assessment, which generates a series of photographs using standard, ultraviolet and cross-polarized lighting for dyspigmentation evaluation) and palpation with snap and distraction tests [6]. The following descriptions are the skin characteristics of IO according to Fitzpatrick type (Figs. 4.1, 4.2, 4.3, 4.4, 4.5, and 4.6).

The quality of skin should be documented and discussed with the patient, as thin skin with moderate to significant elastosis can predispose to adverse events from filler injections.

Thin skin can cause a "preseptal infraorbital hollow", which are seen commonly in certain ethnicities (South East Asian, Hispanics, etc.) (Fig. 4.6).

Additionally, skin with dyschromia/pigmentation issues as a cause for under-eye darkness, will need topical skin care (cosmeceuticals, chemical peels, etc.) or LASERs (Q Switched, IPL, CO2 and Erbium) or PRP to improve the quality of the skin.

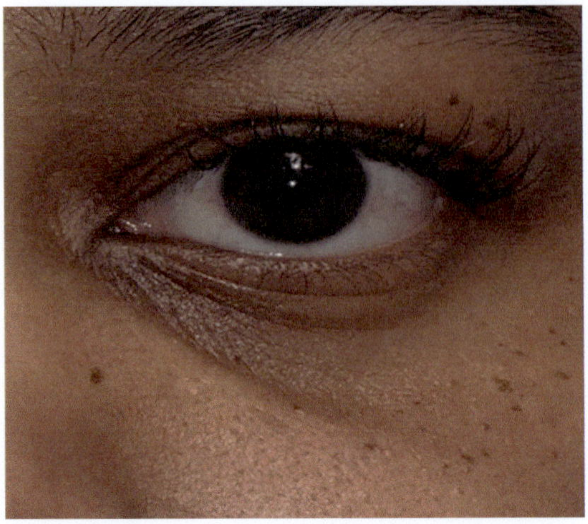

Fig. 4.1 Fitzpatrick type 6: Under-eye hollows due to thin "crepey" skin, with static lines and dyschromia of the skin (brown hyperpigmentation)

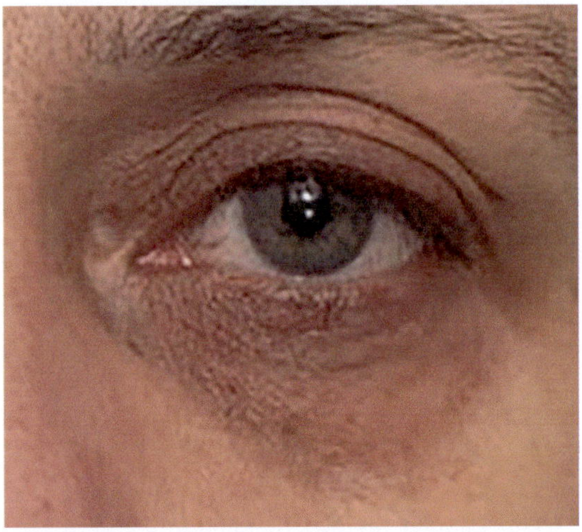

Fig. 4.2 Fitzpatrick 2: Thin "crepey" skin with dyschromia of the skin (grey-brown hyperpigmentation)

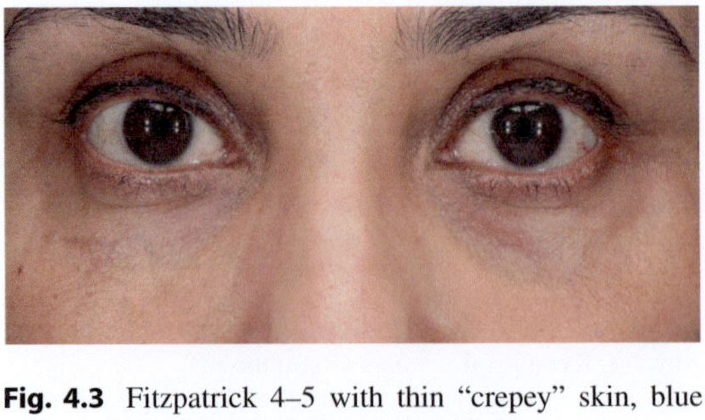

Fig. 4.3 Fitzpatrick 4–5 with thin "crepey" skin, blue veins and dyschromia (brown and reddish)

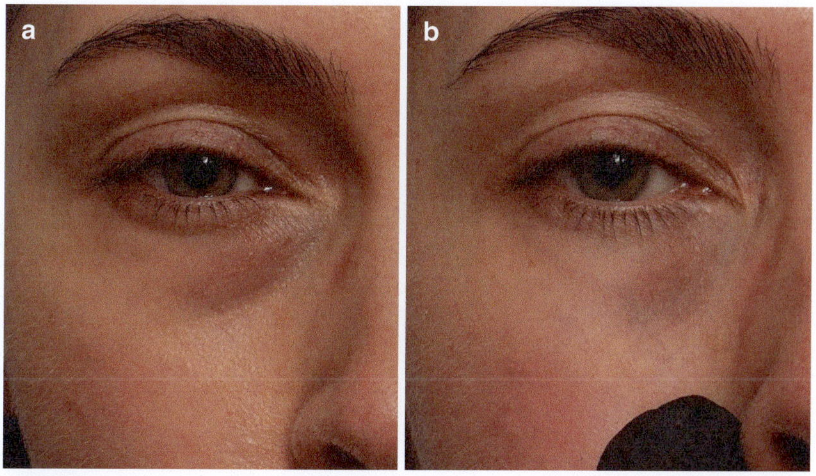

Fig. 4.4 Fitzpatrick 2-3 with haemosiderin staining (**a**) neutral position (**b**) skin pulled down to demonstrate the pigmentation

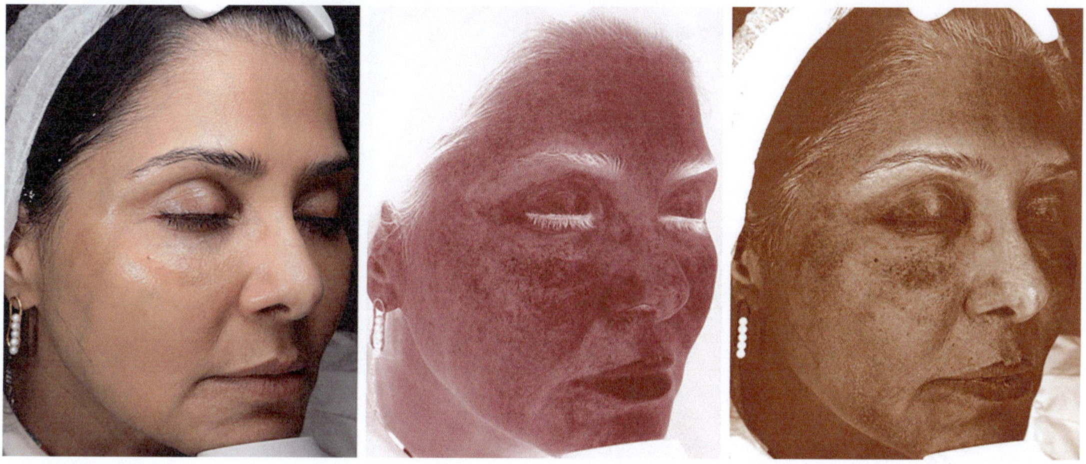

Fig. 4.5 Fitzpatrick 4–5 with VISIA® skin analysis system displaying pigmentation

4.2.2 Orbicularis Oculi Muscle (OOM)

The OOM is a sphincteric muscle responsible for eyelid closure and blinking. It undergoes several age-related changes, and as it lies just below the dermis of the skin, it affects the skin texture. Repetitive movements like smiling and squinting result in more prominent fine lines and wrinkles, especially dynamic wrinkles like crow's feet, with ageing.

The OOM provides muscular support and has two defined sections from the outside: the orbital and palpebral parts. The palpebral part is further subdivided into preseptal and pretarsal parts (Fig. 4.7). The inferior border of the orbicularis oculi corresponds to the nasojugal groove medially, whilst the tear trough is located between the orbital and palpebral parts of the OOM. Voluntary blinking is a function of the orbital and preseptal OOM, whilst involuntary blinking is a function of the pretarsal OOM. The proportion of muscle fibres in the muscle is different in each section [7].

Spontaneously blinking behaviour, which is an index of muscle function of the orbicularis oculi, certainly seems to be affected by ageing. The muscle thickness of the orbicularis oculi tends to be low in older adults [8] and unlike striated skeletal and extraocular muscles, the OOM

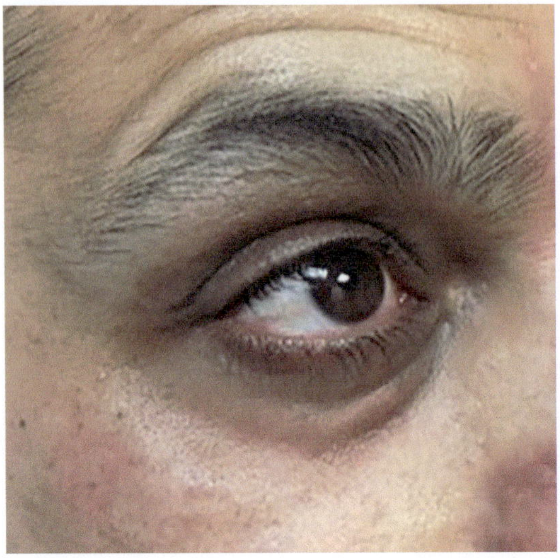

Fig. 4.6 Fitzpatrick type 4–5 with preseptal hollow due to thin skin and hyperpigmented skin

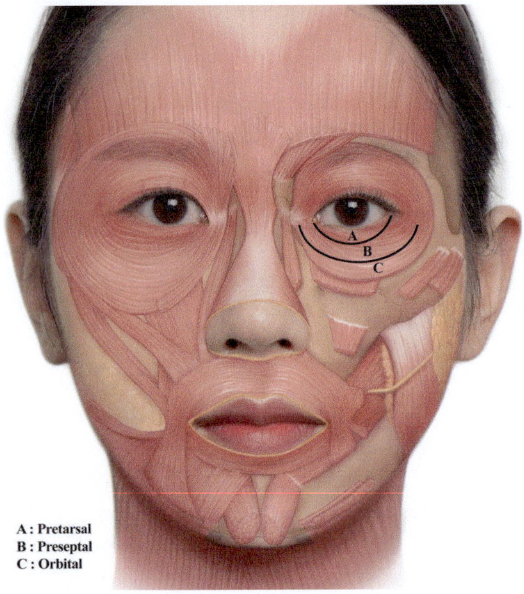

Fig. 4.7 Orbicularis oculi muscle

displays unique ultrastructural features. Ageing diminishes the functional capacity of the orbicularis, as evidenced by reduced contraction strength (Table 4.2) [9]. With time the OOM becomes thinner due to loss of muscle fibres, reduction in muscle mass and decreased contractility, which results in weaker eyelid closure. As orbicularis oculi tone reduces, it contributes to lower eyelid laxity, which can lead to sagging ectropion or increased inferior scleral show and redundant muscle folds (orbicularis roll) in the lower eyelid and descent of midface structures, exacerbating malar bags or festoons (Fig. 4.8). Assessment of OOM should be performed before any injection procedure (Fig. 4.9).

Table 4.2 Assessment of orbicularis oculi muscle

Presence of inferior scleral show
Gentle vs forced eyelid closure
Smile test and laxity/hypertrophic muscle roll on smiling

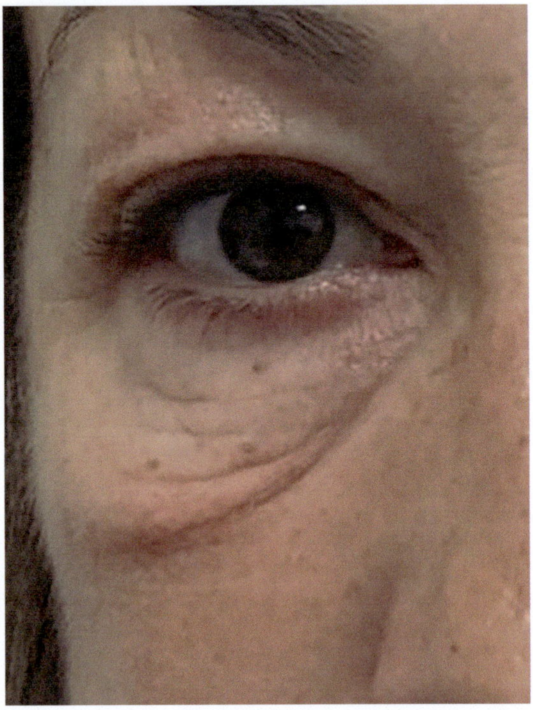

Fig. 4.8 Descent of midface structures with malar bags or festoons due to orbicularis and skin laxity

4.2.3 Orbital Fat Pad

With ageing, weakening of the orbital septum (a fibrous structure which attaches the inferior border of tarsal plate to the arcus marginalis of the orbital rim) causes the orbital fat to protrude forward, creating puffy under-eye bags. There are three fat compartments in the lower eyelid:

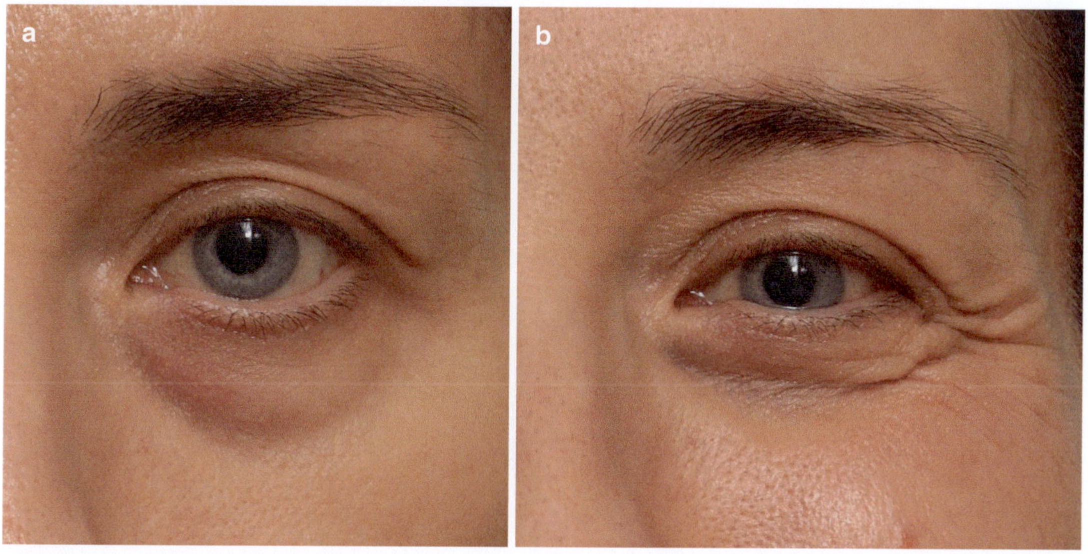

Fig. 4.9 Assessment of OOM. (**a**) Presence of increased inferior scleral show, (**b**) laxity/hypertrophic muscle roll on smiling

Table 4.3 Assessment of the orbital fat pads

Documentation of which fat pads are prominent
Grading them as mild, moderate or severe
Evaluation the fat pads, with face in neutral position and eyes in up gaze or using the tilt test

medial, central and lateral. The fat protrusion occurs especially in the nasal and central compartments (Table 4.3, Fig. 4.10).

4.2.4 Superficial and Deep Fat Pads

The infraorbital and midface also has superficial and deep fat pads.

The superficial fat pad of the eyelid, also known as subcutaneous fat, is located immediately beneath the thin skin and in front of the OOM and orbital septum. This fat is minimal in the eyelids compared to other body areas and is confined to the area just below the orbital rim. The superficial malar fat pad is closely associated with the lower eyelid and extends onto the upper cheek. Due to its location, the infraorbital superficial malar fat pad plays a key role in supporting the lower eyelid and maintaining the smooth transition between the eyelid and the cheek (Fig. 4.11). The superficial fat pads of the midface include the nasolabial, medial, middle and lateral fat pads and they too lie above the OOM.

The deep fat compartments of the midface lie below the OOM and include the medial SOOF (suborbicularis oculi fat), the lateral SOOF and deep medial cheek fat (DMCF).

In the malar region, the SOOF is divided into superior and inferior compartments by a fascial structure called the malar septum. The malar septum is considered to be an impermeable membrane that defines the boundaries of malar mounds, oedema and festoons between the infraorbital and mid cheek region.

Subcutaneous, deep fat (SOOF and DMCF) loss and midfacial deflationary descent lead to worsening tear trough, palpebromalar groove hollows and mid-cheek grooves, with a loss of the fullness of the contours of the lid cheek junction (Fig. 4.12). Malar fat descent along with OOM laxity and loss of ligamentous support due to aging also leads to festoons and malar mounds (Fig. 4.8). Therefore, understanding the reasons for the formation of grooves and hollows is essential for appropriate treatment (Table 4.4).

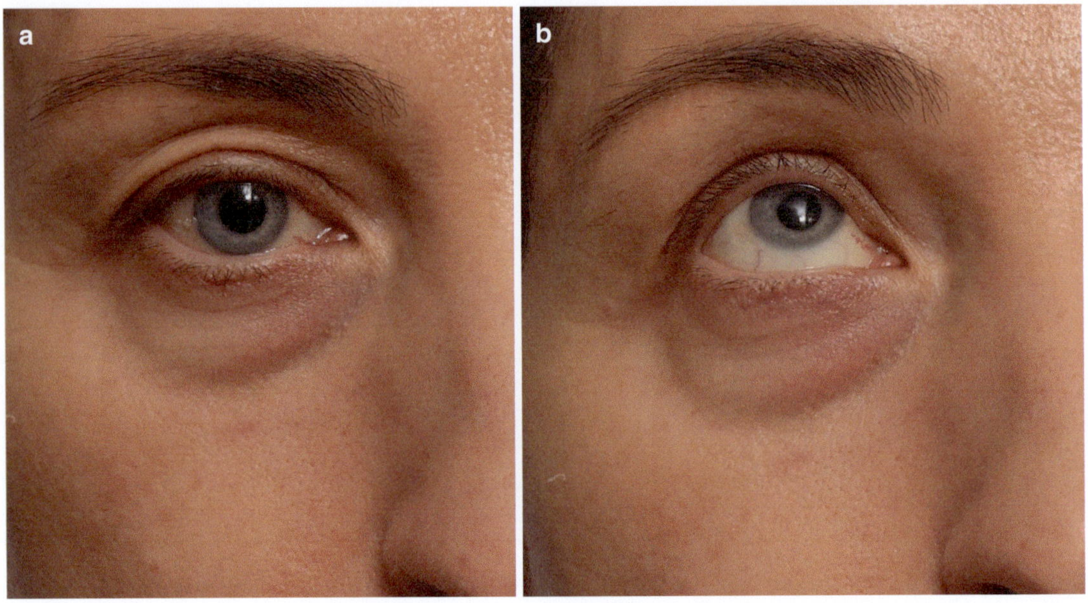

Fig. 4.10 Evaluation of the eye pads, with face in neutral position (**a**) and then in up gaze (**b**)

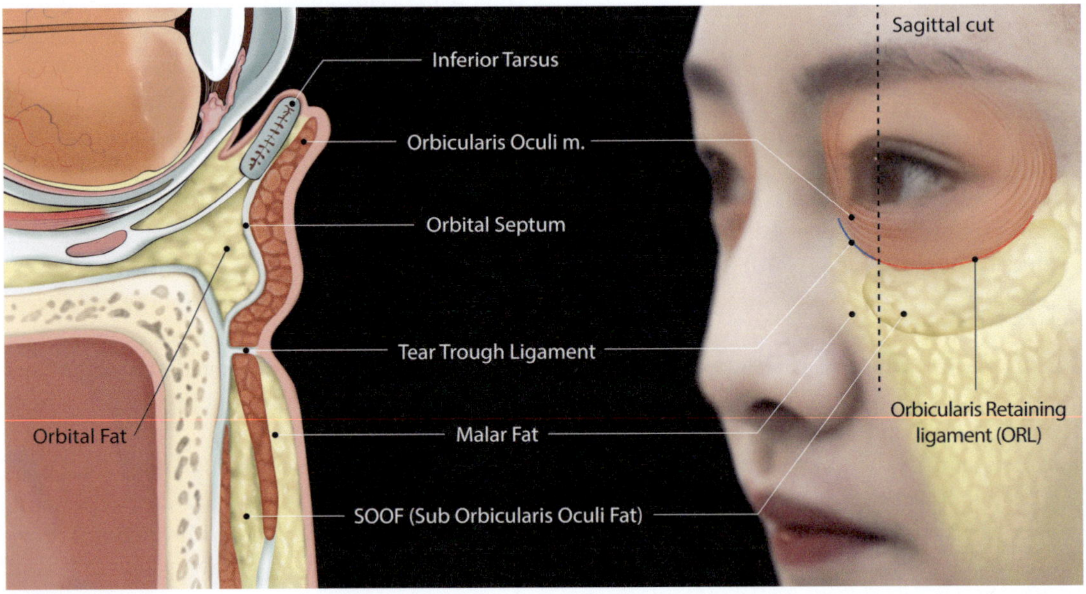

Fig. 4.11 Schematic diagram of midface fat pad

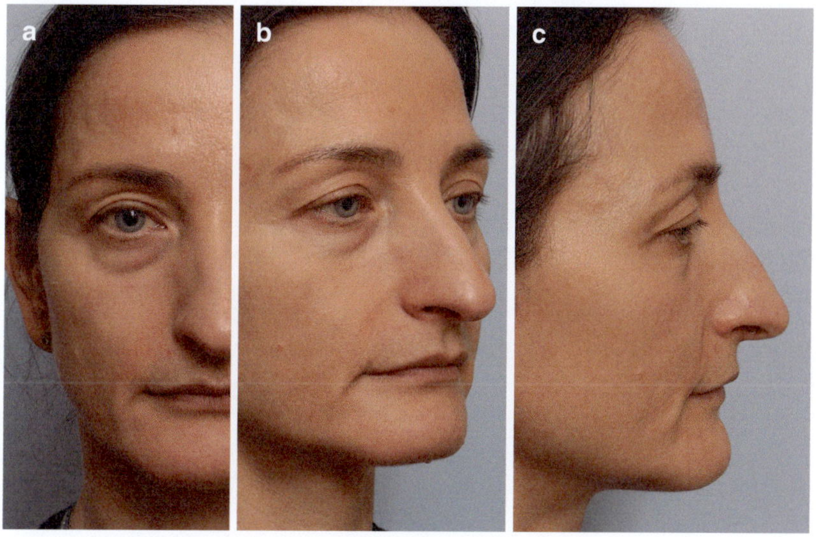

Fig. 4.12 Assess for volume loss in the infra orbital area. (**a**) Frontal view. (**b**) Three quarter view. (**c**) Lateral views

Table 4.4 Assessment of IO grooves and fluid retention

Preseptal
Medial (tear trough groove)
Lateral (palpebromalar groove)
Midfacial (negative vector, mid-cheek groove and loss of ogee curve)
Fluid/oedema over the lid or malar area (pitting on pressure)
Push test to estimate gel volume replacement

4.2.5 Bones and Ligaments

The infraorbital rim is composed of the maxilla medially. The maxilla is the structural support of the bony anterior midface. Located about 6–10 mm below the inferior orbital rim, often aligning vertically with the mid-pupillary line, lies the infraorbital foramen, which serves as the exit point for the infraorbital nerve and vessels.

The zygomatic or malar bone forms the infraorbital rim laterally and supports the lateral aspect of the orbital floor and gives the prominence of the "cheekbone". It houses the zygomaticofacial foramen, approx. 6 mm beneath the infraorbital rim at the inferior lateral orbital notch. This contains the zygomaticofacial vessels and nerve [10].

Infraorbital hollows may occur due to preexisting structural changes of maxillary hypoplasia and age-related orbital bone resorption, creating a negative vector. As the bony orbital floor descends with age, and the facial skeleton undergoes angular rotation due to patterns of resorption, there is recession of the infraorbital rim, with a loss of soft tissue support, which increases the vertical length of the lower lid.

Periorbital ligaments include the orbicularis retaining ligament (ORL) and the zygomatic cutaneous ligament (ZCL). The ORL defines the superior border of the SOOF and the ZCL the inferior edge of the SOOF [11]. The ORL is an osseocutaneous ligament, which is the main periorbital retaining ligament. It originates from the periosteum of the orbital rim inserting into the skin of the lid-cheek junction. The medial part of the ORL is the tear trough ligament (TTL). The angular rotation of the bony skeleton with aging may stretch and weaken facial fascia and ligamentous attachments, inducing mid facial ptosis and fat prolapse of the inferior fat pad.

4.2.6 Blood Vessels

The infraorbital area is supplied by the following arteries: angular artery, zygomaticofacial artery and infraorbital artery (Fig. 4.13).

In the majority of cases, there are no major arteries directly on the infraorbital rim. Some detouring patterns of the angular artery have been

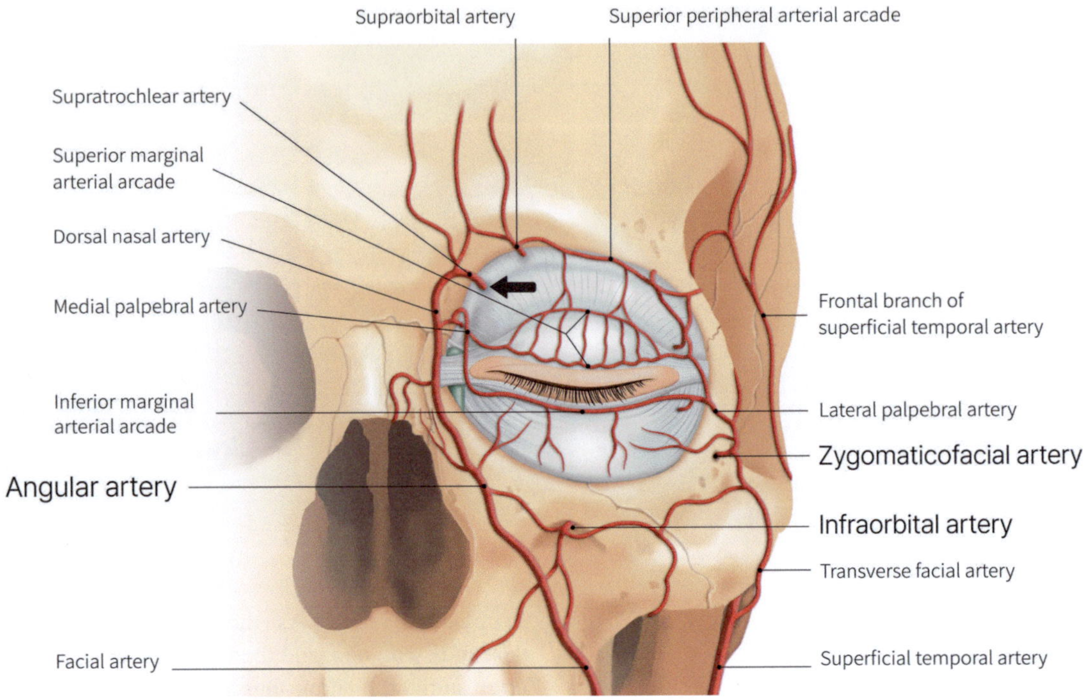

Fig. 4.13 Periorbital arterial supply

Fig. 4.14 Inferior palpebral vein

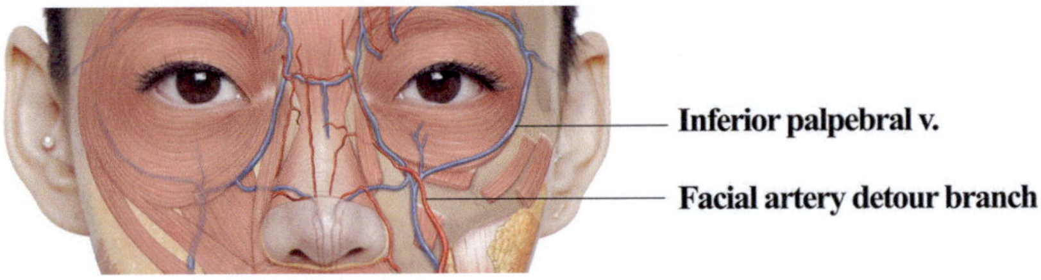

observed in 30% of Asians, where the position of the angular artery is shifted laterally, very close to the infraorbital rim [12]. In some cases, the infraorbital artery can anastomose with the angular artery [13], these variations and anastomose are a risk for potential vascular embolism and haemorrhage.

Over the orbital rim, and superficial to the OOM, there are several small vertical veins. As the vasculature is predominantly over the OOM, use of needles to perform treatments increases the risk of bruising. The inferior palpebral vein (IPV) typically runs from the lateral canthal area in the inferomedial direction to anastomose with the angular vein [14]; however, three more patterns have been described (22% undeveloped, 12% located beneath inferior part of IPV, 8% origin of IPV located beneath both the lateral and inferior parts of OOM), which can pose a risk for haemorrhage and bruises (Fig. 4.14).

4.2.7 Lymphatic Vessels

The periorbital and midface lymphatics drain into the pre-auricular and submandibular lymph nodes, via a dual system of superficial and deep lymphatic vessels. The vessels of the superficial system drain the conjunctiva and eyelid skin, near the medial and lateral canthi and travel above the preseptal OOM. They connect to the deep lymphatic system within the preseptal

OOM. The deep lymphatic system drains the conjunctiva directly from vessels in the tarsal plate and meibomian glands and travels below the preseptal OOM to drain in the preauricular lymph nodes. These vessels have fewer valves compared to the lymphatic system in the limbs, thus predisposing these vessels to obstruction [15].

4.3 Patient Selection

Patient selection is vital as certain patient and anatomical factors can place the candidate at a higher fall risk for adverse events. Patients being considered for hyaluronic acid filler injections to treat their infraorbital hollows need to be categorised as suitable or not (based on Table 4.5).

Patient medical history should include aesthetic expectations and budget. HA fillers are contraindicated in patients who are pregnant, breastfeeding and hypersensitive or allergic to filler materials or lidocaine. Relative contraindications are patients with a history of hypertrophic scarring or keloid formation, autoimmune conditions and patient with one seeing eye.

The ideal patient has no medical contraindications, realistic expectations, with thick skin, negligible skin laxity, mild to no eye bags and a well-defined infraorbital hollow. Patients with thin, translucent skin and a preseptal hollow are more challenging to treat with traditional preperiosteal placed HA fillers.

Patients with "dark circles" due to skin hyperpigmentation, where the colour does not contribute to the depth of the IO hollow, should be informed that hyperpigmentation will still remain post HA fillers and that they would need to consider concomitant topical skin care, peels or LASER to manage the pigment.

Patients with past history of fillers and retained infraorbital fillers, having repeat treatments, may be predisposed to Tyndall effect, lumps, irregularities [16] and malar oedema.

If the retained filler is lumpy with contour irregularities or Tyndall effect, hyaluronidase to dissolve this should be considered 1–2 weeks prior to retreatment. If there is Malar oedema, hyaluronidase to dissolve the underlying filler and review is advised. Any retreatment with HA fillers is appropriate if the malar oedema completely resolves and there is no residual malar festoon, as these patients would be better managed by surgical blepharoplasty or energy-based interventions.

4.4 Types of HA Fillers Suitable for Infraorbital Hollows

Hyaluronic acid fillers remain the gold standard for infraorbital augmentation based on a strong body of clinical evidence. Their reversibility and favourable safety profile make them especially suited to the tear trough area. Other fillers such as poly-L lactic acid (PLLA), calcium hydroxyapatite (CaHA) and polymethyl methacrylate (PMMA) and autologous fat have niche applications but come with caveats regarding consistency and safety; however, the most commonly used filler for infraorbital rejuvenation is hyaluronic acid.

Multiple case series and retrospective studies have shown that low to moderately cross-linked HA fillers (e.g. Belotero Balance, Restylane, Volbella and Redensity2) provide a smooth correction of tear trough deformities with high patient satisfaction. Only two HA fillers are currently approved by the United States Food and Drug Administration for this indication; these are Restylane Eyelight (20 mg/ml HA) and Juvéderm Volbella XC (VYC-15 L, 15 mg/ml HA; Allergan Aesthetics, an AbbVie Company, Irvine, CA.)

In general, an HA filler with lower elasticity and firmness is recommended for treating infraorbital hollows.

4.5 Techniques

Aseptic preparations with facial cleansing prior to injections is standard.

It is not required to apply topical anaesthesia to the infraorbital area prior to treatment.

Injections should be performed with the patient in a sitting position, with the eyes open

Table 4.5 Suitable vs not suitable candidates for IO HA filler injections

Patient factors	Suitable candidate	Not suitable candidate
Expectations	Realistic	Unrealistic
Skin thickness	Thick	Thin skin
Skin laxity	None or mild	Moderate to severe
Skin pigmentation	None to mild hyperpigmentation with IO hollows	Moderate to severe hyper-pigmentation with no IO hollow
Fat pad	None to mild fat pad prolapse	Moderate to severe fat pad prolapse
OOM	Good tone/snap	Poor tone/snap
Lymphatics	No history of fluid retention or malar oedema	Malar oedema, festoons
IO hollow	Present	Absent
Previous IO filler treatments	Smooth	Lumpy retained IO filler

Table 4.6 Infraorbital hollow HA filler injection techniques

Direct treatment for a tear trough hollow (Fig. 4.15)
Treatment for a preseptal hollow (Fig. 4.16)
Direct treatment for an infraorbital hollow (Fig. 4.17)
Indirect treatment of an infraorbital hollow (Fig. 4.18)

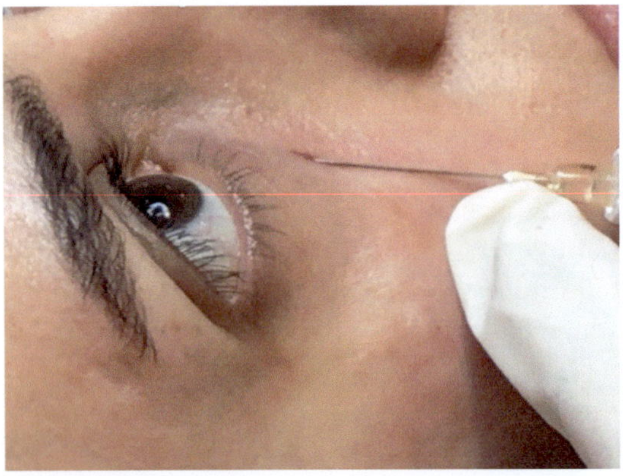

Fig. 4.15 25G 38 mm cannula being used for direct injection of the tear trough, by the author

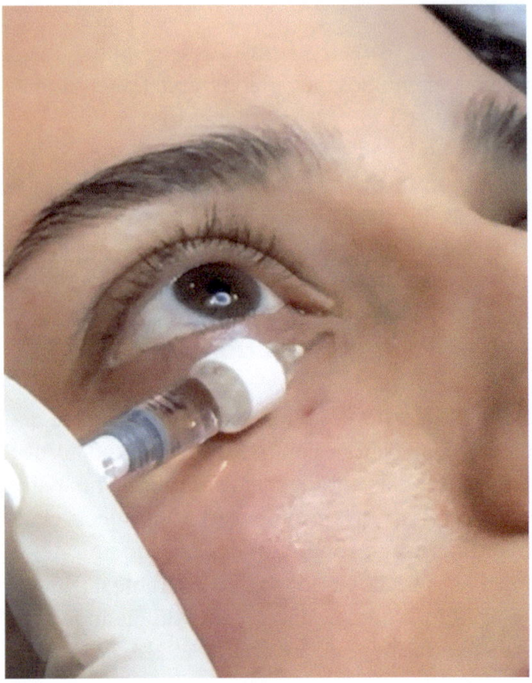

Fig. 4.16 The author using an invisible needle to inject microdroplets of Restylane Skinboosters Vital Light (HA_{SBVL}), subdermally within the preseptal hollow

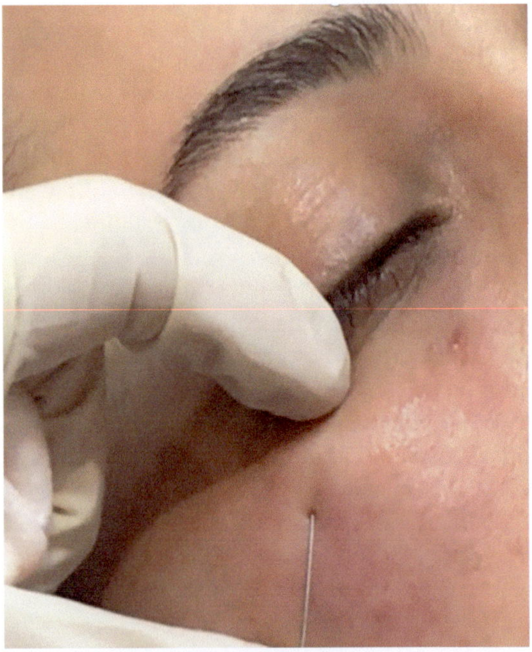

Fig. 4.17 The author using a 25G 38 mm cannula to inject the palpebromalar groove below the ORL. Note use of noninjecting finger on the infraorbital rim to prevent inadvertent entry of cannula into the post septal space, when using the cannula obliquely or vertically

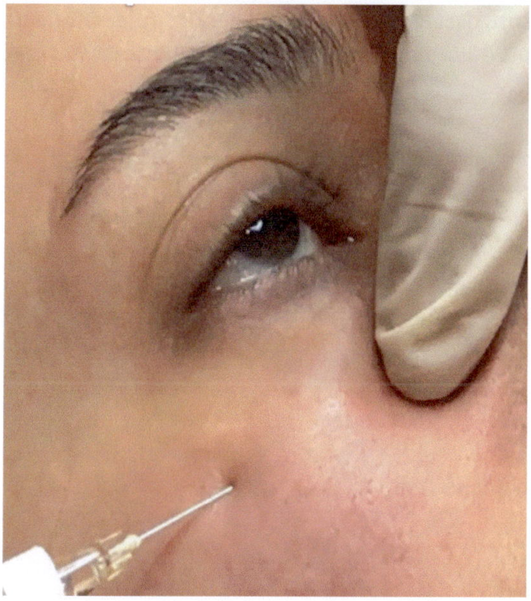

Fig. 4.18 The author using a 25G 38 mm cannula to inject the SOOF and DMCF in the pre-zygomatic space, below the ORL

for good visualization of the infraorbital area, without distortion of the anatomy. If the patient wants to close their eyes, it is recommended to consider marking the superior border of the infraorbital rim with a marker pencil, so that the injector does not lose anatomical landmarks.

Techniques are generally divided into four techniques (Table 4.6).

4.5.1 Direct Approach for the Tear Trough

This is only indicated in patients with a tear trough hollow, thick skin and a negligible or mild eye bag. A 25 G cannula is recommended and plane of injection should be supraperiosteal. Entry points of the cannula depends on the injector's preference. Cadaver studies have shown that the filler is deposited in an intramuscular plane, as there are only three layers in the true tear trough (skin, muscle and bone). Here a technique of pre-injection tear trough ligament stretching (TTLS-I) leading to its release [17] has been described. These techniques are advised to be reserved for advanced injectors, given the risk of vascular adverse events.

TIPS to minimize adverse events

(a) Use a cannula between 22 and 25G.
(b) Use an HA filler approved for use in this area.
(c) Inject the lower part of the tear trough groove, and avoid taking the cannula all the way up to the medial canthus, given the risk of injury to angular artery and vein.
(d) Expert groups do not recommend >0.5 ml volume in each tear trough and a more recent publication reported an average volume of 0.26 (0.1) cc [range: 0.08–0.32], to avoid overfilling [18].

4.5.2 Treatment of the Preseptal Hollow

Microdroplet subdermal placement of filler in the preseptal tear trough has been used by the author, in certain candidates with preseptal hollows, with good outcomes, although all patients initially had small bumps for the first few days post treatment [19]. Restylane Skinboosters Vital Light (HA_{SBVL}) has also been used for treating fine, superficial peri-orbital wrinkles, small volume touch ups or used in a layering technique in patients with deep tear troughs and a tight tear trough ligament. However given the high risk of Tyndall effect and swelling, it was recommended that the superficial use of HA_{SBVL} for treatment of the tear troughs only be attempted by advanced injectors [19].

TIPS to minimize adverse events

(a) Use a fine needle for subdermal placement.
(b) Use very low volumes for each injection as there is a risk of Tyndall effect.
(c) Inject the upper part of the preseptal hollow and tear trough groove, and avoid the small vertical veins in the eyelid skin and injecting closer to the lid cheek junction.
(d) Only for advanced injectors.

4.5.3 Direct Treatment of the Infraorbital Hollow

The direct approach to the IO area is indicated when patients present with a deeper palpebromalar groove due to suborbicularis oculi fat pad (SOOF) volume loss. The treatment approach consists of using a needle or blunt tip cannula, injecting small bolus of HA filler in front of the orbital septum at supraperiosteal level, between the orbicularis retaining ligament and the zygomatic cutaneous ligament. The specialist must be aware of the infraorbital artery branches and of the angular artery and vein. Expert groups do not recommend >1 ml volume in each palpebromalar groove as the volume injected is thought to be a more important factor affecting swelling compared to the brand of filler. As the volume significantly affected short-term post-procedure swelling with more swelling occurring with larger volumes, recommendations are between 0.5 and 1 ml volume initially. If larger amounts are needed it is recommended spacing out treatments with less at each subsequent visit [20].

TIPS to minimize adverse events

(a) Use a cannula between 22 and 25G.
(b) Use an HA filler approved for use in this area.
(c) Entry is 3 cm below the lateral canthus, and inject below the ORL in the pre-zygomatic space. Be mindful of backflow from needle or cannula inadvertently depositing HA filler above the malar septum.
(d) Expert groups do not recommend >1 ml volume to avoid overfilling [18].

4.5.4 Indirect Treatment of the Infraorbital Hollow

This is indicated for patients with a negative vector and an infraorbital hollow. Here injecting the deep fat pads of the midface (SOOF and DMCF) has an indirect impact of supporting the tissues of the anterior cheek and improving the appearance of infraorbital hollows [21]. The product and volumes used are customized based on individual soft tissue volume loss. The HA filler products used are not those used to directly treat the tear trough or infraorbital hollow.

4.6 Adverse Events with Infraorbital HA Filler

Most early adverse events from HA filler injections are transient and mild, although they may seem severe to the patients (Table 4.7). These include bruising, swelling, contour irregularities and Tyndall effect [22]. They are listed in Table 4.8 with recommendations for management.

4.6.1 Bruising and Ecchymosis (Fig. 4.19)

Cause: Injury to superficial blood vessels during injection.

Prevention: Care with patient on oral anticoagulants and NSAIDs prior to treatment. Consider avoiding injection under topical anaesthesia, as it promotes vasodilatation that increases the chances of redness and bruising. Use a blunt tipped cannula rather than needle.

Management: Apply ice and compression immediately. Use heparin or vitamin K creams to

Table 4.7 Adverse events with infraorbital HA filler

	Common	Uncommon
Acute (Table 4.8)	Bruising and ecchymosis	Acute infection
	Lumps and contour irregularity	Acute inflammatory nodules
	Tyndall effect	Post septal filler
	Acute swelling/malar oedema	Visual impairment/blindness/stroke
		Haemosiderin staining
Chronic	Delayed swelling/malar oedema	
	Delayed inflammatory nodules	
	Xanthelasma-like reaction	
	Delayed migration or displacement of filler	
	Discolouration	

Table 4.8 Acute adverse events: prevention and management strategies

Acute AE	Prevention	Management
Pain	Topical anaesthesia	Ice post injection
Bruising	Avoid alcohol, anticoagulants, anti-inflammatories pre-injection	Ice, camouflage makeup, topical vit K/pulse dye LASER within first 24–48 h
Lumps/contour irregularity	Avoid large boluses, superficial filler, correct placement (deep) and small progressive volumes in candidates with thin skin	Massage, hyaluronidase
Swelling/malar oedema	Appropriate patient selection, low volumes, progressive treatments over many sessions	Ice, use of oral steroids or intralesional low dose triamcinolone
Tyndall effect	Avoid large boluses, superficial filler	Hyaluronidase
Visual impairment/ blindness	Inject slowly, small bolus, use cannulas gently, use ultrasound to map vascular anatomy	Contact ophthalmic A&E or multidisciplinary management with interventional neurologist and neurologist
Acute infection	Appropriate patient selection, use aseptic techniques, avoid makeup post injection	Systemic antibiotics may need radiological assessment and hyaluronidase
Acute inflammatory nodules	Do not inject for 2 weeks pre and post vaccine, dental procedures and be aware of patients' immune system	Steroids and oral antibiotics
Post septal filler	Correct placement	Ultrasound-guided hyaluronidase
Haemosiderin staining	Avoid needles, especially in darker skin types	Alexandrite LASER

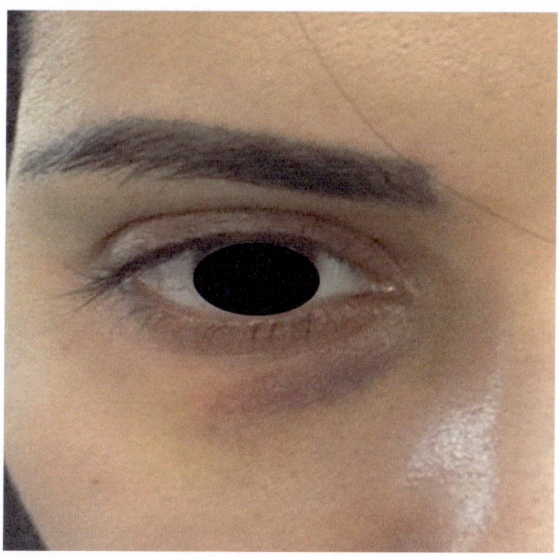

Fig. 4.19 Bruising 1 day after filler injection

reduce discolouration. Wear camouflage makeup. In severe cases, consider pulsed dye laser therapy within 24–48 h to prevent haemosiderin staining.

4.6.2 Lumps or Contour Irregularity (Fig. 4.20)

Cause: Large boluses of filler in one location or one session, superficial filler and incorrect product.

Prevention: Avoid large boluses in one place/session, place filler deep, and choose the correct product for the IO area.

Management: Mould or massage the product after injection, if it does not settle in

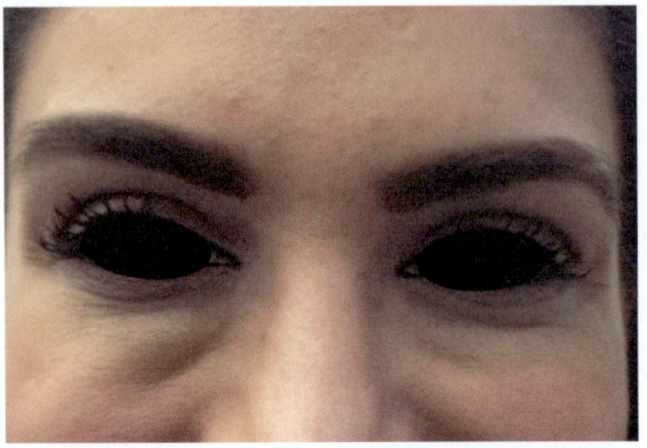

Fig. 4.20 Contour irregularity from overfilling and superficial placement of TT filler

2–4 weeks, consider hyaluronidase to dissolve the lump and smooth the contour.

4.6.3 Tyndall Effect: Bluish Discolouration from the Filler under the Skin (Fig. 4.21)

Cause: Superficial placement of hyaluronic acid fillers.

Prevention: Place filler pre- or supraperiosteal and avoid large bolus in patients with thin skin.

Management: Hyaluronidase to breakdown superficially placed filler.

4.6.4 Acute Swelling/Malar Oedema

This can occur quite commonly after HA filler injection and generally improves over a few weeks (Figs. 4.22 and 4.23).

Cause: Overfilling, improper choice of filler, placement of filler above malar septum or fluid retention. Patients wearing tight swim goggles or ski goggles for 4 weeks post IO treatment.

Prevention: Do not inject patients with preexisting lymphatic stasis/festoons, use appropriate fillers for the IO area, and do not use large volumes.

Management: Administer oral antihistamines or corticosteroids, encourage lymphatic mas-

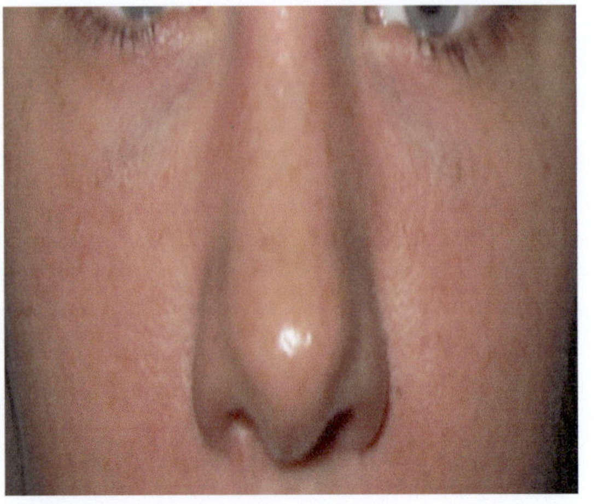

Fig. 4.21 Tyndall effect

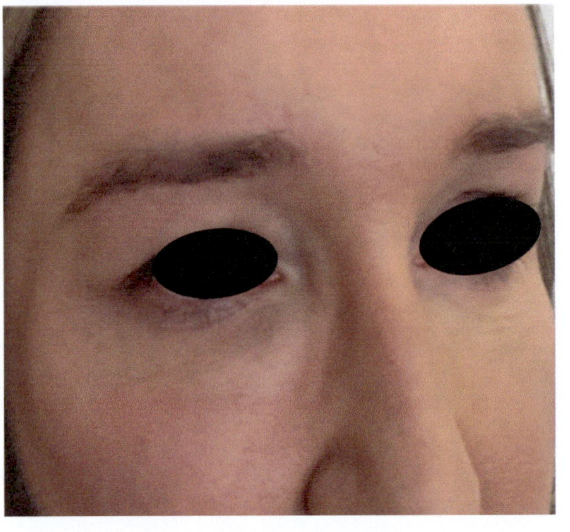

Fig. 4.22 Acute swelling

sage, use hyaluronidase to dissolve excess filler in cases of overcorrection or where the swelling is not settling with conservative management or causing patient emotional/social distress.

4.6.5 Acute Infection

Cause: Poor techniques, injecting patients with acute skin infection (e.g. active pustular acne or cold sores). Not removing or applying makeup immediately pre- or post-procedure.

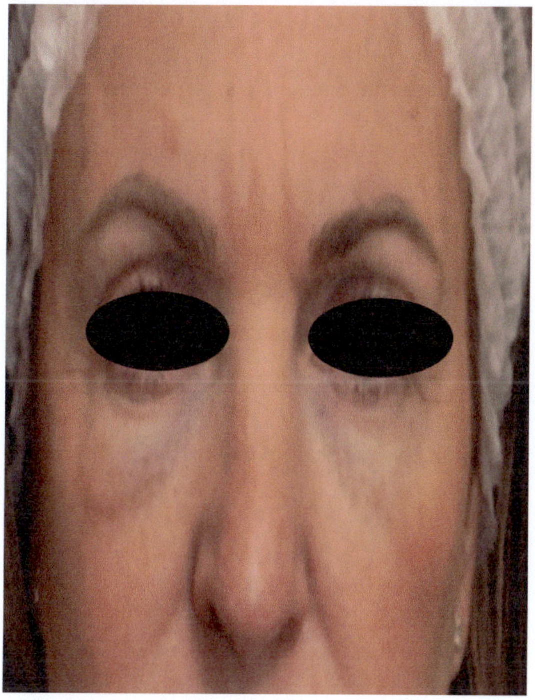

Fig. 4.23 Malar oedema

Prevention: Take a full medical history and appropriate patient selection, aseptic techniques, avoid makeup post injection.

Management: Antibiotic or antiviral cover as appropriate, may need radiological investigations and hyaluronidase dissolving once acute infection resolves.

4.6.6 Acute Inflammatory Nodules

Cause: Immune-mediated reaction to the filler material.

Prevention: Take a full medical history, and do not inject patient's undergoing dental procedures or vaccinations within 2 weeks of scheduled treatment.

Management: May need radiological investigations, dissolving with hyaluronidase, may need antibiotic cover, and may need intralesional corticosteroids or 5-fluorouracil or oral steroids.

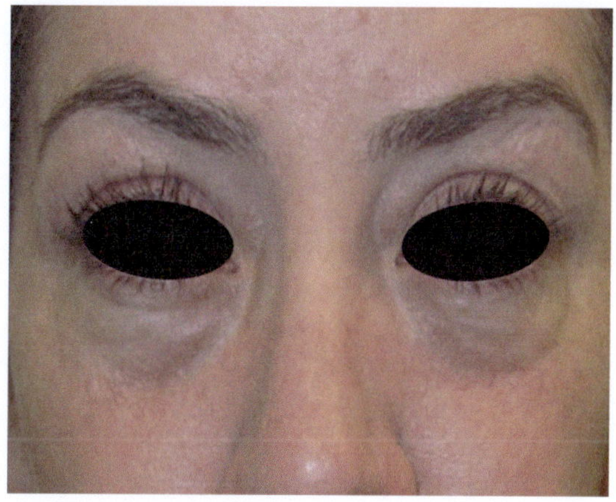

Fig. 4.24 Post septal filler

4.6.7 Post Septal Filler (Fig. 4.24)

Cause: Inadvertent placement of HA filler in the post septal space.

Prevention: Gentle manipulation of the needle or cannula and placement of filler below the ORL in the pre-zygomatic space.

Management: Radiological investigation to confirm diagnosis and ultrasound guided dissolving by an experienced aesthetic practitioner, preferably an oculoplastic surgeon.

4.6.8 Visual Impairment/Blindness/Stroke

Cause: Retrograde embolism of filler material into the ophthalmic artery.

Prevention: Use ultrasound to map the vascular anatomy, use a blunt tipped cannula instead of a needle, very slow extrusion force and small bolus injections.

Management: Stop injecting, document vision and extraocular motility. Immediate office based manoeuvres include the following: getting patient to breathe into a paper bag, immediate use of high dose hyaluronidase to dissolve filler and use of topical timolol drops. The current recommendation is to transfer the patient to an ophthalmologist/oculoplastic surgeon and further management with a team that includes a neurologist and interventional radiologist for consideration of more invasive salvage.

4.6.9 Vascular Occlusion (Fig. 4.25)

Cause: Vascular occlusion by HA filler.
Prevention: Similar to prevention of ocular complication.
Management: Hyaluronidase injection.

4.6.10 Haemosiderin Staining

Cause: significant bruising haematoma can leave temporary or permanent haemosiderin deposits, especially in Fitzpatrick skin types 4 ~ 6.
Prevention: Avoid using needle for treatment, gentle manipulation of blunt tipped cannula, immediate compression of a haematoma, caution injecting patients on oral anticoagulants.
Management: Alexandrite LASER.

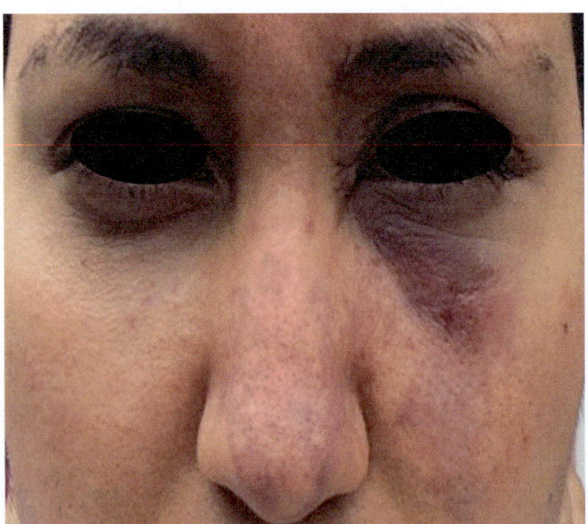

Fig. 4.25 Left IO vascular occlusion, note livedo reticularis on nose and cheek, which is challenging to identify vs a bruise, in darker skin individuals

4.7 Delayed Adverse Events

Delayed adverse events like chronic lower eyelid and malar oedema have been increasingly reported to occur in recent literature. A systematic review in 2022 [23] reported the most common delayed complication with any dermal filler was swelling (42.3%) followed by lumps or nodules (25%). Xanthelasma-like reaction (17.3%), migration (7.7%) and discolouration (3%) also occurred. The average time of onset of any complication was 16.8 months with xanthelasma-like reaction appearing soonest (mean: 10 months) and discolouration appearing latest (mean: 52 months).

4.7.1 Delayed Swelling/Malar Oedema

This can occur a few months to years after IO HA filler injection and can worsen over time (Fig. 4.26).

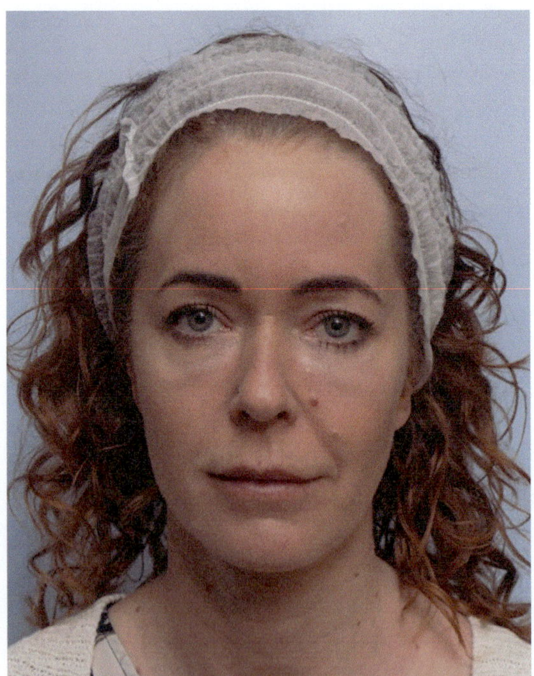

Fig. 4.26 Delayed swelling with malar bags

Cause: The cause of delayed oedema is unclear and thought to be due to injecting filler superficial to the malar septum (either due to inappropriate injection techniques or backflow using needles or cannulas). This can affect the lymphatic drainage resulting in fluid accumulation [15]. Imaging and anatomic studies have confirmed that supraperiosteal injections of HA can lie within the muscle fibres. These results suggest that HA filler can be displaced from deep to superficial, through gaps in OOM resulting in periorbital oedema [24, 25].

Prevention: Do not inject patients with preexisting lymphatic stasis/festoons, use appropriate fillers for the IO area, and do not use large volumes. Care needs to be taken whilst injecting the fat pad that lies between the bilaminar subfascial membrane of the ORL, as this may result in an oblong mass under the eye that is difficult to correct [26].

Management: Administer oral antihistamines or corticosteroids, encourage lymphatic massage, use hyaluronidase to dissolve excess filler in cases of overcorrection, and tighten the lax or stretched eyelid skin. Note multiple dissolving sessions may be required.

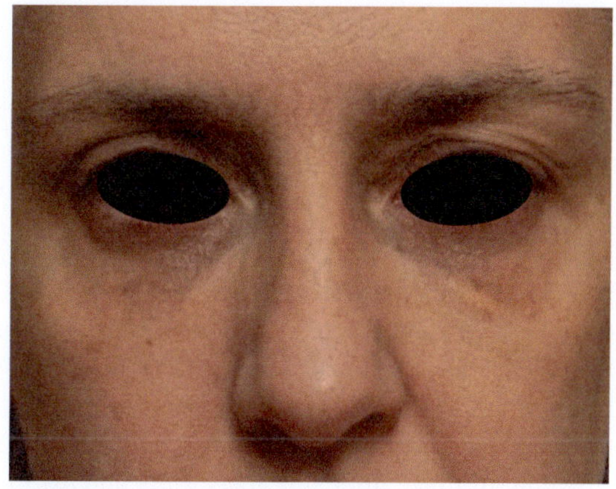

Fig. 4.27 Xanthelasma-like reaction

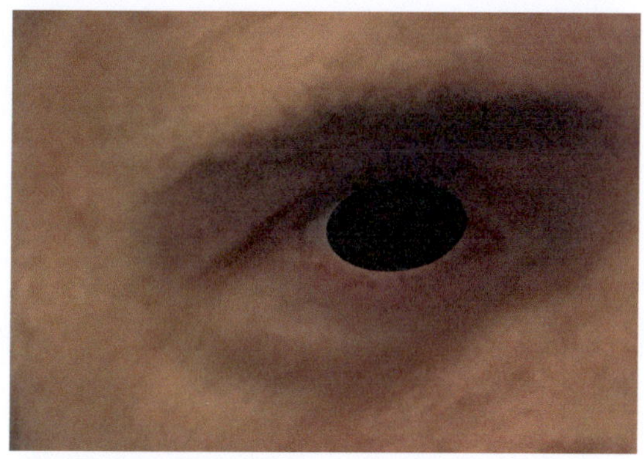

Fig. 4.28 Migrated filler

4.7.2 Delayed Inflammatory Nodules

Cause: Immune-mediated reaction to the filler material.

Prevention: Take a full medical history including recent dental procedures or vaccination.

Management: Need radiological investigations with ultrasound or MRI, dissolving with hyaluronidase, may need antibiotic cover, may need intralesional corticosteroids or 5-fluorouracil or oral steroids [27].

4.7.3 Xanthelasma-Like Reaction (Fig. 4.27)

Cause: Poorly understood, as a few case reports and histology showed nonspecific findings with rare histiocytes present in the papillary dermis. A possible mechanism may be related to binding of low-density lipoprotein and internalization by macrophages [28].

Prevention: No current recommendations.

Management: Check for hyperlipidaemia, consider hyaluronidase, steroid or 5 FU injections or LASER or direct excision of the xanthelasma-like lesion.

4.7.4 Delayed Migration or Displacement of Filler (Fig. 4.28)

Cause: The OOM can gradually push filler over time, if the filler was placed superficially or overfilled.

Prevention: Place filler supraperiosteal and avoid large bolus/overfilling. Avoid vigorous massage to avoid unintended migration.
Management: Dissolve the displaced filler with hyaluronidase.

4.7.5 Discolouration

Cause: As the filler can lie intramuscularly, over time, there is a blue-grey discolouration appearance, especially due to the thin eyelid skin.
Prevention: Place filler supraperiosteal and avoid large bolus in patients with thin skin.
Management: Dissolve the displaced filler with hyaluronidase.

4.8 Summary

Numerous studies report both objective and subjective aesthetic improvements with HA filler injections [29]. A systemic review of periocular HA filler reported patient satisfaction rates of 83.6% in the short term and 76.7% in the long term [30].

Most adverse effects observed with IO HA filler injection are mild, temporary and reversible; however, there is no uniformly successful treatment for filler-induced vision loss.

The most frequent acute complication in the literature is early swelling or oedema, which seems to be predominantly associated with poor selection of product, injection techniques and volumes used. Large volumes and superficial injections are also causally linked to Tyndall effect and contour irregularities.

Whilst acute bruising is seen more commonly with needles, a systematic review found that HA injection with needles or cannulas in tear trough did not significantly differ in patient safety or outcomes.

The most frequent delayed adverse event is delayed eyelid oedema/malar oedema, which has been attributed to orbicularis muscle anatomy and inadequate lymphatic pump function.

Excessive HA volume in the IO area gives rise to unnatural aesthetic results over time.

Current recommendations to improve reduce adverse events from IO HA fillers are the following:

1. Detailed medical history prior to treatment, including autoimmune conditions, medicines and allergies.
2. Thorough assessment of the IO area to customize the treatment.
3. Counsel unsuitable patients regarding alternative treatment options.
4. Perform IO HA filler treatment with the patient seated as the IO anatomy is better visualized in this position.
5. Use low-viscosity instead of high-viscosity hyaluronic acid (HA), which are less hydrophilic.
6. Avoid high-risk zones, such as directly over the infraorbital foramen.
7. Avoid superficial injections to prevent the Tyndall effect.
8. Supraperiosteal injections are preferred as it reduces the occurrence of contour irregularity as well as reduces the risk of accidental vascular injection since few arteries run over the periosteum in this region.
9. Both a needle and a cannula can be used with good results, but blunt-tipped cannulas may be safer due to the reduced chance of damaging vessels and nerves.
10. Employ slow, low-pressure injection techniques.
11. Under correct rather than overcorrect the IO area (volumes between 0.2 and 1 ml).
12. The patients must be informed that they ought to avoid any makeup immediately after treatment.
13. The patients must be informed to avoid strong or extended pressure to the area treated like massage or swim/ski goggles post treatment.
14. The patients must be informed of acute and delayed adverse events, so that they can be managed appropriately.

4.9 Conclusion

Infraorbital filler injections offer significant aesthetic benefits but carry a range of potential adverse effects. By understanding the anatomy, adhering to best practices and employing evidence-based management strategies, practitioners can minimize risks and address complications effectively.

References

1. Iera M. Treatment of infraorbital skin depressions using the hyaluronic acid filler VYC-15L based on the MD codes approach: a retrospective analysis. J Clin Exp Dermatol Res. 2020;11(4):526.
2. Narurkar V, et al. Facial treatment preferences in aesthetically aware women. Dermatologic Surg. 2015;41:S153–60.
3. Palermo E, Costa. Anatomy of the periorbital region. Surg Cosmet Dermatol. 2013;5(3):245–56.
4. Chopra K, Calva D, Sosin M, Tadisina KK, Banda A, De La Cruz C, Chaudhry MR, Legesse T, Drachenberg CB, Manson PN, Christy MR. A comprehensive examination of topographic thickness of skin in the human face. Aesthet Surg J. 2015;35(8):1007–13.
5. Vashi NA, De Castro Maymone MB, Kundu RV. Aging differences in ethnic skin. J Clin Aesthet Dermatol. 2016;9(1):31.
6. Peng PH, Peng JH. Treating the tear trough: a new classification system, a 6-step evaluation procedure, hyaluronic acid injection algorithm, and treatment sequences. J Cosmet Dermatol. 2018;17(3):333–9.
7. Cheng NC, Liao SL, Wang IJ, Lin IC, Tang YB. Fiber type and myosin heavy chain compositions of adult pretarsal orbicularis oculi muscle. J Mol Histol. 2007;38:177–82.
8. Abe T, Loenneke JP. Orbicularis oculi muscle size and function: exploring the influence of aging and exercise training. Cosmetics. 2021;8(2):29.
9. Krajewska-Węglewicz L, Felczak P, Dorobek M. Effects of aging on orbicularis oculi muscle strength and ultrastructure in dermatochalasis: a pilot study. J Clin Med. 2025;14(1):162.
10. Woodward J. Review of periorbital and upper face: pertinent anatomy, aging, injection techniques, prevention, and management of complications of facial fillers. J Drugs Dermatol. 2016;15(12):1524–31.
11. Woodward JA. Periocular fillers and related anatomy. Cutis. 2016;98(5):330–5.
12. Funt DK. Avoiding malar edema during midface/cheek augmentation with dermal fillers. J Clin Aesthet Dermatol. 2011;4(12):32.
13. Kaya TI. Clinical anatomy of the face for filler and botulinum toxin injection. Turk Dermatoloji Derg. 2016;10(3):135.
14. Lee SH, et al. Novel anatomic description of the course of the inferior palpebral vein for minimally invasive aesthetic treatments. Dermatologic Surg. 2016;42(5):618–23.
15. Shoukath S, et al. The lymphatic anatomy of the lower eyelid and conjunctiva and correlation with postoperative chemosis and edema. Plast Reconstr Surg. 2017;139(3):628e–37e.
16. Anido J, et al. Recommendations for the treatment of tear trough deformity with cross-linked hyaluronic acid filler. J Cosmet Dermatol. 2021;20(1):6–17.
17. Berros P, et al. Novel treatment protocol for combined tear trough ligament stretching and injection. Plast Reconstr Surg. 2023;152(5):808e–16e.
18. Bernardini FP, et al. Bridging the gap rather than filling the entire valley—anatomic insights when treating the medial infraorbital region. J Cosmet Dermatol. 2025;24(1):e16582.
19. Metelitsa A, et al. Simplifying the injector's armamentarium: an international consensus regarding the use of gel science to differentiate hyaluronic acid fillers and guide treatment recommendations. J Cosmet Dermatol. 2024;23(5):1604–12.
20. Siperstein R, Montes JR, Speranza AM. A retrospective review of the safety and efficacy of low-dose triamcinolone mixed with hyaluronic acid fillers to reduce post-injection infraorbital swelling. J Clin Aesthet Dermatol. 2022;15(4):13.
21. Raspaldo H, et al. Global, 3-dimensional approach to natural rejuvenation: part 1–recommendations for volume restoration and the periocular area. J Cosmet Dermatol. 2012;11(4):279–89.
22. Funt D, Pavicic T. Dermal fillers in aesthetics: an overview of adverse events and treatment approaches. Plast Aesthet Nurs. 2015;35(1):13–32.
23. Trinh LN, McGuigan KC, Gupta A. Delayed complications following dermal filler for tear trough augmentation: a systematic review. Facial Plast Surg. 2022;38(3):250–9.
24. Griepentrog GJ, et al. Anatomical position of hyaluronic acid gel following injection to the infraorbital hollows. Ophthalmic Plast Reconstr Surg. 2013;29(1):35–9.
25. De Pasquale A, et al. Hyaluronic acid filler injections for tear-trough deformity: injection technique and high-frequency ultrasound follow-up evaluation. Aesth Plast Surg. 2013;37:587–91.
26. Pessa JE. SMAS fusion zones determine the subfascial and subcutaneous anatomy of the human face:

fascial spaces, fat compartments, and models of facial aging. Aesthet Surg J. 2016;36(5):515–26.
27. Philipp-Dormston WG, et al. Global approaches to the prevention and management of delayed-onset adverse reactions with hyaluronic acid-based fillers. Plast Reconstr Surg Glob Open. 2020;8(4):e2730.
28. Or L, Eviatar JA, Massry GG, Bernardini FP, Hartstein ME. Xanthelasma-like reaction to filler injection. Ophthalmic Plast Reconstr Surg. 2017;33(4):244–7.
29. Liu X, et al. The efficacy and safety of hyaluronic acid injection in tear trough deformity: a systematic review and meta-analysis. Aesth Plast Surg. 2024;48(3):478–90.
30. Gorbea E, Kidwai S, Rosenberg J. Nonsurgical tear trough volumization: a systematic review of patient satisfaction. Aesthet Surg J. 2021;41(8):NP1053–60.

Lower Face Contouring and Rejuvenation with HA Fillers

5

Juyoung Go and Won Lee

5.1 Introduction

The contour of the lower third of the face from a frontal view and the profile of the jaw and neck line are crucial elements that determine overall facial harmony and impression [1]. The structural integrity and smoothness of this area play a pivotal role in creating a youthful appearance and achieving harmonious aesthetic balance [2]. A well-defined jawline, characterized by a distinct line extending from the mandibular angle to the chin, clearly demarcates the boundary between the face and neck, adding definition and contributing to a refined appearance (Fig. 5.1).

For individuals whose lower facial contours are compromised due to factors such as a congenitally small chin, previous orthognathic surgery, or the aging process, fundamental treatment typically involves surgical interventions like chin implants, face lifts, or neck lifts. However, driven by the growing interest and demand for non-surgical rejuvenation and aesthetic enhancement,

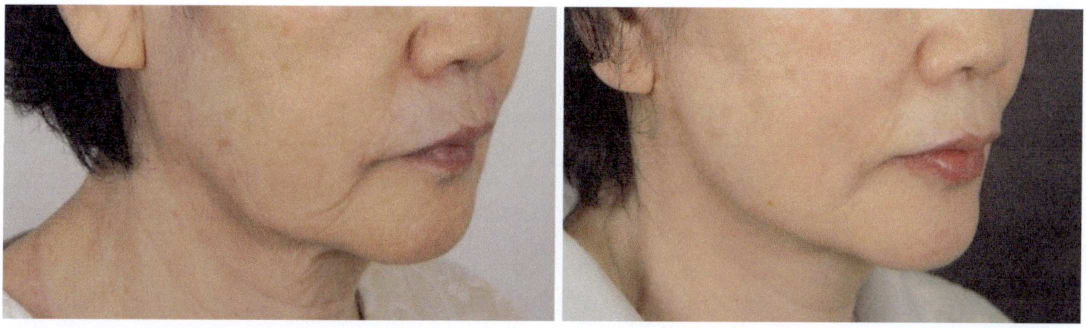

Fig. 5.1 Importance of the jawline: before and after photographs of a 70-year-old patient who underwent face and neck lift and lip filler procedures. Comparison between baseline (pre-procedure) and 3 weeks post-procedure

J. Go
Atelier Plastic Surgery, Seoul, Republic of Korea

W. Lee (✉)
Yonsei E1 Plastic Surgery Clinic,
Anyang, Kyonggi-do, Korea (Republic of)

W. Lee (ed.), *Innovative Injectable Techniques in Minimally Invasive Aesthetics*,
https://doi.org/10.1007/978-981-95-2161-6_5

a variety of therapeutic approaches are now employed, either independently or adjunctively with surgery.

Technologies such as ultrasound, ablative and non-ablative lasers, radiofrequency, botulinum toxin, and fillers are clinically applied, each utilized to address specific manifestations of aging and aesthetic concerns [3, 4]. Among these, hyaluronic acid (HA) fillers have become established as a highly effective method for redefining the contours of the jawline and chin, improving marionette lines, and achieving soft tissue lifting, thereby restoring facial balance and harmony.

Achieving aesthetically satisfactory and safe outcomes necessitates a precise facial assessment and a thorough understanding of the relevant anatomy. Furthermore, a tailored approach that considers the individual anatomical characteristics of each patient is crucial. This chapter will discuss the essential anatomical concepts of the lower face, the associated aging processes, and methods for clinical assessment. We will also share clinical experiences and treatment strategies for enhancing the contours of the chin, marionette lines, prejowl sulcus, and jawline using hyaluronic acid (HA) fillers.

5.2 Anatomy and Aging Process of the Lower Face

The lower face is a crucial region determining the overall balance and contour of the face. Anatomically, it comprises the mandible, soft tissues (including muscles, fat, and skin), vasculature and nerves, and the parotid gland. As aging progresses, these structures undergo complex changes, leading to alterations in facial contours and the development of skin sagging.

5.2.1 Mandible

The mandible is the primary skeletal component forming the structure of the lower face, consisting of a horseshoe-shaped inferior body and vertical mandibular rami. A congenitally small or recessed chin can contribute to an earlier loss of jawline definition.

Bone resorption typically occurs with aging, particularly affecting the mandible. This involves a flattening of the mandibular angle, a decrease in overall mandibular length, and changes such as chin recession or protrusion. These age-related bony changes can be exacerbated by tooth loss [5, 6]. Consequently, the jawline loses definition, and the descent of overlying soft tissues contributes to the formation of jowls (Fig. 5.2).

5.2.2 Soft Tissues: Skin, Fat, Muscles, and Fascia

The soft tissues of the lower face consist of the skin, subcutaneous fat layers, muscles, and fascial layers. The aging process in this region is driven by a complex interplay of structural changes affecting the skin, fat compartments,

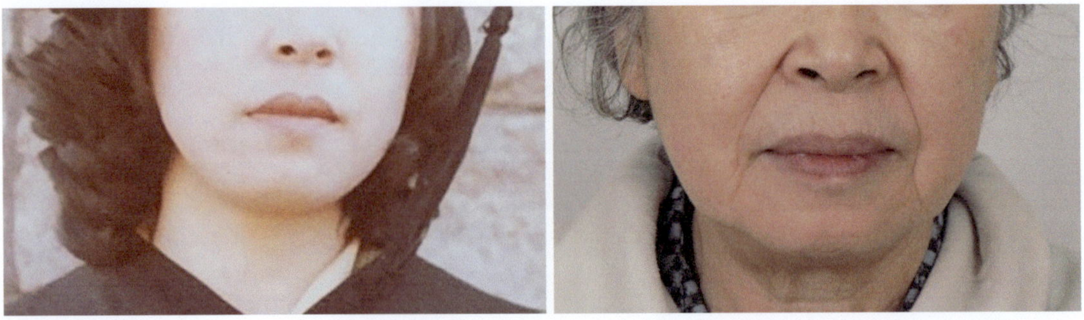

Fig. 5.2 Comparison of lower facial aging in a female patient. Left, Appearance at age 25. Right, Current appearance at age 69

muscles, and retaining ligaments. Factors such as skin atrophy, fat pad redistribution, muscle hyperactivation, and increased ligamentous laxity collectively contribute to alterations in the jawline contour and the formation of jowls. Consequently, a tailored treatment approach is essential, grounded in a thorough understanding of the interactions among these anatomical components.

5.2.2.1 Skin

The skin overlying the mandible is relatively thin posteriorly and progressively thickens toward the anterior aspect, reaching its maximum thickness over the chin. Age-related reduction in collagen and elastin fibers leads to decreased skin elasticity and wrinkle formation. Consequently, the jawline loses definition, jowls and the prejowl sulcus become more pronounced, and generalized sagging develops due to increased skin laxity. These changes are frequently accompanied by the appearance of marionette lines, which extend downward from the oral commissures toward the mandibular border [7, 8] (Fig. 5.3).

5.2.2.2 Fat Layers

The subcutaneous fat in the mandibular region is compartmentalized into several distinct pads. These include the superior and inferior mandibular fat pads, the fat overlying the parotid-masseteric fascia, the submandibular fat compartment, and the lateral lower lip fat compartment [9, 10].

Age-related decline in soft tissue elasticity facilitates both atrophy and redistribution of these fat compartments. The superior and inferior mandibular fat pads tend to atrophy over time. Coupled with laxity of the supporting facial ligaments, this allows for the inferior displacement of fat, contributing significantly to jowl formation. Additionally, atrophy within the lateral lower lip fat compartment accentuates the appearance of marionette lines [7, 8] (Fig. 5.4).

5.2.2.3 Muscles and Fascia

The arrangement of muscles and fascia in the mandibular region exhibits structural differences anterior and posterior to the labiomandibular sulcus. Posteriorly, the platysma muscle is situated beneath the superficial subcutaneous fat. Deep to this fat layer, the parotid-masseteric fascia envelops the masseter muscle [11]. Age-related weakening of the platysma's attachment to the mandible can exacerbate jowl formation [12].

Anteriorly, beneath the subcutaneous fat, muscles such as the depressor anguli oris (DAO), platysma, depressor labii inferioris (DLI), and mentalis modulate mandibular movements and facial expressions. With aging, the downward pull exerted by the DLI, DAO, and platysma contributes to the blunting of the jawline definition

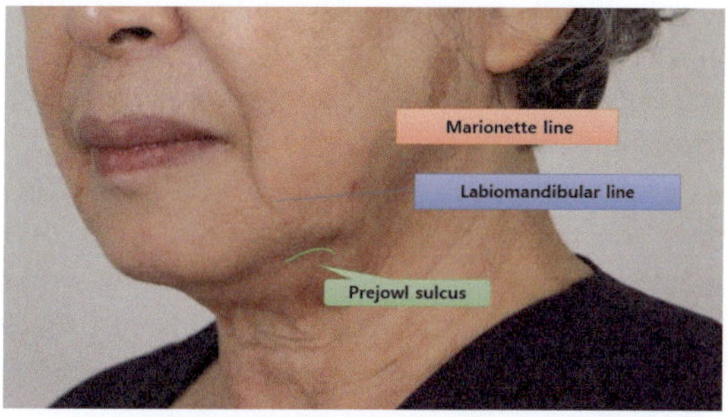

Fig. 5.3 Manifestations of lower facial skin aging

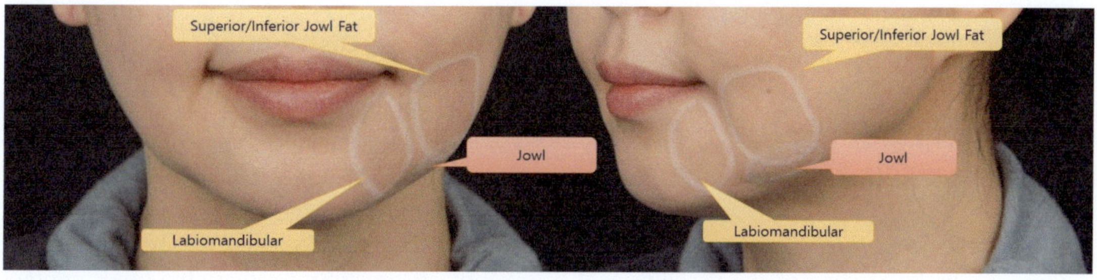

Fig. 5.4 Fat compartments of the lower face: illustrating the components and locations of the subcutaneous fat layers

and the descent of the oral commissures (mouth corners).

Located more deeply in the lower anterior face are the deep labiomandibular and deep mental fat compartments. Atrophy within these deep fat pads can further accelerate age-related contour deformities.

5.2.2.4 Anatomical Boundaries and the Effects of Aging

The superficial anatomical boundary between the cheek and the chin region, often referred to as the labiomandibular fold or cheek-chin crease, becomes more prominent as the difference in tissue thickness across this transition zone increases [13]. In the lateral labiomandibular area, the skin has relatively loose attachments to the underlying musculoaponeurotic structures, making this area susceptible to sagging (ptosis). Conversely, medial attachments are firmer, resulting in comparatively less descent.

The mandibular ligament, situated along the inferior margin of the labiomandibular sulcus and anterior to the jowl proper, functions as a key retaining structure for the lower facial soft tissues. With aging, however, the supportive strength of this ligament decreases. This attenuation, combined with the effects of gravity on overlying fat and soft tissues, leads to more pronounced jowl formation adjacent to the ligament's insertion.

Progressive volume loss and skin ptosis further accentuate the labiomandibular fold and increase the tendency for drooping of the oral commissures. In advanced aging, this fold may deepen and extend toward the mandibular border, contributing to the formation of the prejowl sulcus. This depression, adjacent to the chin, often evolves into distinct marionette lines, which are considered prominent hallmarks of lower facial aging [14] (Table 5.1).

Table 5.1 Contributing factors to marionette lines

Maxillary and mandibular bone resorption
Gravitational descent of soft tissues
Volume loss and redistribution of superficial fat pads (e.g., jowl formation)
Atrophy of deep fat compartments (e.g., deep labiomandibular fat)
Hyperactivity of depressor muscles (e.g., depressor anguli oris)
Tethering effect of the mandibular ligament
Tethering effect of the mandibular ligament

5.2.3 Vasculature and Nerve Distribution

5.2.3.1 Vasculature

A thorough understanding of the vascular anatomy in the mandibular region is crucial for preventing vascular complications during filler injections. The facial artery, the primary blood supply to the face, branches from the external carotid artery. It ascends onto the face by crossing the inferior border of the mandible just anterior to the masseter muscle's insertion. Along its course, it runs deep within the buccal fat pad and branches into the superior and inferior labial arteries near the modiolus. Subsequently, it courses more superficially near the nasolabial sulcus, continuing as the angular artery [15]. The facial vein generally runs lateral and often deeper to the facial artery, typically situated deep to the platysma muscle.

Furthermore, the mental artery, a terminal branch of the inferior alveolar artery, emerges through the mental foramen to supply the chin region. Care must be taken during filler injections near the mental foramen to prevent injury to this vessel. The submental artery, branching from the facial artery in the neck, runs along the mylohyoid muscle before crossing the mandible [16]. Given the significant anatomical variations in the course and branching patterns of these arteries, a thorough understanding of safe injection techniques is essential (Fig. 5.5).

5.2.3.2 Nerve Distribution

Key nerves in the mandibular region relevant to filler injections include the mental nerve and branches of the facial nerve. The mental nerve originates from the mandibular nerve (V3), itself a division of the trigeminal nerve (CN V). It emerges through the mental foramen to provide sensory innervation to the chin and prejowl region [17]. Particular care must be exercised

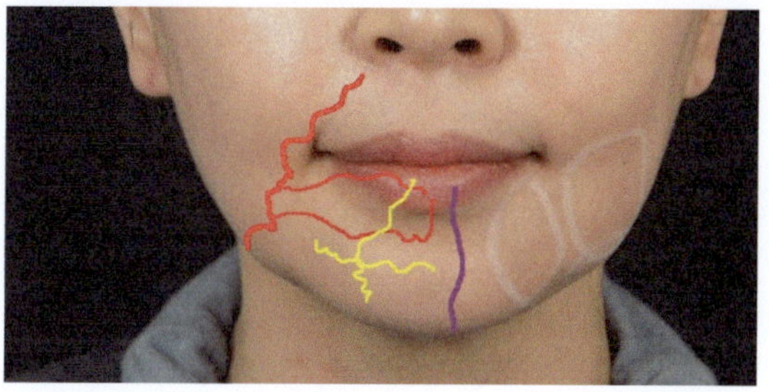

Fig. 5.5 Arterial supply of the lower face. Red lines: Inferior labial artery and horizontal labiomental branches (originating from the facial artery). Yellow line: Mental artery. Purple line: Ascending mental branch (originating from the submental artery)

during injections near the mental foramen to prevent injury to this nerve.

The marginal mandibular branch of the facial nerve innervates muscles responsible for depressing the lower lip. Anterior to the masseter, it typically runs superior to the mandibular border. However, posterior to the anterior edge of the masseter, this nerve branch frequently courses 1–2 cm inferior to the mandibular border. Awareness of this anatomical path is crucial during filler injections to avoid iatrogenic nerve injury [18].

Conversely, the subdermal plane directly overlying the platysma along the jawline is typically devoid of major neurovascular structures and is therefore considered a relatively safe plane for filler placement.

5.2.4 Parotid Gland

The parotid gland is situated in the preauricular area, superior and posterior to the masseter muscle. The parotid duct (Stensen's duct) arises from the anterior aspect of the gland, travels horizontally across the superficial surface of the masseter muscle, and pierces the buccinator muscle to enter the oral cavity. Its path typically aligns with a line drawn from the tragus of the ear towards the midpoint between the nasal ala and the oral commissure. Caution is required during filler injections in this vicinity to avoid damaging the duct [11].

5.3 Clinical Assessment for Lower Face Contouring

Assessment of the lower face contour requires consideration of the overall balance and proportions of the entire face. It is crucial to analyze specific contour concerns through both static and dynamic evaluations. Key elements to assess include the definition and volume of the jawline, mandibular angle, and chin. Additionally, the influence of soft tissue dynamics and muscle activity on the mandibular outline must be carefully evaluated. This comprehensive approach enables the clinician to set realistic patient expectations and formulate an optimal treatment strategy [19–21].

5.3.1 Patient Assessment Methods

5.3.1.1 Static Assessment

Static assessment involves analyzing facial proportions, skeletal structure, and soft tissue conditions while the face is immobile. Typically, this evaluation utilizes standardized photographs taken from frontal, lateral, and oblique (45°) perspectives. The face is assessed in thirds (upper, middle, lower) to evaluate overall harmony and balance.

Analysis of facial proportions determines if the lower third is in harmony with the overall face and assesses the structural definition of the jawline and mandibular angles. The underlying skeletal framework and overlying soft tissues are inspected for evidence of bone resorption or volume deficits attributable to congenital factors or aging processes. Skin elasticity and the degree of ptosis are also evaluated to guide the decision between non-surgical interventions (such as fillers or thread lifts) and surgical options (like facelift or genioplasty) [22, 23].

The interplay between the midface and lower face requires careful consideration. In cases of midface volume deficiency, addressing this deficit often yields a more natural enhancement of the jawline contour compared to treating the lower face in isolation. Furthermore, when significant midface ptosis is present, the efficacy of lower face treatments alone may be limited. This interdependence should be factored into the treatment planning process [24].

5.3.1.2 Dynamic Assessment

Dynamic assessment focuses on observing how facial expressions and muscle activity influence the contour of the lower face. This evaluation extends beyond static assessment of bone and soft tissue by analyzing the functional impact of muscle movement on the lower facial appearance.

Muscle movement analysis involves assessing the activity of key muscles, including the depressor anguli oris (DAO), depressor labii inferioris (DLI), mentalis, and platysma. The goal is to determine how hyperactivation of specific muscles contributes to alterations in the lower facial contour. Particular attention should be paid to changes in the jawline definition during speech and smiling, and whether dynamic movements exacerbate skin ptosis or wrinkling [25].

Furthermore, it is important to observe changes in jawline definition during active chin movement and assess the dynamic elasticity of the skin and soft tissues. Analyzing whether jowls become more pronounced with specific facial expressions helps determine the suitability of non-surgical interventions such as fillers or thread lifting.

Additionally, as dental alignment and occlusion can significantly influence lower facial contours, evaluating for underlying orthognathic or odontological issues is also an important part of the assessment [26] (Fig. 5.6).

5.3.2 Key Assessment Indicators

5.3.2.1 Jawline Definition

The jawline is a fundamental element for the structural balance of the lower face and serves as a critical indicator for aesthetic enhancement. Evaluation should focus on whether the jawline maintains clear definition or appears indistinct due to skin ptosis. Skeletal deficiencies can result in inadequate mandibular support, leading to a poorly defined jawline. Specifically, a flattened mandibular angle or a congenitally small mandible provides insufficient structural scaffolding, increasing the susceptibility to downward displacement of soft tissues [27] (Fig. 5.7).

5.3.2.2 Severity of Marionette Lines and Prejowl Sulcus

Marionette lines and the prejowl sulcus represent key manifestations of aging in the lower face. Assessment involves determining the extent of the marionette lines (i.e., whether they reach the mandibular border from the oral commissures) and evaluating the presence and depth of the prejowl sulcus in conjunction with soft tissue ptosis.

When drooping of the oral commissures (mouth corners) coexists, the improvement achievable with fillers alone may be limited; combining fillers with soft tissue lifting procedures can often yield more effective results. Additionally, restoring volume to a deficient lateral lower lip fat compartment can help soften the appearance of marionette lines and may provide a

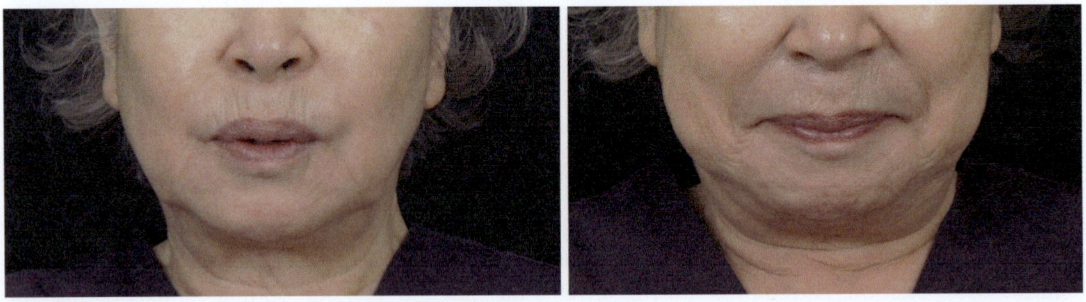

Fig. 5.6 Dynamic assessment of the lower face: analyzing the influence of facial expressions and muscle activity on the mandibular contour

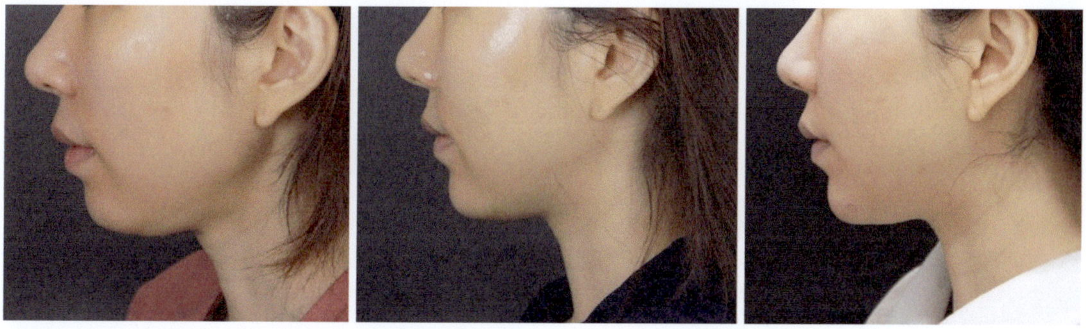

Fig. 5.7 Lower face changes before and after filler treatment. Lateral views of a 35-year-old patient treated with fillers in the nasolabial folds (NLF), lips, chin, and jawline. Left, Before. Middle, 1 week post-procedure. Right, 6 months post-procedure

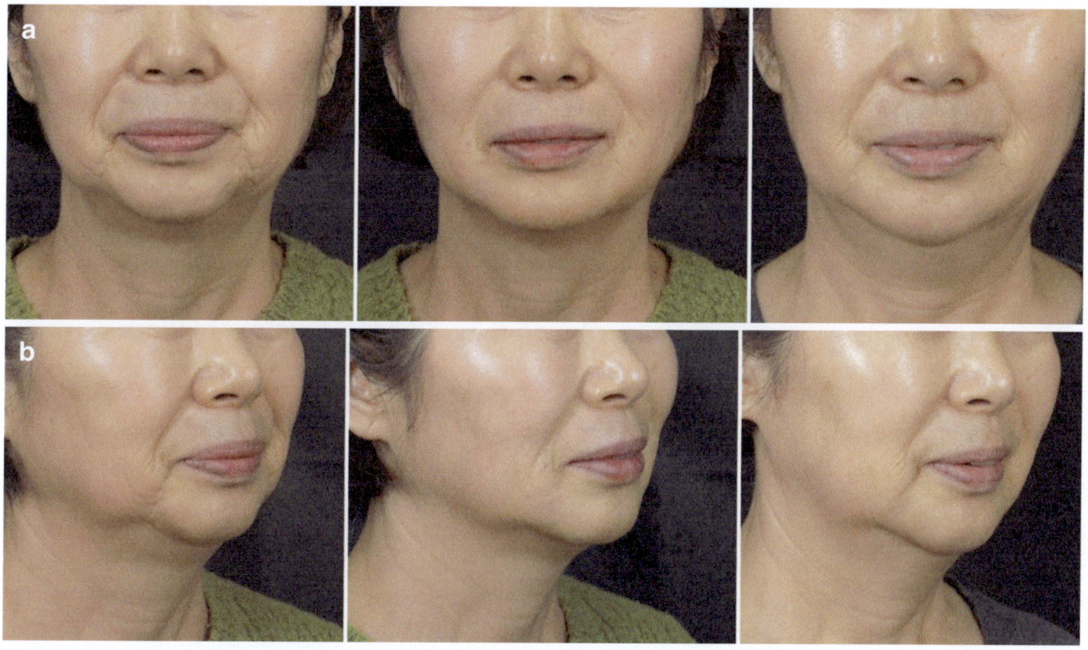

Fig. 5.8 Lower face changes before and after filler treatment. A 64-year-old patient treated with fillers in the nasolabial folds (NLF), prejowl sulcus, chin, and marionette lines. Left, Before. Middle, Immediately post-procedure. Right, 6 months post-procedure. (**a**) Frontal views. (**b**) oblique views

secondary lifting effect on the oral commissures [28] (Fig. 5.8).

5.3.2.3 Anteroposterior Position and Projection of the Chin

The anteroposterior position and projection of the chin significantly influence the balance of the lower face. In cases of mandibular recession (retrogenia), the chin may appear disproportionate to the overall facial profile. Such cases often benefit from augmentation using fillers or surgical implants [29].

The condition of the overlying soft tissues and skin of the chin is also critical. If soft tissue deficiency or skin ptosis is evident, treatment should incorporate both appropriate volume restoration and lifting techniques. Chin length and width must also be assessed to achieve an optimal con-

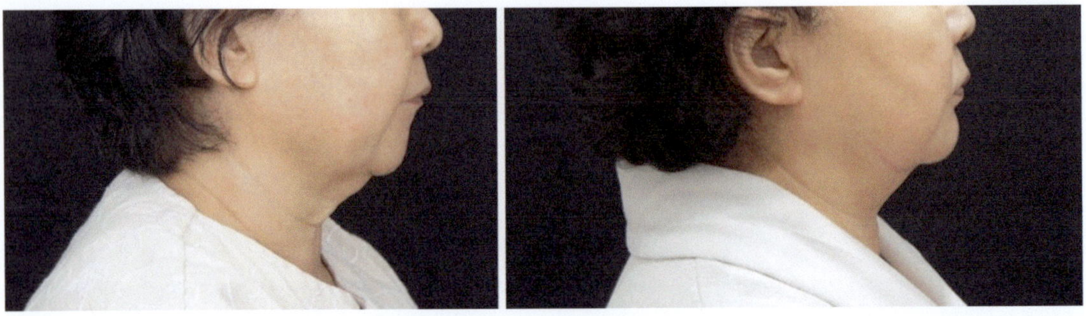

Fig. 5.9 Changes before and after neck lift and filler treatment. Lateral views of a 73-year-old patient who underwent neck lift surgery combined with filler injections to the chin and prejowl sulcus. Left: Before. Right: 6 months post-procedure

tour that harmonizes with the overall proportions of the lower face [30] (Fig. 5.9).

5.3.2.4 Skin Elasticity and Soft Tissue Volume Status

Evaluating skin elasticity and the status of soft tissue volume is essential for planning lower face contouring. When skin elasticity is reduced, non-surgical options like fillers or thread lifting may offer effective improvement. Concurrently, assessment for fat pad atrophy is also necessary [31].

Gravitational descent can cause soft tissue migration, leading to apparent volume excess in some areas and deficits in others. Therefore, assessing the impact of this age-related fat redistribution on the overall lower facial contour is crucial. In particular, where fat pad atrophy or general soft tissue volume loss has occurred, volume restoration is key to achieving better jawline definition [32, 33].

5.4 Lower Face Contouring Strategy Using HA Fillers

HA filler treatment for the lower third aims to enhance facial contours primarily by reshaping and defining the jawline. This structural enhancement can also create an apparent lifting effect relative to the neck. Through careful selection of appropriate fillers and the use of precise injection techniques, clinicians can improve jawline definition, modulate chin volume and projection, and ameliorate aging signs like marionette lines and the prejowl sulcus. Achieving optimal outcomes requires choosing products based on their rheological characteristics and employing injection strategies grounded in a thorough understanding of the relevant anatomy [13, 30].

5.4.1 Characteristics of Fillers and Selection Criteria

5.4.1.1 Properties of HA Fillers

In lower face filler treatments, it is essential to select the appropriate product by considering the elasticity (G') and viscosity (G'') of hyaluronic acid (HA) fillers. The elastic modulus (G') represents the material's ability to resist compression, while the complex modulus (G^*) measures firmness or hardness—specifically, the energy required to deform the filler.

Fillers with a low G^* value are suitable for superficial filling, whereas those with a high G^* value are preferred for deep volume restoration [34, 35] (Table 5.2). High G' fillers provide strong structural support within the tissue, making them effective for reshaping the jawline, while fillers with higher viscosity blend naturally with the soft tissue, facilitating more natural volume restoration. Additionally, the *retention* of the filler plays a critical role in maintaining stable contours after injection, depending on the treated area [34, 35] (Table 5.3).

Table 5.2 Rheological and physicochemical properties of hyaluronic acid (HA) fillers

parameter	Description
Elastic modulus (G')	Storage modulus, restoration of deformation by external stress Unit: Pascals, pas High G' has high potency for restore from deformation
Viscous modulus (G'')	Loss modulus of external stress High G'' higher power is needed to extrude from needle
Tan delta (tan δ)	Relative ratio of viscous modulus and elastic modulus (G''/G') High elastic gel (e.g., gelatin), tan δ is near 0 High viscous gel (e.g., honey), tan δ is near 1
Complex modulus (G^*)	Total energy for not to deform $G^* = \sqrt{(G')^2 + (G'')^2}$ Most HA filler $G' > G''$ Most HA filler G^* is near G'
Gel cohesion	Aggregation property not dispersing by external force Attractive force by each molecules Low cohesiveness filler disperse easily
Concentration (mg/mL)	Total hyaluronic acid mount at 1 mL product Cross-linked HA maintain shape at human body Pendant linked HA or free HA degrades faster at human body

Elastic modulus (G'), viscous modulus (G''), complex modulus (G^*), and other material properties of HA fillers measured in vitro [35].

Filler Selection Guide by Injection Site

- *Jawline → High Elasticity Fillers ($G' > 400$ Pa, 0.1 Hz)*

  To enhance the structural definition of the jawline, fillers with high elasticity suitable for injection into the supraperiosteal plane are required.

  High G' fillers demonstrate excellent shape retention within the tissue and are ideal for sculpting a more defined mandibular contour.
- *Chin → Fillers with Balanced Viscoelastic Properties (G' 200–400 Pa, 0.1 Hz)*

  The chin must harmonize with the jawline while maintaining appropriate projection and volume.
  Therefore, fillers with moderate elasticity and viscosity should be selected.
  Using excessively firm fillers may lead to unnatural results, making it essential to choose products that blend well with the surrounding soft tissues.
- *Marionette lines → Softer fillers ($G' < 200$ Pa, 0.1 Hz)*

  Since the marionette lines require both wrinkle correction and natural soft tissue volume restoration, a softer filler with high viscosity is appropriate.

  Using fillers that are too firm may cause unnatural expressions during dynamic facial movements; therefore, selecting a product that integrates smoothly with the soft tissue is crucial [36] (Fig. 5.10, Table 5.3).

A comparative graph showing the changes in elastic modulus (G') of various hyaluronic acid (HA) fillers according to frequency variations [34].

5.4.2 Filler Injection Techniques

5.4.2.1 Jawline and Mandibular Angle Enhancement

The jawline and mandibular angle are critical areas that define the lower facial contour. To create a sharper and more structured appearance, it is effective to inject filler into the supraperiosteal layer to enhance structural support. This technique improves the definition of the jawline and maximizes the lifting effect on both the neck and the cheek.

Sagging (ptosis) and excessive volume in the jowl area are not treated directly. Instead, the target zone extends from posterior to the jowl toward the mandibular angle. Filler is injected parallel to the inferior border of the mandible, within a range of approximately 1.5 cm [13, 37] (Figs. 5.11 and 5.12).

Fig. 5.10 Changes in elastic modulus (G') of hyaluronic acid fillers by frequency

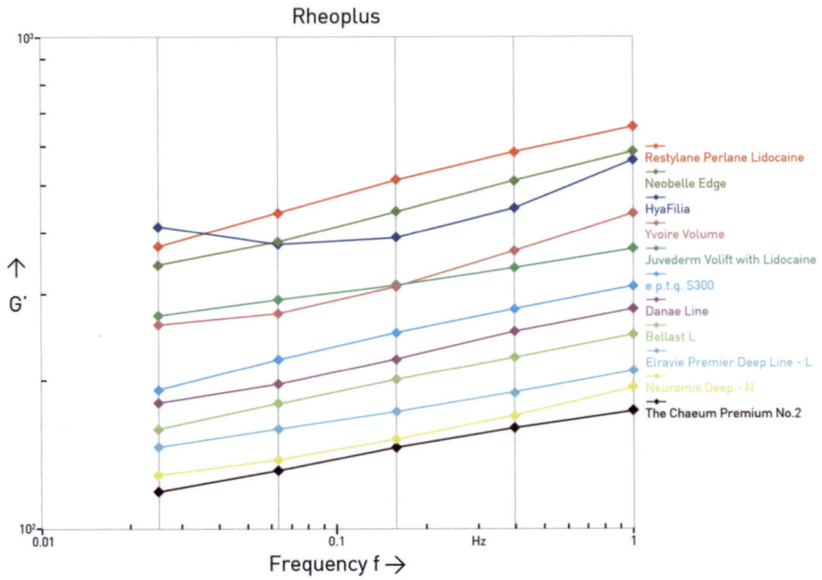

Table 5.3 Rheological data of various hyaluronic acid (HA) fillers

Product	G' (Pa)	G'' (Pa)	Complex modulus	Tan delta	Complex viscosity (η)	Cohesiveness (N)	Particle size (μm/mL)	Injection force (N)
Restylane	349	145	378	0.4180	3,011,188	0.3509	547 ± 280	8
Perlane	411	199	457	0.4849	3,637,022	0.2869	1024 ± 547	16
Restylane SubQ	768	245	806	0.3190	6,420,375	0.3387	1393 ± 757	25
NeobelleSkin	372	136	396	0.3667	3,157,278	1.0296	241 ± 117	12
NeobelleBasic	365	116	383	0.3182	3,048,961	0.9481	447 ± 215	15
NeobelleEdge	374	110	390	0.2936	3,106,528	0.9183	941 ± 499	16
NeobelleContour	387	111	403	0.2884	3,207,126	0.9019	1472 ± 796	18
HyafiliaPetit	247	85	261	0.343	2,080,246	0.5536	227 ± 124	10
HyafiliaClassic	345	101	359	0.294	2,858,186	0.6038	488 ± 267	12
HyafiliaGrand	407	166	440	0.407	3,499,743	0.5185	991 ± 525	15
ClevielPrime	372	180	413	0.485	3,291,663	0.8778	284[a]	16.6
ClevielContour	857	694	1103	0.81	8,774,267	1.536	243[a]	20
YvoireClassic	286	103	304	0.3624	2,424,107	0.2894	693 ± 344	9.8
YvoireVolume	253	73	263	0.2910	2,097,766	0.3567	1036 ± 581	12.7
YvoireContour	484	157	509	0.3245	4,049,358	0.2867	1258 ± 742	19
CutegelMax	701	286	757	0.41	6,024,716	0.57	1106 ± 689[a]	20
JuvedermVolbella	99	21	101	0.2189	814,593	0.3046	634 ± 255	8
JuvedermVolift	179	42	184	0.2343	1,468,502	0.3417	644 ± 303	10
JuvedermVoluma	284	58	290	0.2066	2,309,805	0.4043	703 ± 389	25
E.p.t.q.S100	37	15	40	0.4269	323,859	0.4184	UD	19.6
E.p.t.q.S300	128	27	131	0.2137	1,048,864	0.6102	UD	29.4
E.p.t.q.S500	224	57	231	0.2551	1,847,607	0.8776	296 ± 168	31
Danae Original	154	81	174	0.5279	1,389,716	0.5531	646 ± 352	9.8
Danae Line	260	100	279	0.3869	2,222,574	0.3785	1162 ± 668	19
Danae Contour	469	134	488	0.2873	3,887,740	0.46	1291 ± 762	37.2

(continued)

Table 5.3 (continued)

Product	G' (Pa)	G'' (Pa)	Complex modulus	Tan delta	Complex viscosity (η)	Cohesiveness (N)	Particle size (µm/mL)	Injection force (N)
BellastVital	128	72	147	0.5636	1,170,954	0.2362	685 ± 386	15
BellastSoft L	94	22	97	0.2400	775,485	0.2285	683 ± 321	12
Bellast L	119	25	122	0.2135	969,817	0.2880	684 ± 242	16
BellastPlus	87	18	89	0.2062	714,771	0.5093	652 ± 319	32.3
BellastVolume	106	23	108	0.215	866,658	0.4458	685 ± 313	33
ElraviePremiumLight	140	34	144	0.2431	1,151,729	0.5260	UD	23
ElraviePremiumDeep line	159	39	164	0.2486	1,309,982	0.5874	UD	25
ElraviePremiumUltra volume	198	59	207	0.2985	1,646,177	0.8478	UD	24.5
Neuramis Light	4	4	6	1.0530	51,271	0.2049	322 ± 133	8
Neuramis	57	24	133	0.4284	499,532	0.4532	433 ± 178	12.7
Neuramis deep	127	38	133	0.3000	1,061,307	0.5998	411 ± 171	16.6
Neuramis volume	281	71	290	0.2551	2,309,230	0.8003	402 ± 175	22.5
Chaeum No. 1	76	28	81	0.3733	651,115	0.4888	480 ± 204	14.7
Chaeum No. 2	146	29	149	0.2036	1,193,756	0.6716	473 ± 242	34.3
Chaeum No. 3	232	52	238	0.2200	1,896,742	0.7474	596 ± 291	37.2
Chaeum No. 4	340	68	347	0.2013	2,766,277	0.9180	664 ± 348	54.8
Lorient No2	203	41	207	0.20	1,673,007	0.4401	UD	UD
Lorient No4	338	95	351	0.28	2,795,776	0.4237	UD	UD
Lorient No6	413	121	430	0.29	3,423,232	0.4454	UD	UD
Belotero Soft L	2.66	2.76	3.9	1.03	30,620	UD	UD	UD
Belotero Balance L	21.7	10.4	23.9	0.479	191,817	UD	UD	UD
Belotero Intense L	78	23.7	81.5	0.3040	650,018	UD	UD	UD
Belotero Volume L	168	42.5	173.3	0.2525	1,383,440	UD	UD	UD

A comparison of the rheological properties (G', G'', G^*) and physicochemical data of various hyaluronic acid fillers [34]
MCR 301 rheometer (Anton Paar Co, Austria), Frequency 0.02 Hz
[a]Median, *SD* standard deviation, *UD* undetermined

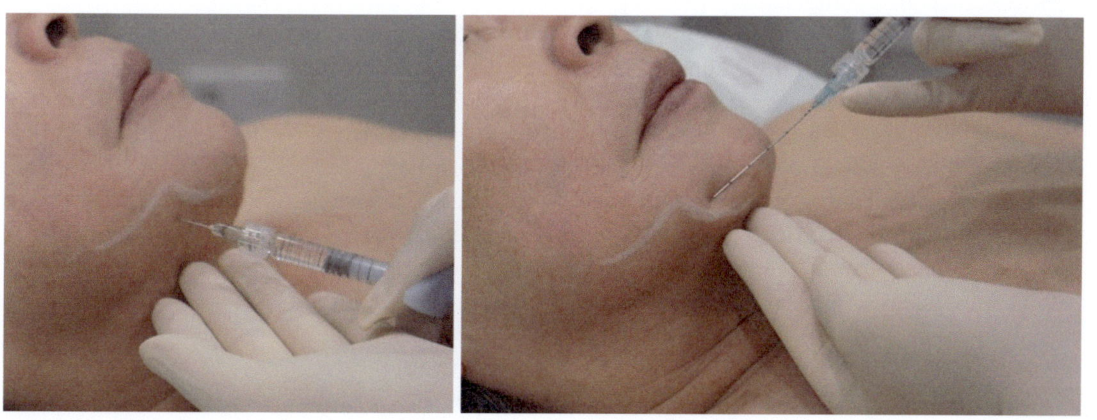

Fig. 5.11 Filler injection approaches for the jawline. Two techniques used in jawline filler procedures: needle approach (left) and cannula approach (right)

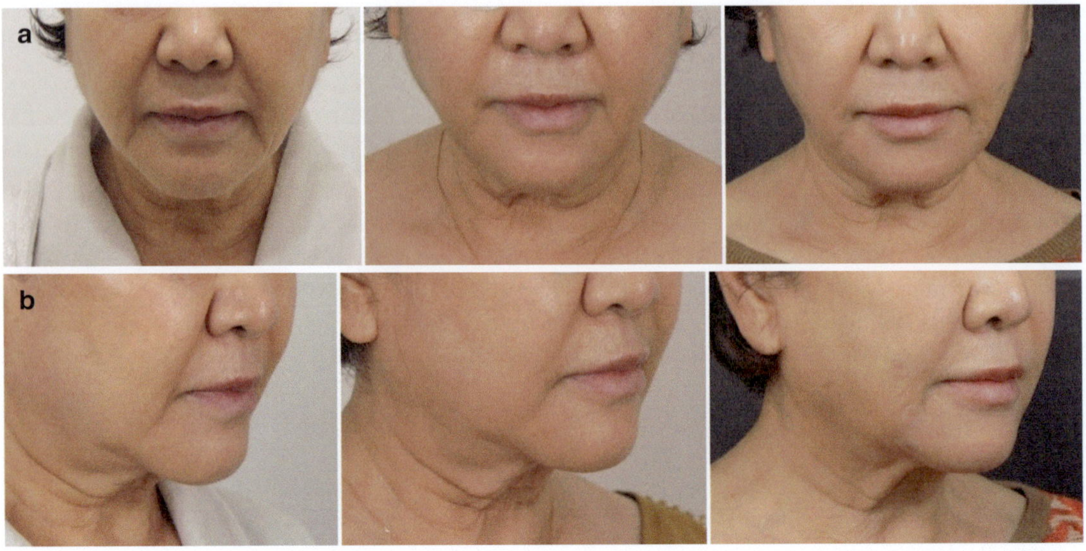

Fig. 5.12 Changes after corner of the mouth, chin botox, and filler treatments. Pre- and post-treatment photographs of a 64-year-old patient following corner of the mouth botox, chin botox, HIFU, and filler injections to the chin, marionette lines, prejowl, and lips. Photos were taken before treatment (left), 2 weeks after treatment (center), and 1.5 years after touch-up (right). (**a**) Frontal view; (**b**) oblique view

- *Cannula vs. needle approaches*
  - *Cannula*:
    Cannulas are suitable for volumizing larger areas and help minimize the risk of vascular injury. Typically, a 20G or 22G blunt-tipped cannula with a length of 40–50 mm is used. This technique allows treatment of a broad area through a single entry point, reducing the risk of bruising, vascular injuries, and other complications [38, 39].
  - *Needle*:
    Needles allow for direct supraperiosteal injections, making them effective for creating strong, well-defined contours [40].

5.4.2.2 Layering Technique and Natural Contour Formation

It is ideal to first inject filler into the deep plane (supraperiosteal layer) to establish structural support, followed by fine volume adjustments in the superficial plane as needed. A linear threading technique along the jawline is employed to achieve clear definition [41].

The cannula entry point is positioned at the prejowl point along the inferior border of the mandible. Using a retrograde injection technique in the superficial subcutaneous plane, fillers are carefully deposited. This approach is effective for correcting hollowing of the anterior border of the mandible, which often results from volume loss around the premasseteric ligament and adjacent muscles.

After filler placement, moderate pressure is applied manually to shape the area and achieve a natural contour [13].

5.4.2.3 Adjustment of Chin Volume and Projection

Adjusting chin volume and projection is essential for achieving overall balance of the lower face. Injection techniques must be tailored based on the patient's muscular and skeletal structures. In cases of retrogenia (recessed mandible), filler is injected into the supraperiosteal plane to enhance chin projection [29].

The ideal chin width is determined anatomically:

For women, it should correspond to the medial intercanthal distance;

For men, it should match the mouth width.

Regarding ideal chin projection, in men, the chin should align with the lower lip, while in women, the lower lip should project 1–2 mm beyond the chin [42]. A semicircular marking is drawn on the chin according to the ideal male or female chin width, assessing symmetry between both sides of the symphysis area using the mentalis muscles as landmarks.

The cannula entry point is located laterally at the prejowl area, approximately 5 mm above the jawline. By pinching the treatment area during injection, filler can be more easily delivered beneath the mentalis muscle. Typically, 0.2–0.5 mL of filler is injected per side depending on patient needs and treatment goals [43].

To create a softer contour, additional filler can be injected into the subcutaneous layer through the same entry point. In this case, approximately 0.1 mL of filler is retroinjected per side. After removing the cannula, firm and precise manual molding is performed to shape the treated area.

For improving chin projection, filler should primarily be placed at the pogonion (anterior chin point). Conversely, to lengthen the chin, filler is injected inferiorly into the menton area (lower border of the mandible). Considering the activity of the depressor labii inferioris and mentalis muscles, botulinum toxin may be used adjunctively in cases of strong muscle movement to achieve more natural results. Filler must be evenly distributed across the midline and lateral areas to avoid unnatural projection [41] (Figs. 5.13 and 5.14).

5.4.2.4 Correction of Prejowl Hollowing and Marionette Lines

Prejowl hollowing and marionette lines can diminish the definition of the jawline, and filler-based volume restoration combined with lifting techniques can serve as an effective treatment option [37]. For marionette lines, restoring support to the oral commissure is crucial, and a soft filler should be used to achieve a natural correction.

In the prejowl sulcus area, a combined injection strategy into both the supraperiosteal plane and the subcutaneous fat plane effectively restores lost volume. Particularly in female patients, caution must be taken to avoid overfilling, as excessive volume can create the appearance of a broader chin [44]. Injecting fillers into both the submuscular layer and the superficial subcutaneous layer helps achieve natural volume restoration (Figs. 5.15 and 5.16).

When soft tissue laxity is present, filler treatment alone may have limitations. In such cases, adjunctive procedures such as thread lifting or botulinum toxin injections can be beneficial. Additionally, combining various skin boosters can help improve skin quality and achieve satisfying outcomes while minimizing the amount of filler required [45, 46] (Figs. 5.17 and 5.18).

Treatment of the lower face with hyaluronic acid (HA) fillers aims not merely to replenish

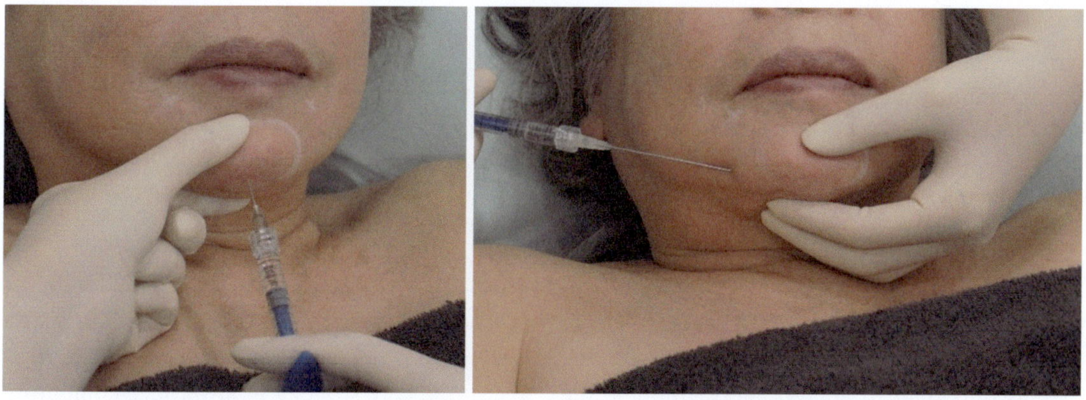

Fig. 5.13 Filler injection approaches for the chin: two techniques used in chin filler procedures: needle approach (left) and cannula approach (right)

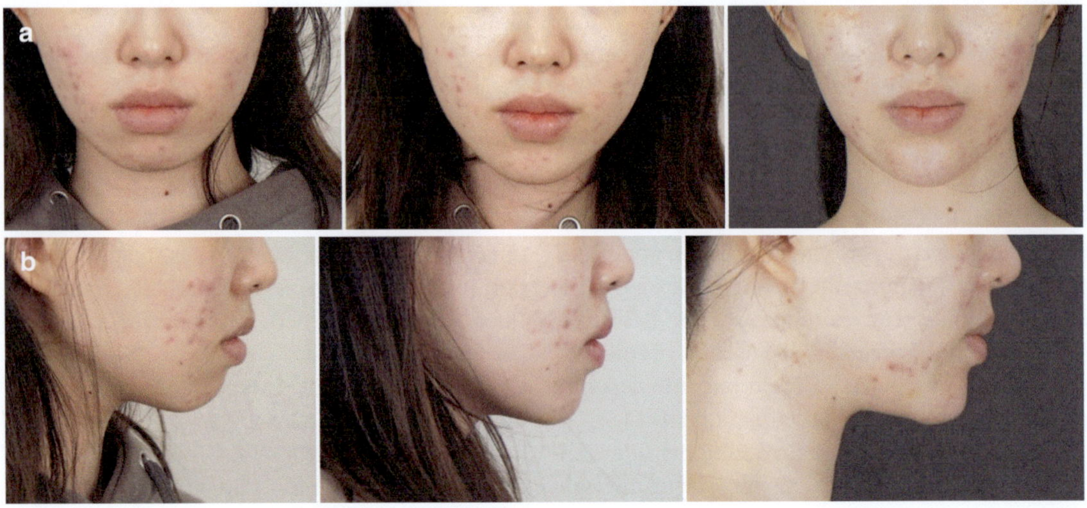

Fig. 5.14 Changes after chin botulinum toxin and filler treatments. Pre- and post-treatment photographs of a 26-year-old patient following chin botulinum toxin and filler injections. Photos were taken before treatment, 3 days after initial treatment, and 3 months after additional filler injection. (**a**) Frontal view; (**b**) lateral view

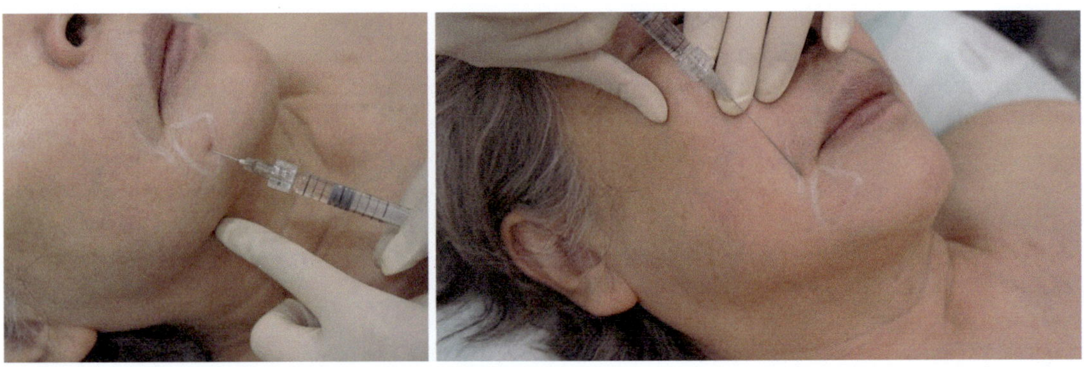

Fig. 5.15 Filler injection approaches for prejowl hollowing and marionette lines. Two techniques used for treating prejowl hollowing and marionette lines: needle approach (left) and cannula approach (right)

volume but to reshape the jawline, enhance facial contours, and provide a lifting effect to the cheeks and neck. To achieve these goals, filler selection and injection strategies must be customized for each target area. High-elasticity fillers should be used along the jawline and chin to create clear definition, while softer fillers are appropriate for natural volume restoration in the marionette lines and prejowl sulcus [41].

It is important to appropriately combine the use of cannulas and needles during filler injection and apply a layering technique to promote natural outcomes. Considering the underlying muscular and skeletal structures, adjunctive treatments such as botulinum toxin injections or thread lifting can further optimize the effects of filler therapy [47].

Through individualized treatments tailored to the patient's anatomical characteristics, contouring of the lower face can be significantly improved, achieving optimal overall facial balance—the core strategy in lower face contouring with HA fillers [48].

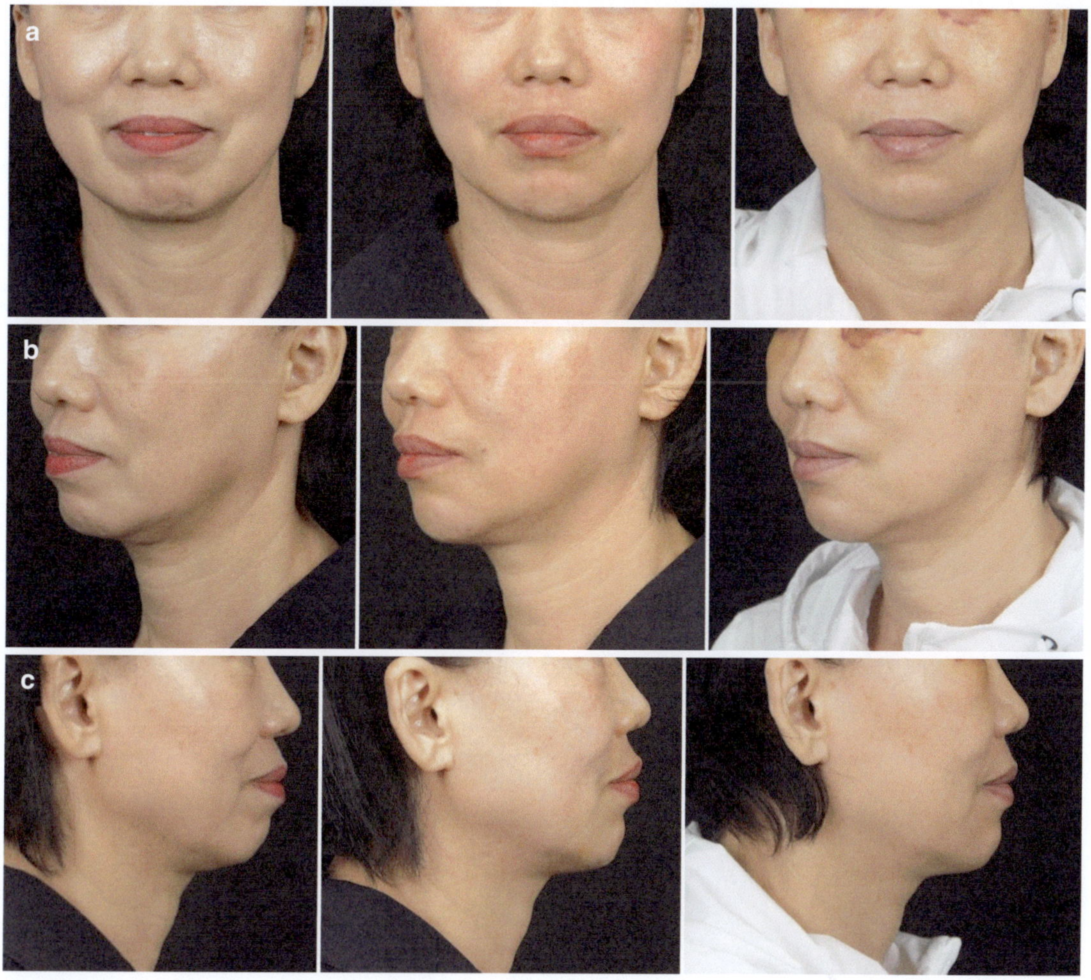

Fig. 5.16 Pre- and post-treatment photographs of a 57-year-old patient after chin botulinum toxin and filler injections: Photos showing treatment results after chin botulinum toxin and filler injections to the chin, marionette lines, and philtrum. Images were taken before treatment (left), immediately after treatment (center), and 3 months post-treatment (right). (**a**) Frontal view; (**b**) oblique view; (**c**) lateral view

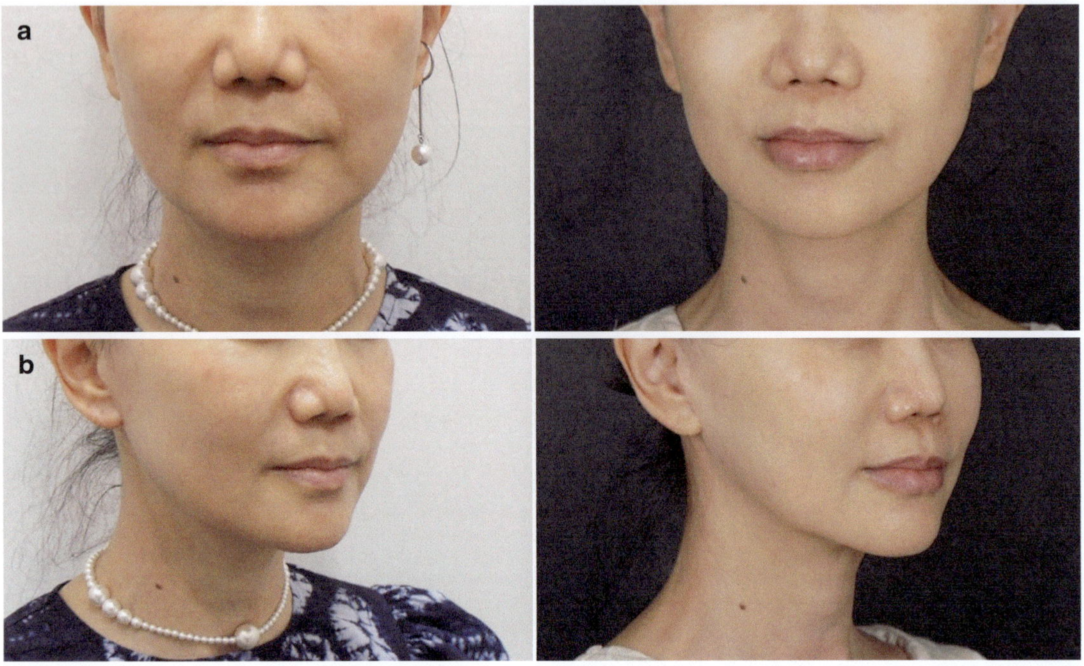

Fig. 5.17 Pre- and post-treatment photographs of a 59-year-old patient after skin botox, exosome skin booster, HIFU, and filler injections: Photos showing results after treatments including skin botox, exosome skin booster, HIFU, and filler injections to the chin, marionette lines, prejowl, and lips. Images were taken before treatment (left) and 1 year after treatment (right). (**a**) Frontal view; (**b**) oblique view

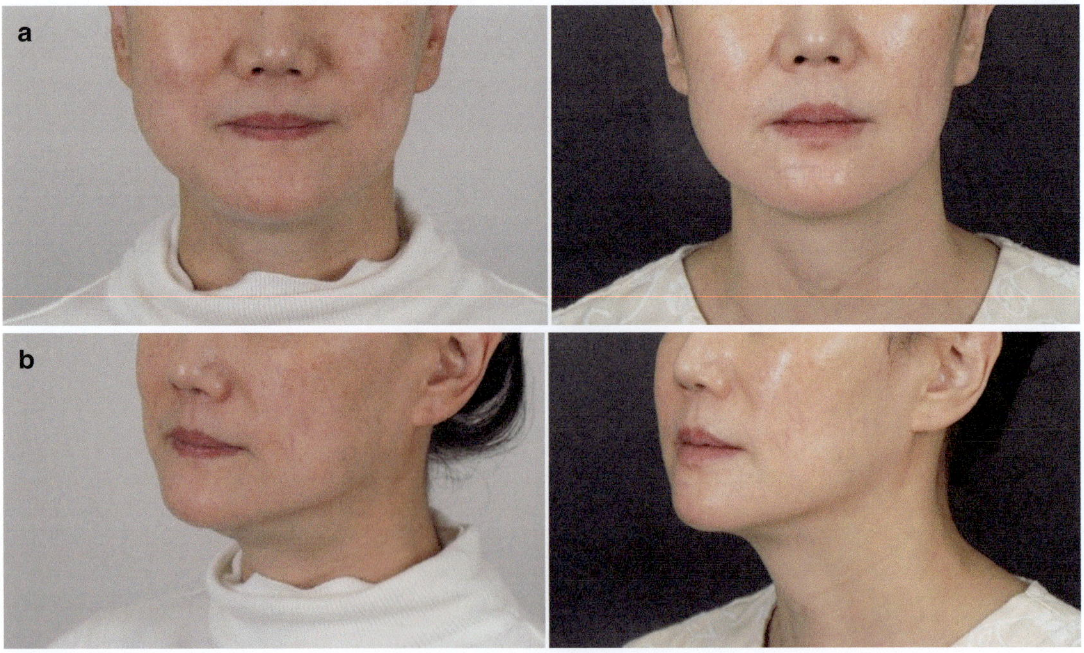

Fig. 5.18 Pre- and post-treatment photographs of a 55-year-old patient after skin botox, PRP, HIFU, and filler injections: Photos showing results after treatments including skin botox, PRP, HIFU, and filler injections to the chin, nasolabial folds (NLF), marionette lines, prejowl, and lips. Images were taken before treatment (left) and 1 year after treatment (right). (**a**) Frontal view; (**b**) oblique view

5.5 Post-Treatment Care and Complication Prevention

Appropriate post-procedure care and complication prevention are essential to achieve optimal outcomes following lower face HA filler treatments. Since fillers require time to stabilize within the tissues, patients should be properly informed about potential immediate post-treatment symptoms such as swelling, bruising, and temporary discomfort. Particularly, systematic management plans are necessary to prevent and respond promptly to serious adverse events, including vascular occlusion—the most severe complication associated with filler injections [49, 50].

5.5.1 Patient Education After Treatment

Early complications related to filler injections are typically mild and self-limiting. Common post-procedure reactions include erythema, swelling, and bruising, which usually resolve spontaneously within a few days. Rare adverse effects such as infection, nodules, or foreign body granulomas may occur, and patients should be adequately informed about these possibilities before treatment. To minimize complications and promote faster recovery, patients should be advised on the following precautions [51]:

- *Cold compresses to reduce swelling*:
  Intermittent application of cold compresses during the first 24 h can help reduce swelling and mitigate the progression of bruising.
  However, direct pressure on the treated areas should be avoided.
- *Restriction of activities that induce vasodilation*:
  Patients should avoid saunas, hot baths, and strenuous exercise for 48 h after treatment to minimize the risk of vascular dilation and associated complications.
- *Avoidance of massage and pressure*:
  Massage should be avoided for the first 2 weeks after filler injections, as this is the period during which the filler is stabilizing within the tissue.
  External pressure during this time can lead to asymmetry or displacement of the filler.
- *Limiting the use of anticoagulants and anti-inflammatories*:
  Medications such as aspirin and NSAIDs (e.g., ibuprofen) may increase the risk of bleeding and bruising.
  Patients should consult with their physician regarding the use of these medications if necessary.
- *Patient education regarding differences between initial and final results*:
  Immediately after treatment, patients may notice differences between their initial appearance and the final desired outcome due to swelling and transient tissue expansion.
  Clear pre-procedure counseling is essential to reduce unnecessary anxiety.
  Contours may appear exaggerated immediately post-injection but typically normalize over the next 1–2 weeks.

Additionally, HA fillers gradually integrate with surrounding tissues, and the final results are usually visible within 2–4 weeks. Patients should also be informed that, due to individual filler absorption rates and anatomical differences, additional touch-up treatments may sometimes be necessary [52].

5.5.2 Management of Adverse Events and Complications

5.5.2.1 Prevention and Treatment of Vascular Occlusion

One of the most serious complications associated with filler injections is vascular occlusion. This occurs when the filler compresses or obstructs a blood vessel, leading to an interruption of blood flow. Early detection and prompt intervention are critical in managing vascular occlusion [53, 54].

A thorough understanding of vascular anatomy is essential, and the use of a cannula in areas with dense vascular networks may enhance safety. During filler injections, applying low pressure, injecting slowly, and distributing small amounts of filler can help minimize the risk of vascular injury. Aspiration tests may also be performed to check for intravascular placement before injecting the filler [49, 55].

5.5.2.2 Early Signs and Immediate Response to Vascular Occlusion

If sudden blanching or cyanosis occurs immediately after injection, vascular compromise should be suspected. Persistent or increasing pain is another warning sign that vascular occlusion may have occurred. As tissue ischemia can progress to skin necrosis, immediate management is required [56, 57].

5.5.2.3 Management Protocol for Vascular Occlusion

1. *Administration of hyaluronidase*

Upon suspicion of vascular occlusion, hyaluronidase should be promptly injected into the affected area to dissolve the filler.

High-dose, repeated injections may be necessary if required.

2. *Warm compresses and promotion of blood flow*

Warm compresses can be applied to promote local blood circulation, and vasodilators may be considered.

3. *Hyperbaric oxygen therapy (HBOT)*

If tissue ischemia is evident, hyperbaric oxygen therapy can be used to enhance oxygen delivery to the affected tissues [58].

4. *Pharmacologic therapy*

Medications such as aspirin, topical nitroglycerin, and low-molecular-weight heparin may be considered to support vascular recovery.

5.5.2.4 Correction of Filler Imbalance and Asymmetry

After filler treatment, some patients may experience minor volume imbalances or filler migration.

Due to initial swelling and soft tissue changes, slight asymmetries often resolve spontaneously, and reassessment is recommended 2–4 weeks post-procedure [59].

If mild asymmetry persists, it can be corrected by injecting a small additional amount of filler.

Conversely, in cases of overcorrection, small doses of hyaluronidase can be used to partially dissolve the excess filler. Hyaluronidase is an enzyme that effectively degrades hyaluronic acid fillers, allowing for correction of undesired results.

However, temporary swelling or bruising may occur after hyaluronidase administration, and rare allergic reactions are possible, so thorough pre-treatment counseling and caution are necessary. If filler has migrated to a superficial plane or unintended area, gentle massage or manual repositioning may help redistribute the filler. In cases of significant migration, hyaluronidase treatment followed by re-injection may be required [60].

When asymmetry or imbalance is detected, it is crucial to account for swelling and tissue changes over time, reassess appropriately, and perform corrective procedures if necessary [61]. Through such post-treatment management and complication prevention strategies, the safety and patient satisfaction of filler procedures can be maximized.

5.6 Conclusion

The contour of the lower face is shaped through the interaction of various factors, including skeletal structure, soft tissue, muscle dynamics, and skin elasticity. Over time, changes in mandibular bone structure, soft tissue repositioning, and the loss of skin elasticity collectively contribute to the blurring of the jawline, alterations in chin definition, and the appearance of aging signs such as marionette lines and prejowl hollowing. By understanding these aging processes and applying strategic treatments using HA fillers, lower face contouring can be enhanced nonsurgically, leading to natural and harmonious results [28, 62].

In lower face filler procedures, the most important element is a customized approach based on each patient's unique anatomical features and patterns of aging. Since the shape and volume of the jawline, mandibular angle, and chin vary among individuals, a strategic treatment plan focused on overall facial balance—rather than simple volume augmentation—is necessary [13, 24]. Furthermore, analyzing the relationship between the midface and lower face can help refine the final outcome; in some cases, midface volumization should be prioritized to achieve a more natural and balanced lower face contour.

Effective lower face contouring with fillers requires appropriate product selection and precise injection techniques. To enhance jawline and chin definition, high-elasticity (high *G′*) fillers should be injected into the supraperiosteal plane, while softer fillers that blend naturally with soft tissues are ideal for correcting marionette lines and prejowl hollows [13, 41]. Appropriate use of cannulas and needles, along with layering techniques and attention to vascular safety, are critical to minimizing complications and achieving optimal results.

Post-treatment care and complication prevention are essential components of successful filler procedures. Patients must be properly informed about early swelling, bruising, and tissue adaptation processes, and immediate intervention should be available in the event of serious complications such as vascular occlusion [63]. If filler migration or volume imbalance occurs, reassessment after an appropriate period followed by corrective procedures, including the use of hyaluronidase if necessary, should be considered [64].

In conclusion, lower face filler treatments should be approached with a thorough analysis of each patient's individual anatomy and aging patterns. When the correct filler products and injection techniques are applied, lower face contouring can be effectively achieved through nonsurgical methods, providing natural lifting effects and maximizing patient satisfaction.

References

1. Petrusic W, Cronin-Golomb A. The face, beauty, and symmetry: perceiving asymmetry in beautiful faces. Int J Neurosci. 2005;115(8):1165–73. https://doi.org/10.1080/00207450590914464.
2. Galantucci LM, Deli R, Laino A, Di Gioia E, D'Alessio R, Lavecchia F, Percoco G, Savastano C. Three-dimensional anthropometric database of attractive Caucasian women: standards and comparisons. J Craniofac Surg. 2016;27(7):1884–95. https://doi.org/10.1097/SCS.0000000000002933. PMID: 27763980; PMCID: PMC5076491.
3. Tierney EP, Hanke CW, Petersen J. Ablative fractionated carbon dioxide laser treatment of photoaging: a clinical and histologic study. Dermatol Surg. 2012;38(11):1777–89. https://doi.org/10.1111/j.1524-4725.2012.02506.x. PMID: 22958069.
4. Lemperle G, Rullan PP, Gauthier-Hazan N. Avoiding and treating dermal filler complications. Plast Reconstr Surg. 2006;118(3 Suppl):92S–107S. https://doi.org/10.1097/01.prs.0000234915.75005.71. PMID: 16936549.
5. Shaw RB Jr, Katzel EB, Koltz PF, Kahn DM, Girotto JA, Langstein HN. Aging of the mandible and its aesthetic implications. Plast Reconstr Surg. 2010;125(1):332–42. https://doi.org/10.1097/PRS.0b013e3181c2a3f8.
6. Pessa JE, Slice DE. Aging and the shape of the mandible. Plast Reconstr Surg. 2010;125(1):373–7. https://doi.org/10.1097/PRS.0b013e3181c2aabf. PMID: 20048635.
7. Auerbach JD, Weidner Z, Pill SG, Mehta S, Chin KR. The mandibular angle as a landmark for identification of cervical spinal level. Spine (Phila Pa 1976). 2009;34(10):1006–11. https://doi.org/10.1097/BRS.0b013e31819f2a03. PMID: 19404175.
8. Kim SC, Kwon JG, Jeong WS, Na D, Choi JW. One-piece mandibuloplasty compared to conventional mandibuloplasty with narrowing genioplasty. J Craniofac Surg. 2018;29(5):1161–8. https://doi.org/10.1097/SCS.0000000000004458. PMID: 29521758.
9. Gierloff M, Stohring C, Buder T, Wiltfang J, Hakim SG. The role of the fat compartments in aging of the lower face: a computed tomographic study. Plast Reconstr Surg. 2012;129(1):263–73. https://doi.org/10.1097/PRS.0b013e3182362b20. PMID: 21987030.
10. Gierloff M, Stohring C, Buder T, Wiltfang J, Hakim SG. Aging changes of the midfacial fat compartments: a computed tomographic study. Plast Reconstr Surg. 2012;129(3):263e–73e. https://doi.org/10.1097/PRS.0b013e318244227b. PMID: 22395343.
11. Kang MS, Kang HG, Nam YS, Kim IB. Detailed anatomy of the retaining ligaments of the mandible

for facial rejuvenation. J Craniomaxillofac Surg. 2016;44(9):1126–30. https://doi.org/10.1016/j.jcms.2016.06.018. PMID: 27427339.
12. Talei B, Ziai H. Mandibular ligament and the prejowl sulcus explained. Aesthet Surg J. 2024;44(11):1131–9. https://doi.org/10.1093/asj/sjae151. PMID: 39001648.
13. Braz A, Eduardo CCP. Reshaping the lower face using injectable fillers. Indian J Plast Surg. 2020;53(2):207–18. https://doi.org/10.1055/s--0040-1716185. Epub 2020 Aug 29. PMID: 32884187; PMCID: PMC7458843.
14. Hong GW, Wong S, Yoon SE, Wan J, Yi KH. Anatomical-based diagnosis and filler injection techniques: marionette line (static labiomandibular fold). J Dermatolog Treat. 2025;36(1):2452954. https://doi.org/10.1080/09546634.2025.2452954. Epub 2025 Feb 2. PMID: 3989445.
15. Huettner F, Goncalves M, Vasconcelos K, et al. Vascular mapping of the face: implications for safe superficial musculoaponeurotic system elevation. Plast Reconstr Surg. 2020;145(5):1047e–55e. https://doi.org/10.1097/PRS.0000000000006741. PMID: 32332417.
16. Kikuta S, Iwanaga J, Kusukawa J, Tubbs RS. The mental artery: anatomical study and literature review. J Anat. 2020;236(3):564–9. https://doi.org/10.1111/joa.13113. Epub 2019 Nov 6. PMID: 31691967; PMCID: PMC7018628.
17. Standring S, editor. Gray's anatomy: the anatomical basis of clinical practice. 41st ed. Amsterdam: Elsevier; 2016. ISBN: 9780702052309.
18. Batra APS, Mahajan A, Gupta K. Marginal mandibular branch of the facial nerve: an anatomical study. Indian J Plast Surg. 2010;43(1):60–4. https://doi.org/10.4103/0970-0358.63968. PMID: 20924442; PMCID: PMC2938626.
19. Lin Y, Lin H, Lin Q, Zhang J, Zhu P, Lu Y, Zhao Z, Lv J, Lee M, Xu Y. A novel three-dimensional smile analysis based on dynamic evaluation of facial curve contour. Sci Rep. 2016;6:22103. https://doi.org/10.1038/srep22103.
20. Moradi A, Montes JR, Humphrey S, Grunebaum LD, Bertossi D, Dimitrijevic E, Sangha S. A unified approach to facial contours and volume correction: the role of the cheek and the chin. Plast Reconstr Surg Glob Open. 2024;12(10):e6219. https://doi.org/10.1097/GOX.0000000000006219. PMID: 39372878; PMCID: PMC11452099.
21. Tseng FF, Li YH, Chen YW. Hard and soft tissue facial landmarks for mandibular angle reduction: a clinical study. Clin Pract. 2024;14(5):1707–15. https://doi.org/10.3390/clinpract14050136. PMID: 39311286; PMCID: PMC11417696.
22. Gaber A, Taher MF, Abdel Wahed M, Shalaby NM, Gaber S. Comprehensive assessment of facial paralysis based on facial animation units. PLoS One. 2022;17(12):e0277297. https://doi.org/10.1371/journal.pone.0277297. PMID: 36516130; PMCID: PMC9750034.
23. Azuma T, Fuchigami T, Nakamura K, Kondo E, Sato G, Kitamura Y, Takeda N. New method to evaluate sequelae of static facial asymmetry in patients with facial palsy using three-dimensional scanning analysis. Auris Nasus Larynx. 2022;49(5):755–61. https://doi.org/10.1016/j.anl.2022.01.007. Epub 2022 Jan 31. PMID: 35105501.
24. Trévidic P, Kaufman-Janette J, Weinkle S, Wu R, Dhillon B, Antunes S, Macé E, Maffert P. Injection guidelines for treating midface volume deficiency with hyaluronic acid fillers: the ATP approach (anatomy, techniques, products). Aesthet Surg J. 2022;42(8):920–34. https://doi.org/10.1093/asj/sjac007. PMID: 35039828; PMCID: PMC9373948.
25. Hwang UJ, Kwon OY, Jung SH, Ahn SH, Gwak GT. Effect of a facial muscle exercise device on facial rejuvenation. Aesthet Surg J. 2018;38(5):463–76. https://doi.org/10.1093/asj/sjx238. PMID: 29365050; PMCID: PMC5888959.
26. de Almeida ART, Romiti A, Carruthers JDA. The facial platysma and its underappreciated role in lower face dynamics and contour. Dermatol Surg. 2017;43(8):1042–9. https://doi.org/10.1097/DSS.0000000000001135. PMID: 28394862.
27. Viscomi B, Faria G, Hernandez CA, Perez L, Spada J, De la Fuente V, Muniz M. Contouring plus: a comprehensive approach of the lower third of the face with calcium hydroxylapatite and hyaluronic acid. Clin Cosmet Investig Dermatol. 2023;16:911–24. https://doi.org/10.2147/CCID.S400605. PMID: 37041818; PMCID: PMC10083035.
28. Yi KH, Park SY. Marionette lines correction with volumizing threads. J Cosmet Dermatol. 2024;23(12):3871–7. https://doi.org/10.1111/jocd.16490. Epub 2024 Jul 23.
29. Chen B, Ma L, Wang J. Chin augmentation with hyaluronic acid: an injection technique based on anatomical morphology. Dermatol Surg. 2022;48(7):747–51. https://doi.org/10.1097/DSS.0000000000003459. Epub 2022 Apr 25. PMID: 35482662; PMCID: PMC9241653.
30. Rauso R, Rugge L, Chirico F, Nicoletti GF, Fragola R, Bove P, Zerbinati N, Giudice GL. Nonsurgical reshaping of the lower jaw with hyaluronic acid fillers: a retrospective case series. Dermatol Pract Concept. 2022;12(3):e2022095. https://doi.org/10.5826/dpc.1203a95. PMID: 36159131; PMCID: PMC9464529.
31. Li K, Meng F, Li YR, Tian Y, Chen H, Jia Q, Cai H, Jiang HB. Application of nonsurgical modalities in improving facial aging. Int J Dent. 2022;2022:8332631. https://doi.org/10.1155/2022/8332631. PMID: 35251183; PMCID: PMC8894069.
32. Chang CS, Kang GC. Achieving ideal lower face aesthetic contours: combination of tridimensional fat grafting to the chin with masseter botulinum toxin injection. Aesthet Surg J. 2016;36(10):1093–100. https://doi.org/10.1093/asj/sjw082. Epub 2016 May 18. PMID: 27193172.

33. Shridharani SM. Novel surface anatomic landmarks of the jowl to guide treatment with ATX-101. Plast Reconstr Surg Glob Open. 2019;7(10):e2459. https://doi.org/10.1097/GOX.0000000000002459. PMID: 31772888; PMCID: PMC6846303.
34. Lee W, Hwang SG, Oh W, Kim CY, Lee JL, Yang EJ. Practical guidelines for hyaluronic acid soft-tissue filler use in facial rejuvenation. Dermatol Surg. 2020;46(1):41–9. https://doi.org/10.1097/DSS.0000000000001858. PMID: 30883477.
35. de la Guardia C, Virno A, Musumeci M, Bernardin A, Silberberg MB. Rheologic and physicochemical characteristics of hyaluronic acid fillers: overview and relationship to product performance. Facial Plast Surg. 2022;38(2):116–23. https://doi.org/10.1055/s--0041-1741560. Epub 2022 Feb 3. PMID: 35114708; PMCID: PMC9188840.
36. Guida S, Galadari H. A systematic review of Radiesse/calcium hydroxylapatite and carboxymethylcellulose: evidence and recommendations for treatment of the face. Int J Dermatol. 2024;63(2):150–60. https://doi.org/10.1111/ijd.16888. Epub 2023 Oct 28. PMID: 37897174.
37. Go BC, Frost AS, Friedman O. Using injectable fillers for chin and jawline rejuvenation. World J Otorhinolaryngol Head Neck Surg. 2023;9(2):131–7. https://doi.org/10.1002/wjo2.93. PMID: 37383337; PMCID: PMC10296042.
38. Pavicic T, Frank K, Erlbacher K, Neuner R, Targosinski S, Schenck T, Gotkin RH, Cotofana S. Precision in dermal filling: a comparison between needle and cannula when using soft tissue fillers. J Drugs Dermatol. 2017;16(9):866–72. PMID: 28915281.
39. Hexsel D, Soirefmann M, Porto MD, Siega C, Schilling-Souza J, Brum C. Double-blind, randomized, controlled clinical trial to compare safety and efficacy of a metallic cannula with that of a standard needle for soft tissue augmentation of the nasolabial folds. Dermatol Surg. 2012;38(2):207–14. https://doi.org/10.1111/j.1524-4725.2011.02195.x. Epub 2011 Oct 19. PMID: 22092962.
40. Spada J, Ravera K, Schneider C. Needle versus cannula to treat tear trough: a prospective study comparing both methods. Plast Reconstr Surg Glob Open. 2023;11(11):e5327. https://doi.org/10.1097/GOX.0000000000005327. PMID: 37936826; PMCID: PMC10627584.
41. Clark NW, Pan DR, Barrett DM. Facial fillers: relevant anatomy, injection techniques, and complications. World J Otorhinolaryngol Head Neck Surg. 2023;9(3):227–35. https://doi.org/10.1002/wjo2.126. PMID: 37780674; PMCID: PMC10541169.
42. Fanous N, Yoskovitch A. Estimating implant size in chin augmentation: a simplified approach. Can J Plast Surg. 2003;11(3):161–5. https://doi.org/10.1177/229255030301100305. PMID: 24115862; PMCID: PMC3792756.
43. Holt S, Fronek L, Witfill K. Nonsurgical augmentation of the chin using a lateral to medial approach with hyaluronic acid based filler: a case series. J Clin Aesthet Dermatol. 2023;16(10):40–2. PMID: 37915338; PMCID: PMC10617898.
44. van Loghem J, Sattler S, Casabona G, Cotofana S, Fabi SG, Goldie K, Gout U, Kerscher M, Lim TS, de Sanctis PC, Sattler G, Trindade de Almeida A, Wanitphakdeedecha R, Werschler P, Pavicic T. Consensus on the use of hyaluronic acid fillers from the cohesive polydensified matrix range: best practice in specific facial indications. Clin Cosmet Investig Dermatol. 2021;14:1175–99. https://doi.org/10.2147/CCID.S311017. PMID: 34526796; PMCID: PMC8435881.
45. Moon H, Fundaro SP, Goh CL, Hau KC, Paz-Lao P, Salti G. A review on the combined use of soft tissue filler, suspension threads, and botulinum toxin for facial rejuvenation. J Cutan Aesthet Surg. 2021;14(2):147–55. https://doi.org/10.4103/JCAS.JCAS_119_20. PMID: 34566355; PMCID: PMC8423215.
46. Rho NK, Kim HS, Kim SY, Lee W. Injectable "skin boosters" in aging skin rejuvenation: a current overview. Arch Plast Surg. 2024;51(6):528–41. https://doi.org/10.1055/a-2366-3436. PMID: 39544509; PMCID: PMC11560330.
47. Galadari H, Weinkle SH. Injection techniques for midface volumization using soft tissue hyaluronic acid fillers designed for dynamic facial movement. J Cosmet Dermatol. 2022;21(3):924–32. https://doi.org/10.1111/jocd.14700. Epub 2021 Dec 28. PMID: 34964234; PMCID: PMC9303613.
48. Lipko-Godlewska S, Bolanča Ž, Kalinová L, Kermen I, Onisak B, Papp I, Rebrov M, Valančienė G. Whole-face approach with hyaluronic acid fillers. Clin Cosmet Investig Dermatol. 2021;14:169–78. https://doi.org/10.2147/CCID.S292501. PMID: 33633459; PMCID: PMC7901566.
49. Murray G, Convery C, Walker L, Davies E. Guideline for the management of hyaluronic acid filler-induced vascular occlusion. J Clin Aesthet Dermatol. 2021;14(5):E61–9. Epub 2021 May 1. PMID: 34188752; PMCID: PMC8211329.
50. King M, Walker L, Convery C, Davies E. Management of a vascular occlusion associated with cosmetic injections. J Clin Aesthet Dermatol. 2020;13(1):E53–8. Epub 2020 Jan 1. PMID: 32082474; PMCID: PMC7028373.
51. Kim JH, Ahn DK, Jeong HS, Suh IS. Treatment algorithm of complications after filler injection: based on wound healing process. J Korean Med Sci. 2014;29(Suppl 3):S176–82. https://doi.org/10.3346/jkms.2014.29.S3.S176. Epub 2014 Nov 21. PMID: 25473207; PMCID: PMC4248003.
52. Bhojani-Lynch T. Late-onset inflammatory response to hyaluronic acid dermal fillers. Plast Reconstr Surg Glob Open. 2017;5(12):e1532. https://doi.org/10.1097/GOX.0000000000001532. PMID: 29632758; PMCID: PMC5889432.
53. Wang Z, Jiang L, Hu J. 5-Fluorouracil for the treatment of pustulosis caused by vascular occlusion after receiving filler injection. Aesthet Plast Surg. 2025;49(11):3263–5. https://doi.org/10.1007/

s00266-024-04333-2. Epub ahead of print. PMID: 39174802.

54. Soares DJ, Hynes SD, Yi CH, Shah-Desai S, Irving SC. Cosmetic filler-induced vascular occlusion: a rising threat presenting to emergency departments. Ann Emerg Med. 2024;83(1):59–67. https://doi.org/10.1016/j.annemergmed.2023.07.006. Epub 2023 Aug 11. PMID: 37565956.
55. Lee AL, Chen YF, Yao WT, Liu YC, Yu CM, Tu CP, Huang WC, Tung KY, Tsai MF. Laser Doppler imaging for treating vascular complications from procedures involving dermal fillers: case series and literature review. Diagnostics (Basel). 2021;11(9):1640. https://doi.org/10.3390/diagnostics11091640. PMID: 34573980; PMCID: PMC8468831.
56. Chuchvara N, Alamgir M, John AM, Rao B. Dermal filler-induced vascular occlusion successfully treated with tadalafil, hyaluronidase, and aspirin. Dermatol Surg. 2021;47(8):1160–2. https://doi.org/10.1097/DSS.0000000000002894. PMID: 33867474.
57. Barbarino S, Banker T, Fezza J. Standardized approach to treatment of retinal artery occlusion after intraarterial injection of soft tissue fillers: EYE-CODE. J Am Acad Dermatol. 2022;86(5):1102–8. https://doi.org/10.1016/j.jaad.2020.12.047. Epub 2020 Dec 27. PMID: 33378659.
58. Johnson-Arbor K. Hyperbaric oxygen therapy for treatment of vascular occlusion after permanent dermal filler injection. Undersea Hyperb Med. 2024;51(4):403–6. PMID: 39821769.
59. Blanco Souza TA, Colomé LM, Bender EA, Lemperle G. Brazilian consensus recommendation on the use of polymethylmethacrylate filler in facial and corporal aesthetics. Aesthet Plast Surg. 2018;42(5):1244–51. https://doi.org/10.1007/s00266-018-1167-1. Epub 2018 Jun 5. PMID: 29872906.
60. King M, Convery C, Davies E. This month's guideline: the use of hyaluronidase in aesthetic practice (v2.4). J Clin Aesthet Dermatol. 2018;11(6):E61–8. Epub 2018 Jun 1. PMID: 29942426; PMCID: PMC6011868.
61. Kroumpouzos G, Treacy P. Hyaluronidase for dermal filler complications: review of applications and dosage recommendations. JMIR Dermatol. 2024;7:e50403. https://doi.org/10.2196/50403. PMID: 38231537; PMCID: PMC10836581.
62. Swift A, Liew S, Weinkle S, Garcia JK, Silberberg MB. The facial aging process from the "inside out". Aesthet Surg J. 2021;41(10):1107–19. https://doi.org/10.1093/asj/sjaa339. PMID: 33325497; PMCID: PMC8438644.
63. Philipp-Dormston WG, Goodman GJ, De Boulle K, Swift A, Delorenzi C, Jones D, Heydenrych I, Trindade De Almeida A, Batniji RK. Global approaches to the prevention and management of delayed-onset adverse reactions with hyaluronic acid-based fillers. Plast Reconstr Surg Glob Open. 2020;8(4):e2730. https://doi.org/10.1097/GOX.0000000000002730. PMID: 32440404; PMCID: PMC7209845.
64. Farmer A, Murray G, Croasdell B, Davies E, Convery C, Walker L. Facial vascular events and tissue ischemia: a guide to understanding and optimizing wound care. J Clin Aesthet Dermatol. 2021;14(12 Suppl 1):S39–48. PMID: 35291261; PMCID: PMC8903221.

6 Delayed Inflammatory Reaction Induced by Hyaluronic Acid Filler

Won Lee

6.1 Introduction

Delayed inflammatory reaction refers to symptoms accompanied by inflammatory signs that appear 2–3 weeks after HA filler injection [1]. This side effect has gained more attention with the emergence of the COVID-19 virus, which caused a global pandemic, as cases of delayed onset edema have been reported in patients who had previously received filler injections and subsequently contracted the virus or were administered the vaccine. However, the exact cause has not yet been clearly elucidated. This chapter describes the potential causes and solutions for delayed inflammatory reaction.

6.2 Hyaluronic Acid Filler Itself

Hyaluronic acid fillers are made from hyaluronic acid, which is normally present in our bodies, and cross-linking agents modified for prolonged duration. Strictly speaking, they are foreign substances, and whether they cause foreign body reactions is a crucial factor. Issues with the hyaluronic acid filler itself, such as problems with cross-linking agents or foreign materials, are considered the most significant factors. Additionally, hyaluronic acid molecular weight, endotoxin, and chemical components from the manufacturing process are also being raised as potential issues.

6.2.1 Structural Issues and Cross-Linking Agents of Hyaluronic Acid Fillers

Hyaluronic acid is a disaccharide composed of N-acetylglucosamine and glucuronic acid (Fig. 6.1). Hyaluronic acid fillers are primarily manufactured by mixing hyaluronic acid produced by bacteria with cross-linking agents, the most commonly used of which is 1,4-butanediol diglycidyl ether (BDDE).

BDDE must react with hyaluronic acid to cross-link two hyaluronic acid molecules, creating a hyaluronic acid filler that lasts longer [2]. However, unreacted BDDE sometimes remains; thus BDDE exists in four forms (Fig. 6.2).

Generally, A represents the normally conjugated form, B is the pendant type, C is the free type 1,4-butanediol di-(propan-2,3-diolyl) ether (BDPE), and D is the raw BDDE form with the epoxide group not opened. Therefore, the likelihood of foreign body reactions increases when there are many B, C, and D forms. Consequently, for the cleanest hyaluronic acid filler, there should be a high amount of the well-conjugated A form and ideally no B, C, or D forms of

W. Lee (✉)
Yonsei E1 Plastic Surgery Clinic,
Anyang, Kyonggi-do, Korea (Republic of)

W. Lee (ed.), *Innovative Injectable Techniques in Minimally Invasive Aesthetics*,
https://doi.org/10.1007/978-981-95-2161-6_6

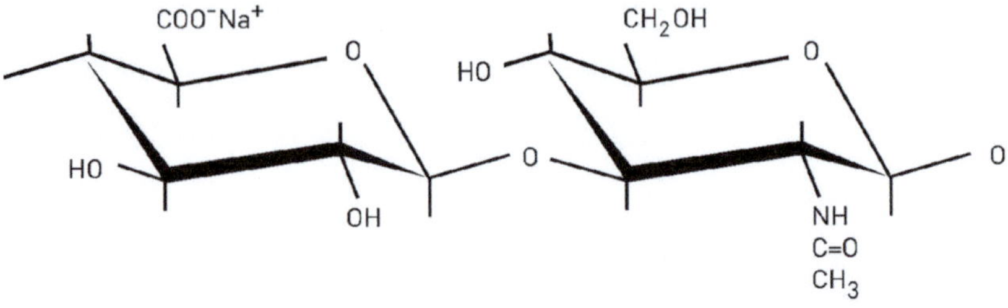

Fig. 6.1 Molecular structure of hyaluronic acid

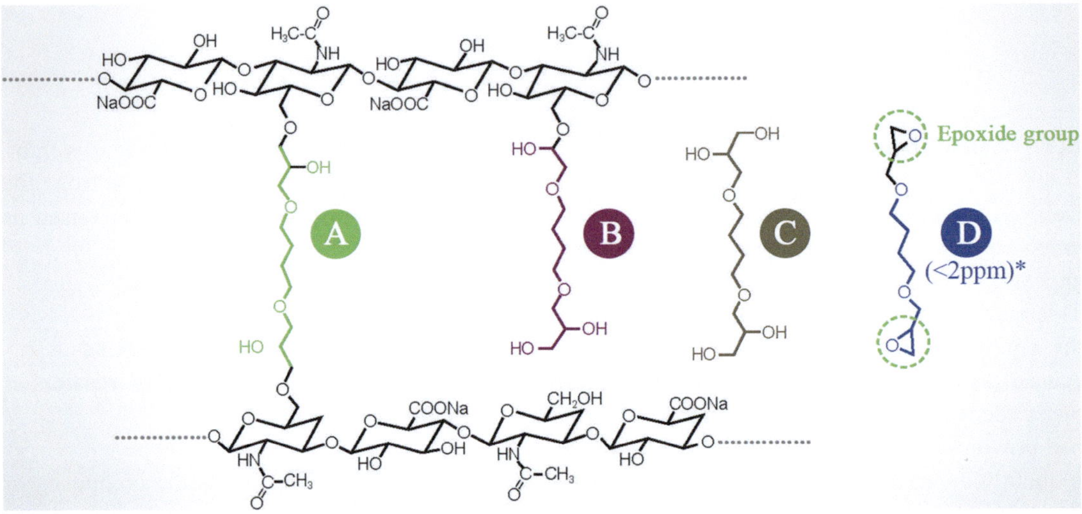

Fig. 6.2 Four forms of BDDE binding with hyaluronic acid. (**a**) well cross-linked BDPE; (**b**) pendant BDPE; (**c**) free BDPE; (**d**) free BDDE

BDDE. For quantitative measurement, nuclear magnetic resonance (NMR) is used.

First, when hyaluronic acid filler is dissolved with chondroitinase, it breaks down into various molecular forms. Among these, the molecular weight and the distribution of H and C atoms differ between BDPE well conjugated with two hyaluronic acid molecules and BDPE conjugated with only one hyaluronic acid molecule on one side. Thus, the structure to be measured can be analyzed using NMR. Measuring based on hydrogen in the molecular structure yields 1H NMR data, and measuring based on carbon yields 13C NMR data.

For the measurement, 13 hyaluronic acid fillers were selected as follows: Restylane Volyme (LOT:17031-1, Galderma, Uppsala, Sweden), Restylane Defyne (LOT:18681-1, Galderma, Uppsala, Sweden), Restylane Lyft (LOT: 19765, Galderma, Uppsala, Sweden), Juvederm Voluma (LOT: 1000561748, Allergan, Irvine, CA), Belotero Volume (LOT: B00016110, Merz Pharmaceuticals, Frankfurt, Germany), Teosyal RHA4 (LOT: 22372DL03128, TEOXANE Laboratories, Geneva, Switzerland), L'orient No. 6 (LOT: J21001, Joonghun Pharmaceutical, Seoul, Republic of Korea), Neuramis Volume (LOT C523010A, Medy-Tox, Seoul, Republic of Korea), The Chaeum Premium No. 4 (LOT: BLD21008, HUGEL, Seoul, Republic of Korea), Elravie Deep (LOT D6016002AA, Humedix, Seoul, Republic of Korea), Eptq S500 (LOT YLC22006, Jetema, Seoul, Republic of Korea), QTfill SubQ (LOT: QPAI21001G, S. THEPHARM, Seoul, Republic of Korea), and Youthfill Shape (LOT: YDE19013, RFBio, Seoul, Republic of Korea). One gram of each hyaluronic acid filler was placed in a phosphate buffer solution and mixed with 100U of chondroitinase ABC. The mixture was dissolved by shaking for 48 h. After lyophilization, a 5mL NMR tube was filled with D2O solution and placed into the NMR instrument. For 13C measurement, each sample was measured for 26 h (Fig. 6.3).

In this way, the amount of BDPE contained in the filler was measured, and this was quantified as MoD (modification of degree). Essentially, it is a value indicating how much the original HA has been modified by the attachment of BDDE. However, as mentioned above, not all BDPE is properly attached. Therefore, the amount of pendant form is also important. The value representing this is CrR (cross-linked ratio). It is the ratio of properly attached cross-linking agents to those that are simply attached. Additionally, CrD (degree of cross-linking) represents the value obtained by multiplying MoD and CrR. These three parameters can be found in previous literature [3].

1. MoD (%, ^{1}H) = $(I^{\delta H1.6}/4)/(I^{\delta H2.0}/3) \times 100$
2. MoD (%, ^{13}C) = $(I^{\delta c25.2}/2)/I^{\delta c1.9\text{-}22.6} \times 100$
3. CrR = $1\text{-}I^{\delta C62.7}/(I^{\delta 25.2}/2)$
4. CrD (%) = (CrR × MoD) × 100

The results of analyzing the 13 hyaluronic acid fillers are shown in Table 6.1.

This can be represented more easily in a diagram (Fig. 6.4). As shown in the figure, a filler is considered proper when BDPE is correctly bonded between hyaluronic acid molecules. If a filler contains many pendant BDPE forms and is

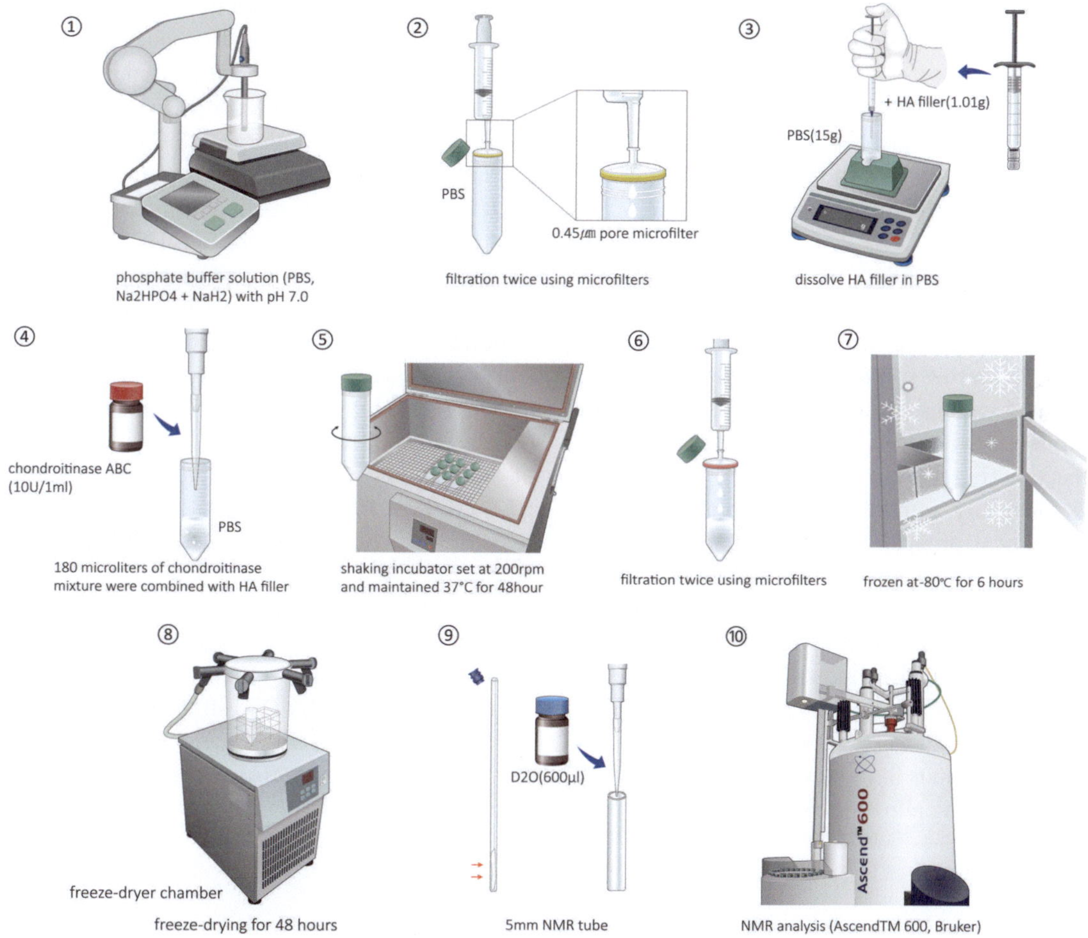

Fig. 6.3 NMR analysis of 13 hyaluronic acid fillers

Table 6.1 MoD and CrR values analyzed for 13 fillers

Product	MoD (%,1H)	MoD (%,13C)	CrR (13C)	CrD (%,13C)	NMR reading date
1 A	11.215	8.187	0.394	3.232	20230724
2 B	10.194	9.723	0.085	0.824	20230425
3 C	2.370	2.112	0.117	0.246	20230918
4 D	8.789	7.103	0.143	1.015	20230819
5 E	17.065	12.567	0.086	1.077	20230803
6 F	6.303	4.915	0.118	0.581	20230807
7 Lorient	2.239	1.947	0.227	0.443	20230914
8 H	14.748	9.904	0.014	0.204	20230804
9 I	14.476	12.101	0.333	4.034	20230728
10 J	10.912	9.269	0.141	1.304	20230726
11 K	4.748	2.999	0.049	0.146	20230725
12 L	8.055	4.747	0.065	0.306	20230731
13 M	7.192	6.147	0.343	2.110	20230820

not properly cross-linked, it is more likely to cause foreign body reactions under similar rheological conditions. It is a natural consequence that the purest fillers cause fewer side effects.

6.2.2 Impurities in Hyaluronic Acid Fillers

Hyaluronic acid fillers are produced through several stages. Therefore, foreign substances can be introduced during the manufacturing process. First, impurities can be present in the raw materials, and various impurities can also be added at different stages during the washing process in the reaction (Fig. 6.5).

Generally, impurities can be present in pharmaceutical products. Even when producing the cleanest product, small amounts can be included, and this has been described by the US Food and Drug Administration [4]. Various impurities that can be contained include silicone, metals, proteins, and dust. The problem is that if the amount is excessive, it can cause various side effects, so acceptable limits have been set. The US FDA [5] has set criteria allowing no more than 600 particles larger than 25 μm and no more than 6000 particles larger than 10 μm per prefilled syringe. Therefore, hyaluronic acid fillers containing a large amount of such foreign substances have the potential to show foreign body reactions.

Particles were measured using a total of 12 fillers: Restylane Volume (LOT 18684-1, Galderma, Uppsala, Sweden), Juvéderm Voluma (LOT VB20A90809, Allergan, Irvine, CA, USA), Belotero Volume (LOT 547253/1, Merz Pharmaceuticals, Frankfurt, Germany), Teosyal RHA4 (LOT TPUL-183815C, TEOXANE Laboratories, Geneva, Switzerland), L'orient No. 6 (LOT J20001, Joonghun Pharmaceutical, Seoul, Republic of Korea), Neuramis Volume (LOT C521007A, Medy-Tox, Seoul, Republic of Korea), The Chaeum Premium No. 3 (LOT BLD21008, HUGEL, Seoul, Republic of Korea), Elravie Deep (LOT D1915001BA, Humedix, Seoul, Republic of Korea), Eptq S500 (LOT YLC18012, Jetema, Seoul, Republic of Korea), QTfill SubQ (QPAI21001G, S. THEPHARM, Seoul, Republic of Korea), Youthfill Deep (LOT YDE19019, RFBio, Seoul, Republic of Korea), and Cleviel Contour (LOT J94118001, PharmaResearch, Seongnam, Republic of Korea).

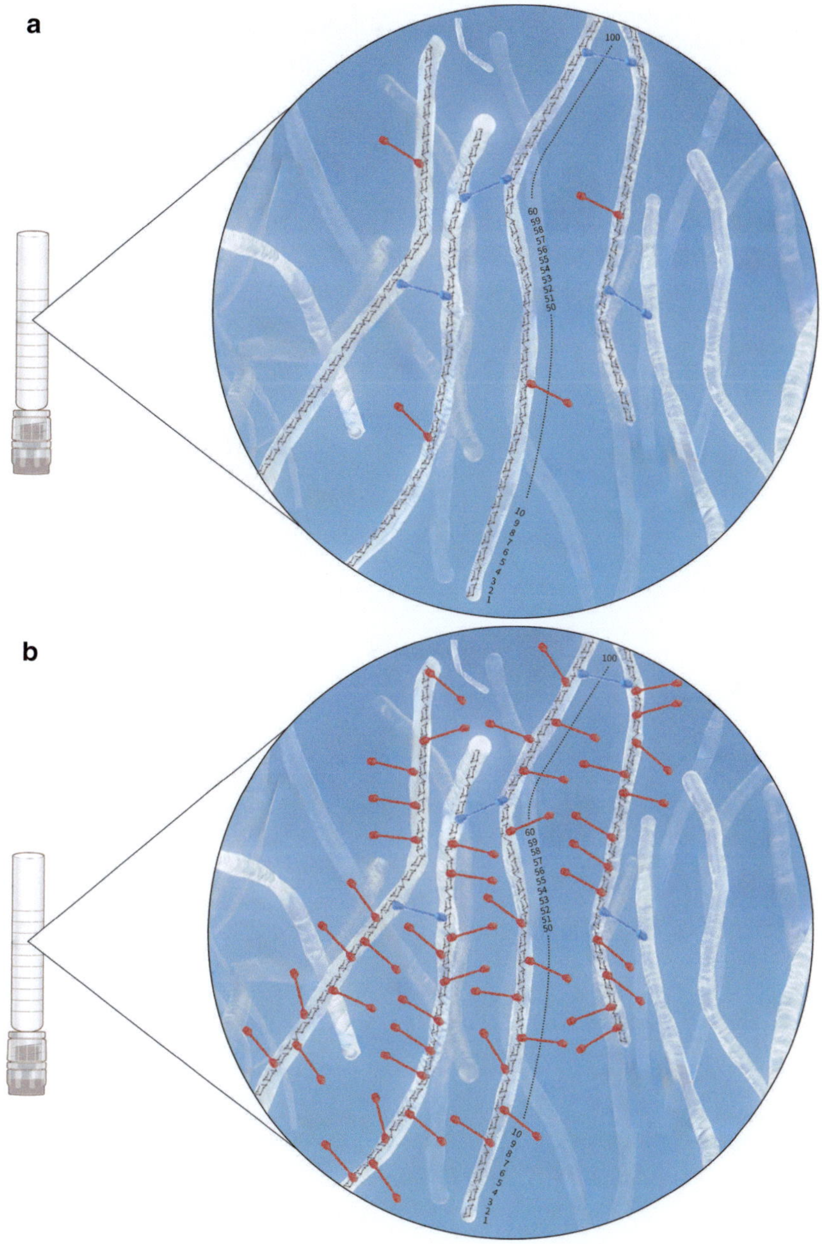

Fig. 6.4 Schematic illustration of hyaluronic acid filler used in the experiment. (**a**) Lorient filler (product 7). (**b**) Product 5 E

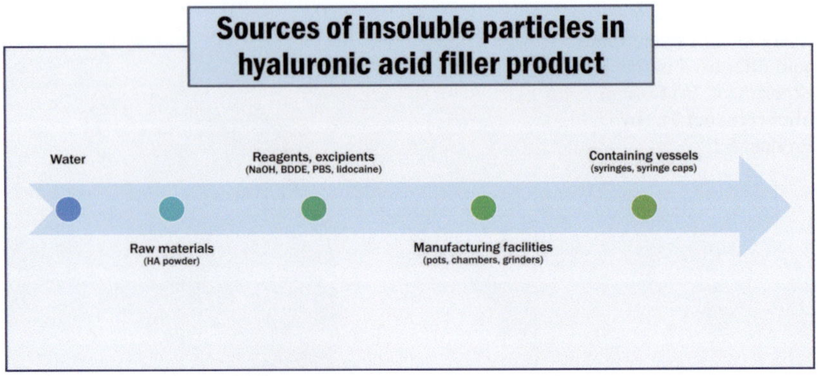

Fig. 6.5 Process during hyaluronic acid filler manufacturing where impurities can occur

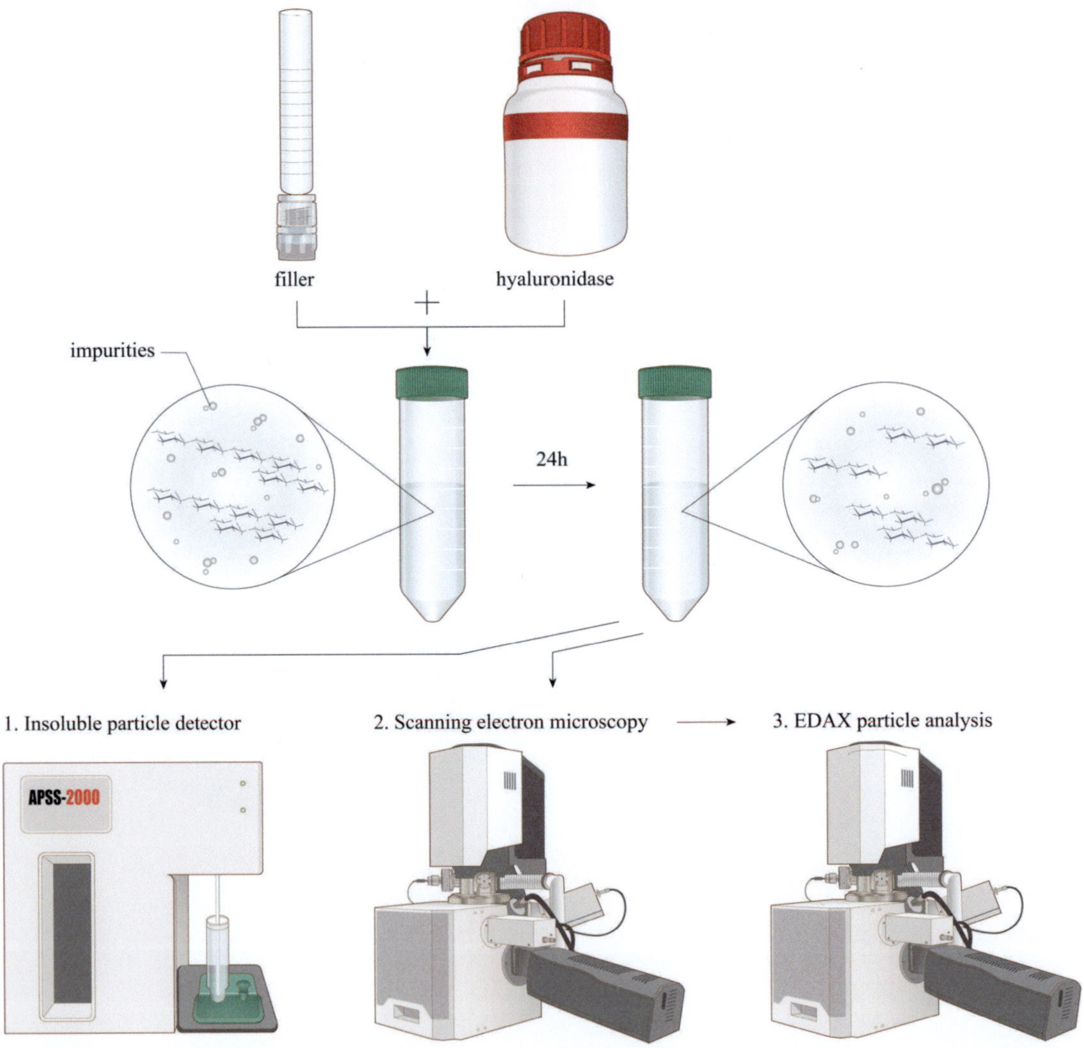

Fig. 6.6 Impurity particle analysis process

Table 6.2 HA filler products with variable counts of insoluble particles

	Larger than 10 μm (count/syringe)				Larger than 25 μm (count/syringe)			
	1st	2nd	3rd	Average	1st	2nd	3rd	Average
A	4048	3012	3528	3529	60	32	72	54
B	1352	1264	1272	1296	156	112	118	128
C	1304	968	828	1033	72	44	28	48
D	3632	3588	3536	3585	28	8	16	17
Lorient	1204	1340	1196	1246	88	72	88	82
F	76,520	79,792	76,588	77,633	812	1044	876	910
G	11,468	10,460	10,804	10,910	312	312	236	286
H	16,264	16,816	17,084	16,721	936	916	936	929
I	121,244	120,184	118,140	119,856	6156	6600	6008	6254
J	27,912	29,712	28,180	28,601	120	84	96	100
K	28,892	25,780	25,480	26,717	896	756	820	824
L	46,408	43,516	40,568	43,497	992	1100	1092	1061
Control	44	32	36	37	20	4	12	12

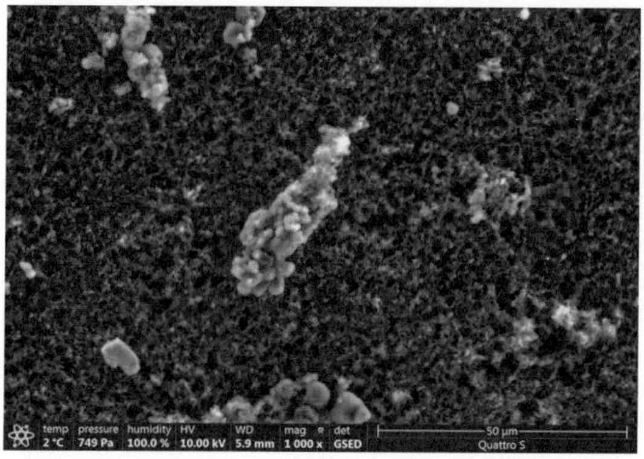

Fig. 6.7 Electron microscopic findings of filler K (1000 X). A 50 μm particle is visible

The experimental method is as follows (Fig. 6.6). First, the hyaluronic acid filler is dissolved in hyaluronidase. It is completely dissolved in a shaking tank for 24 h. Subsequently, the particle count is measured three times using an insoluble particle counter (Table 6.2). The same sample was then placed on filter paper and examined under an electron microscope to observe the shape of the particles. Observations were made using a Quattro S SEM (Fig. 6.7). Elemental composition of the visible particles was then confirmed using energy-dispersive X-ray spectrometer analysis (EDS) (Fig. 6.8).

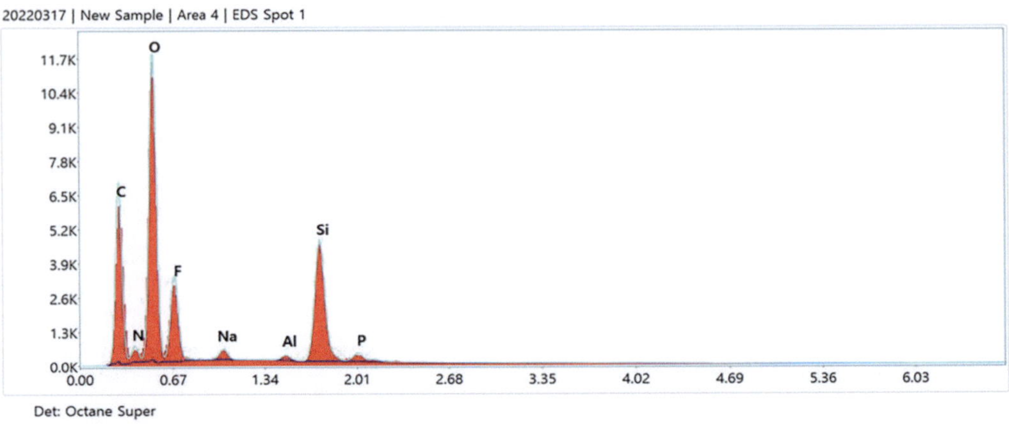

eZAF Quant Result - Analysis Uncertainty: 6.59 %

Element	Weight %	MDL	Atomic %	Net Int.	Error %	R	A	F
C K	39.9	0.22	48.6	1673.3	8.8	0.9347	0.3597	1.0000
N K	6.1	0.38	6.3	153.7	13.1	0.9401	0.2127	1.0000
O K	37.6	0.13	34.4	3194.1	8.6	0.9443	0.3662	1.0000
F K	8.6	0.11	6.6	910.5	9.6	0.9482	0.3388	1.0000
Na K	0.5	0.07	0.3	114.1	12.1	0.9552	0.6288	1.0024
Al K	0.2	0.05	0.1	65.3	12.3	0.9616	0.8364	1.0075
Si K	6.5	0.05	3.4	1700.6	3.8	0.9645	0.8921	1.0040
P K	0.5	0.07	0.3	114.3	8.6	0.9674	0.9085	1.0053

Fig. 6.8 EDAX results of product G. silicon is detected

Foreign substances are detected in the majority of hyaluronic acid fillers, and a high content of these substances increases the likelihood of foreign body reactions. Therefore, this is considered a potential cause of delayed onset edema.

6.3 Patient's Immune Status

Delayed inflammatory reaction frequently appears after the onset of symptoms similar to a cold [6]. Thus, it is recognized that type IV hypersensitivity occurs depending on the patient's condition. Recently, numerous cases of delayed onset edema have been reported during the COVID-19 pandemic. It is believed that in a state of viremia or post-vaccination, the immune response is enhanced, and severe immune reactions occur due to virulent bacteria around the hyaluronic acid filler, among other factors [7]. The spike protein of COVID-19 is thought to act as a trigger, influencing Th1 cells and CD8+ T cells through the angiotensin-converting enzyme receptor. Consequently, there has been an increase in cases treated with the ACE inhibitor lisinopril in such instances. Additionally, delayed inflammatory reaction is treated with steroids, among other medications.

6.4 Infection

Infection is a significant factor in all inflammation. Aseptic technique is one of the most crucial elements when injecting hyaluronic acid fillers. However, normal skin commensal bacteria can be introduced during injection and coexist with the filler. Therefore, thorough disinfection is paramount. Although filler procedures are often perceived as quick, it is essential to completely remove makeup and perform meticulous disinfection. In addition to disinfection, it is important to prepare for infection by checking the patient's history of prior infections and previous filler procedures. Chlorhexidine gluconate and isopropanol are the most commonly recommended disinfectants [8]. Regardless of how simple a filler procedure is perceived, thorough disinfection must be performed, and administering the procedure after removing the patient's makeup is very important.

6.5 Conclusion

The cause of delayed inflammatory reaction due to hyaluronic acid fillers is not certain. However, delayed inflammatory reaction is associated with foreign body reactions and causes persistent inflammation around the hyaluronic acid filler. Therefore, the injected hyaluronic acid filler should be as clean as possible and free from foreign substances. Furthermore, it is most important to inject aseptically, slowly, and in small amounts to avoid foreign body reactions.

References

1. Lemperle G, Gauthier-Hazan N, Wolters M, et al. Foreign body granulomas after all injectable dermal fillers: Part 1. Possible causes. Plast Reconstr Surg. 2009;123(6):1842–63.
2. De Boulle K, Glogau R, Kono T, Nathan M, Tezel A, Roca-Martinez JX, Paliwal S, Stroumpoulis D. A review of the metabolism of 1,4-butanediol diglycidyl ether-crosslinked hyaluronic acid dermal fillers. Dermatol Surg. 2013;39(12):1758–66. https://doi.org/10.1111/dsu.12301.
3. Wende FJ, Gohil S, Nord LI, Helander Kenne A, Sandström C. 1D NMR methods for determination of degree of cross-linking and BDDE substitution positions in HA hydrogels. Carbohydr Polym. 2017;10(157):1525–30. https://doi.org/10.1016/j.carbpol.2016.11.029.
4. Langille SE. Particulate matter in injectable drug products. PDA J Pharm Sci Technol. 2013;67:186–200.
5. US Pharmacopeia. U.S. Pharmacopeia and National Formulary. Rockville: The United States Pharmacopeial Convention, Inc; 2021.
6. Turkmani MG, De Boulle K, Philipp-Dormston WG. Delayed hypersensitivity reaction to hyaluronic acid dermal filler following influenza-like illness. Clin Cosmet Investig Dermatol. 2019;12:277–83.
7. Goodman GJ, McDonald CB, Lim A, et al. Making sense of late tissue nodules associated with hyaluronic acid injections. Aesthet Surg J. 2023;43(6):NP438–48.
8. Philipp-Dormston WG, Goodman GJ, De Boulle K, et al. Global approaches to the prevention and management of delayed-onset adverse reactions with hyaluronic acid-based fillers. Plast Reconstr Surg Glob Open. 2020;8(4):e2730.

Perioral Rejuvenation with Variable Injectables

7

Kyu Hwa Jung and Won Lee

7.1 Introduction

Facial changes associated with aging occur throughout the entire face, but the perioral area is one of the regions where these changes are most prominent (Fig. 7.1). As we age, the lips become thinner, and the surrounding tissues lose elasticity, leading to volume loss and drooping at the corners of the mouth. This area is also characterized by highly dynamic muscle activity, which contributes to the formation of various types of wrinkles. These changes go beyond aesthetic concerns—they also affect a person's overall impression and the expression of emotions.

The perioral region is highly active due to frequent muscle movements. Repetitive facial expressions, external environmental factors (such as UV exposure, smoking, and lifestyle habits), and intrinsic skin aging all act together to bring about visible changes. Therefore, perioral rejuvenation requires a comprehensive approach that goes beyond simple wrinkle reduction to include skin quality improvement, volume restoration, muscle management, and natural three-dimensional contouring.

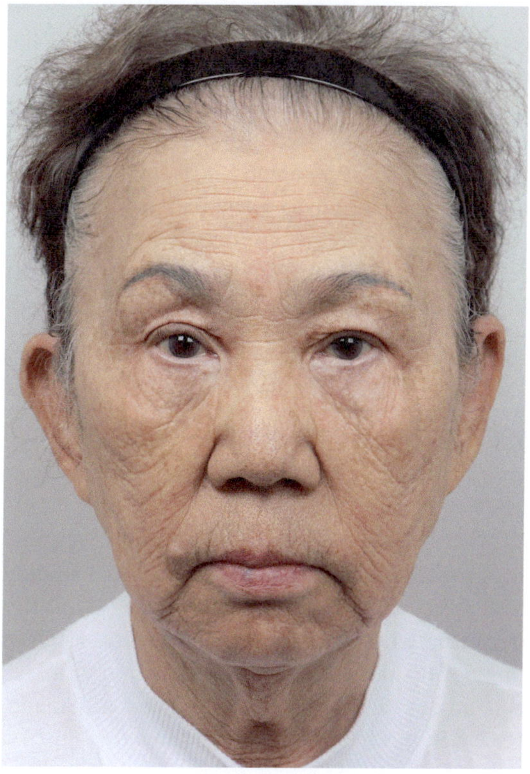

Fig. 7.1 An elderly individual with prominent perioral wrinkles

K. H. Jung
Liting Plastic Surgery, Seoul, Republic of Korea

W. Lee (✉)
Yonsei E1 Plastic Surgery Clinic,
Anyang, Kyonggi-do, Korea (Republic of)

W. Lee (ed.), *Innovative Injectable Techniques in Minimally Invasive Aesthetics*,
https://doi.org/10.1007/978-981-95-2161-6_7

Traditionally, methods like chemical peeling, dermabrasion, and CO_2 laser resurfacing were used to improve skin quality. More recently, microneedle radiofrequency (RF) has been introduced as a method with shorter downtime. Deep structural improvements used to rely mainly on fat grafting, but the development of fillers and biostimulators has expanded treatment options. In addition, combining HIFU and botulinum toxin has allowed for not only wrinkle correction but also prevention. These advances in nonsurgical techniques have enabled more precise and personalized treatments.

This chapter focuses specifically on perioral rejuvenation using injectables. It explores the causes of perioral wrinkles, methods for assessing their severity, the effects and limitations of various injectable options, and techniques for their use. It also emphasizes individualized approaches tailored to each patient's anatomy, age, and expectations. Ultimately, the goal is to present a modern strategy for perioral rejuvenation—one that aims not just for wrinkle correction but for a natural and harmonized result.

7.2 Understanding Perioral Wrinkles

Wrinkles begin as dynamic and progress to static forms over time [1]. A wrinkle refers to a folding line observed on the skin surface, typically occurring with facial muscle movement. Even in individuals in their 20s or 30s, dynamic wrinkles can appear when facial expressions are made. However, these lines disappear when the muscles relax, thanks to the elastic recoil of the epidermis, which is rich in elastin fibers. As aging progresses, the amount and integrity of collagen and elastin fibers diminish, leading to decreased elasticity and increased fragility. As a result, even after facial muscles relax, the skin's ability to return to its original shape declines, and the folds between the epidermis and dermis persist for longer periods [2–4]. This prolonged folding transforms dynamic wrinkles into static ones. Moreover, the process is accelerated by fat atrophy, facial muscle sarcopenia, and bone resorption.

Perioral wrinkles can be categorized into three main types: vertical upper lip lines, lateral mouth corner lines (extending from the nasolabial fold), and marionette lines.

The transition of wrinkles from dynamic to static is influenced by different factors depending on their location. Upper lip wrinkles, which lie directly over the facial expression muscle (orbicularis oris), are formed when the orbicularis oris contracts to pucker the lips, producing accordion-like central compression that creates multiple vertical dynamic lines (Fig. 7.2). Repeated use of this expression causes central vector energy to accumulate in the skin over time.

In younger individuals, not only the dermis and subcutaneous fat but also the viable epidermis (excluding the stratum corneum) function as a cushion that absorbs kinetic energy. As a result, wrinkling is initially limited to the stratum corneum and disappears once the expression is relaxed. However, with aging, changes in the composition of each facial layer degrade the skin's mechanical properties, allowing the effects of motion to penetrate deeper layers. Eventually, wrinkling involves the entire epidermis. When the dermis becomes affected, the wrinkles become visibly pronounced (Fig. 7.3).

While this process typically becomes apparent around the eyes in the 30s, upper lip wrinkles tend to become markedly visible later, generally after the age of 45 [5, 6] (Fig. 7.4). This delayed onset is attributed to the philtrum's high density of sebaceous glands and blood vessels, which are believed to help prevent wrinkle formation. This also explains why men tend to have fewer upper lip wrinkles than women [7].

The lateral wrinkle at the mouth corner is an extension of the nasolabial fold. It forms at the dermal insertion area where the zygomaticus major muscle and the orbicularis oris muscle interconnect. When the zygomaticus major contracts, it moves the orbicularis oris muscle in a superolateral direction. This movement also creates a posterior compressive force in three dimensions, causing the malar fat pad and perioral tissues to be pinched along a defined boundary. With repeated movement, this pinch line becomes a static wrinkle (Fig. 7.5).

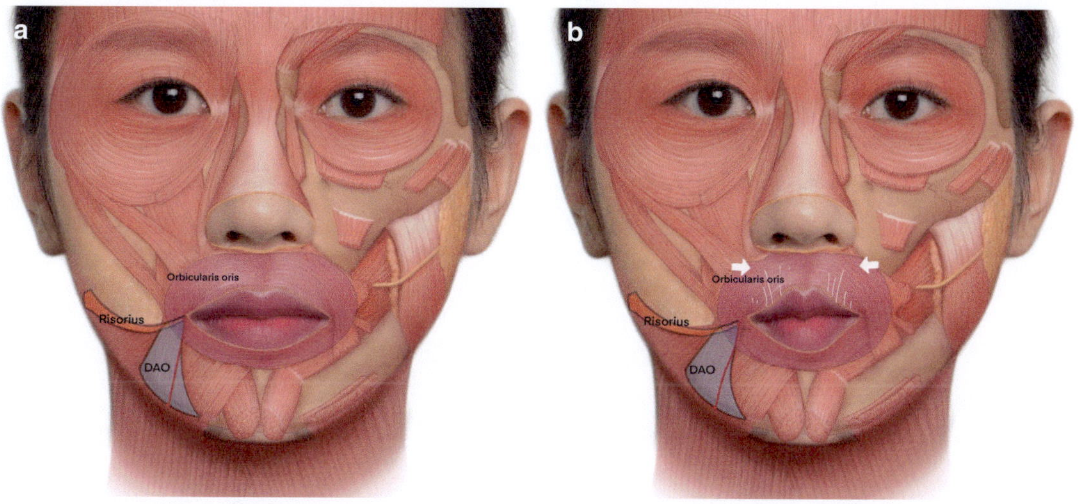

Fig. 7.2 Correlation between the direction of muscle compression during orbicularis oris contraction (puckering of the lips) and the formation of upper lip wrinkles. (**a**) Muscle anatomy. (**b**) During lip puckering

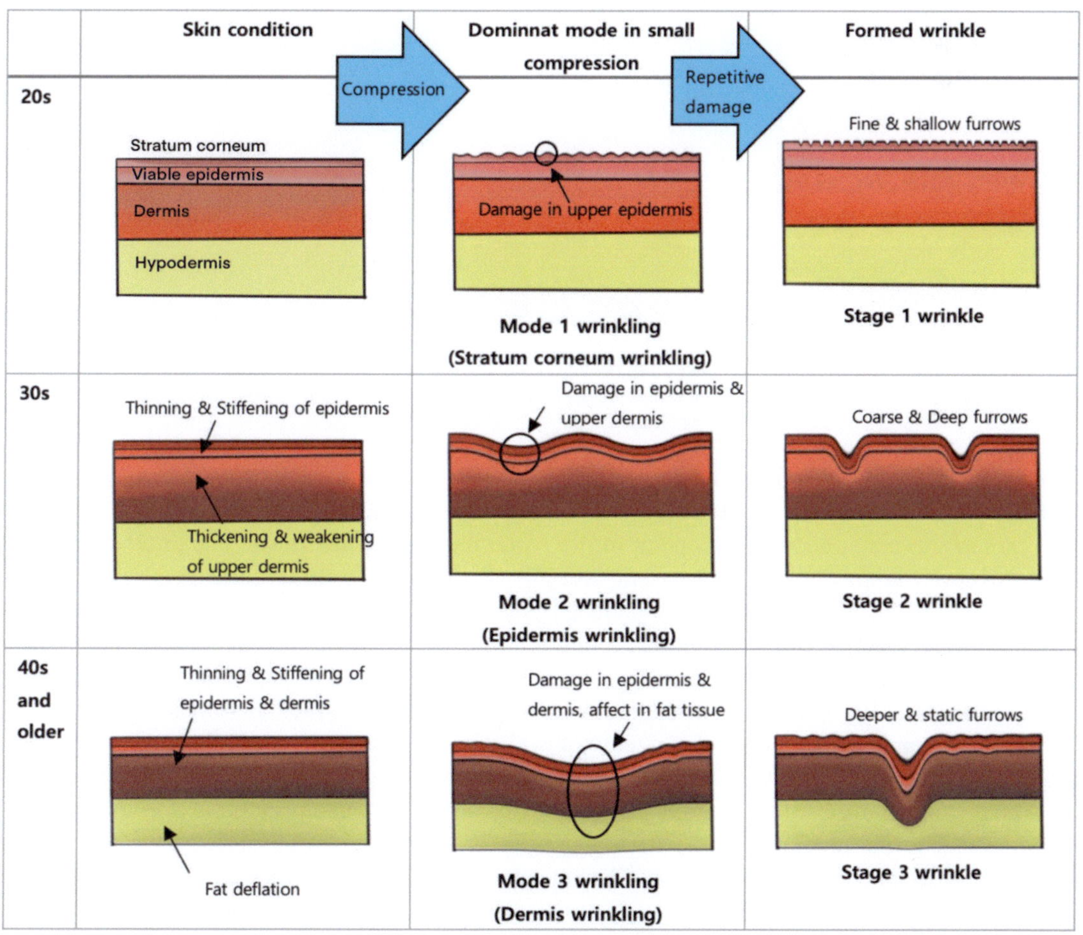

Fig. 7.3 Wrinkling formation mechanism based on multistage wrinkling theory [5]

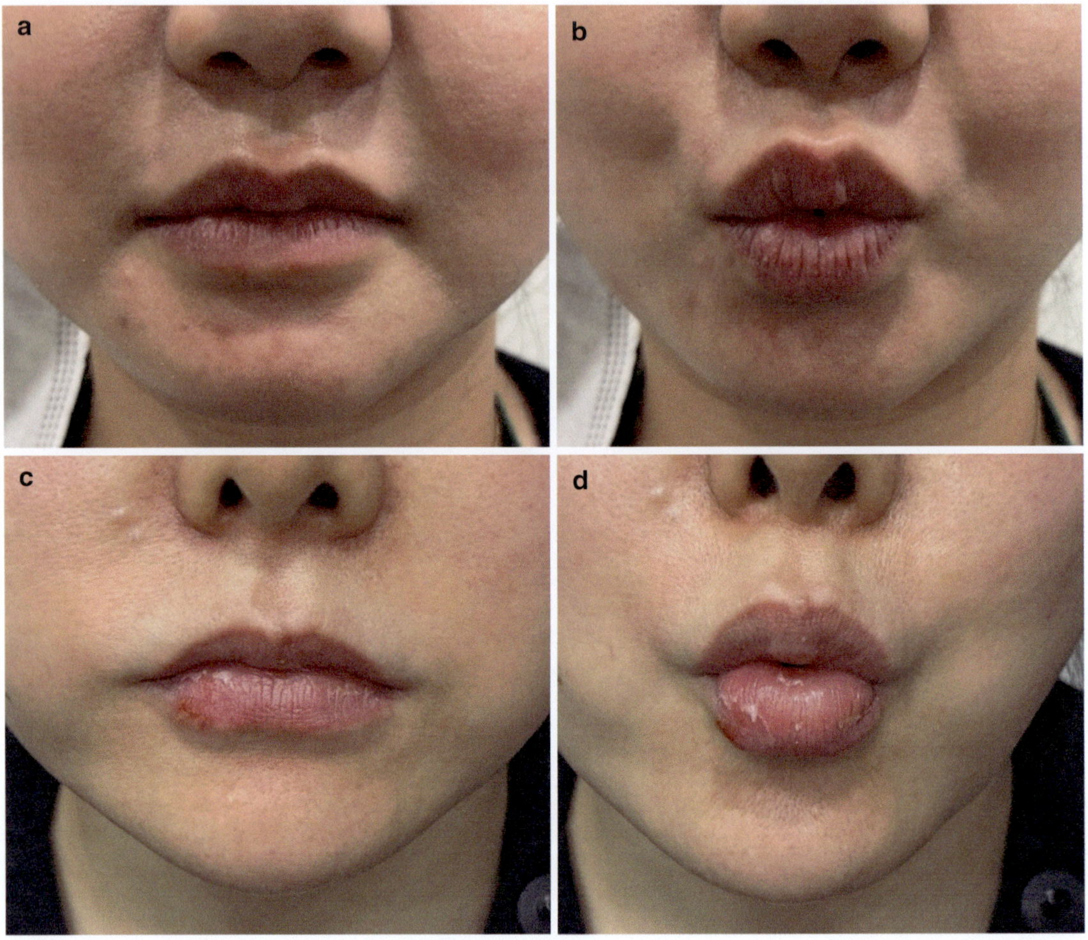

Fig. 7.4 Neutral facial expressions and puckering of the orbicularis oris muscle in individuals of different age groups. (**a**, **b**) Lips in their 30s. (**c**, **d**) Lips in their 40s. Vertical lines on the upper lip are more clearly observed in the 40s group

Therefore, in a lateral view, the greater the horizontal distance between the insertion site of the zygomaticus major and the peak point of the orbicularis oris muscle (i.e., the lips), the stronger the pinching effect. This explains why patients with protruding mouths tend to present with this type of wrinkle more frequently (Fig. 7.6).

The marionette line extends from the modiolus along the medial border of the depressor anguli oris (DAO) muscle to the mandibular border. The upper one-third of the line runs from the mouth corner to the modiolus, while the lower two-thirds is formed along the medial border of the DAO. The modiolus is a tendinous structure composed of fibers from nine facial expression muscles. With aging, the support from these muscles weakens, and fat atrophy occurs, causing the modiolus to descend, which deepens the upper one-third of the marionette line [8, 9] (Fig. 7.7).

The lower two-thirds corresponds to the insertion zone of the DAO's medial border. The DAO originates from the medial tubercle and inserts into the dermis. It is activated when expressing negative emotions such as sadness or depression, pulling the medial border of the DAO posteriorly and deepening the line. As aging progresses, dermal and subcutaneous fat tissues diminish—similar to changes in the nasolabial fold—enhancing the dermal insertion and making the border more defined, eventually becoming a static wrinkle. Descending superficial fat tissue and overlying skin accumulate above the now-static marionette

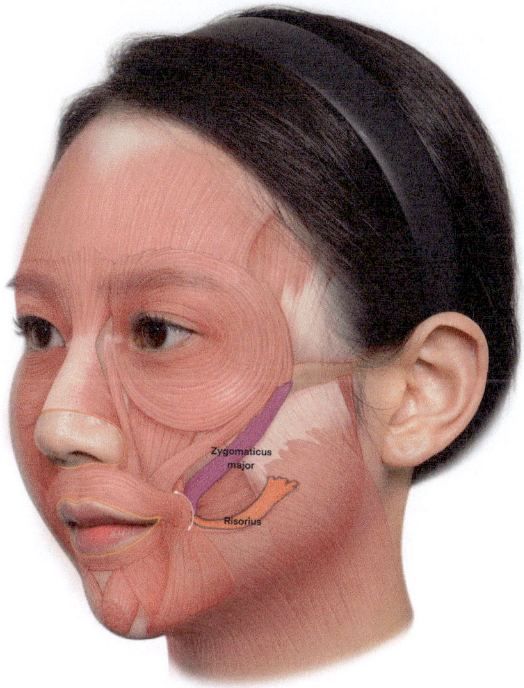

Fig. 7.5 Movement of the orbicularis oris muscle (OOM) caused by the action of the zygomaticus major muscle, leading to the formation of lateral wrinkles at the mouth corner

line, making the crease appear even deeper and more pronounced (Fig. 7.8).

In summary, the causes of perioral wrinkles vary depending on their location, and the factors that exacerbate these wrinkles differ from patient to patient. Therefore, a thorough understanding of the underlying mechanisms is essential prior to treatment in order to determine the most effective therapeutic approach. A common contributing factor is fat atrophy, which normally serves as a cushion. As this cushion diminishes, the movement of facial muscles has a more direct impact on the dermis and epidermis. The resulting thinning and loss of elasticity in the epidermis reduce skin resilience, causing folds to persist longer and leading to the formation of perioral wrinkles. Thus, focusing on improving this aspect and selecting appropriate treatment methods accordingly can lead to favorable outcomes.

In addition to these factors, thinning of the lips results in a loss of vitality; disrupts the aesthetic proportion between the philtrum, lips, and lower face; and blurs the vermilion border—contributing to an aged appearance. Furthermore, the per-

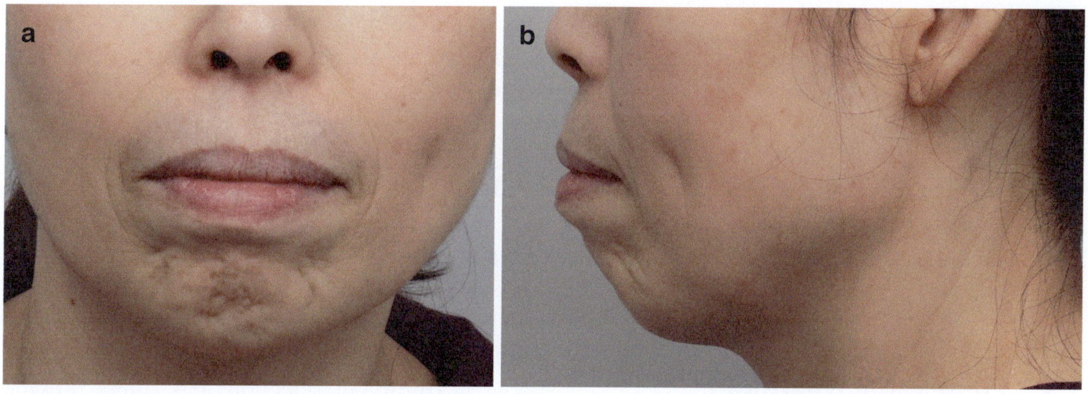

Fig. 7.6 Protruded mouth patient. Individuals with a protruded oral structure are more likely to have structural wrinkles around the mouth. (**a**) Frontal view. (**b**) Lateral view

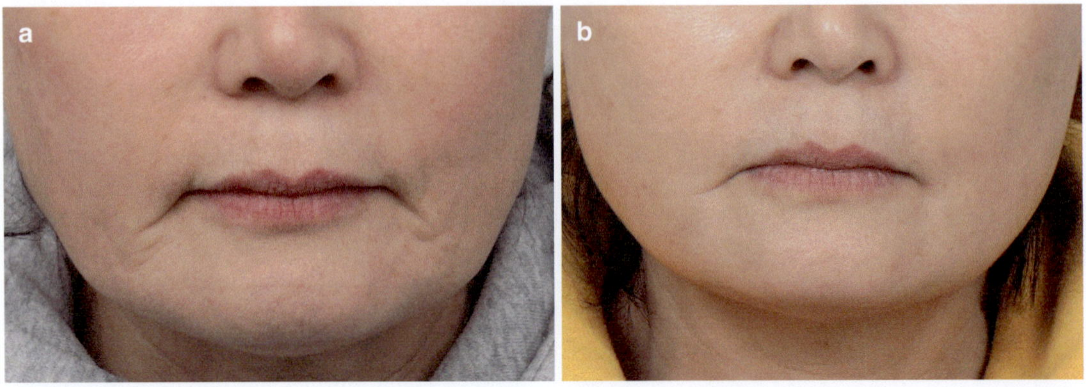

Fig. 7.7 Marionette line. The upper one-third is caused by the downward displacement of the modiolus, while the lower two-thirds primarily result from DAO activation. After DAO botulinum toxin injection, correction is observed only in the lower two-thirds. (**a**) Before botox treatment. (**b**) After treatment

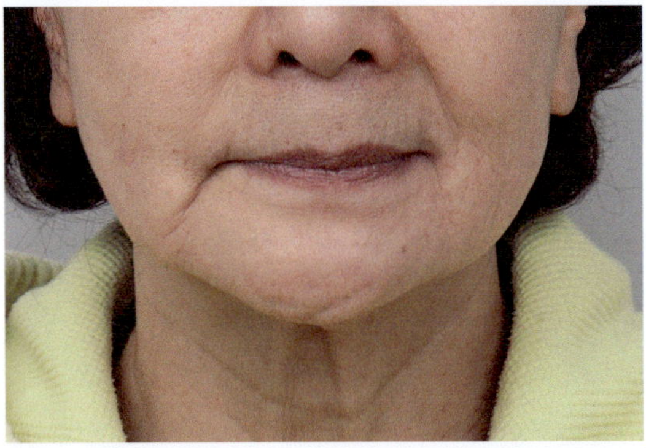

Fig. 7.8 With aging, the marionette line becomes deeper and more static due to the descent of overlying tissues

sistent contraction of the mentalis muscle can cause a cobblestone appearance, which draws visual attention to the mouth area and makes wrinkles more noticeable.

7.3 Injectable Treatment Options

The treatment goal for perioral wrinkles is clear: to minimize the residual kinetic energy on the epidermis generated by facial muscle movements.

1. Restore the dermis to a quality that can absorb and dissipate greater amounts of kinetic energy.
2. Replenish atrophied fat to reduce the transmission of muscular energy to the epidermis.
3. Decrease the amount of kinetic energy generated by the facial expression muscles themselves.

Each type of injectable has different effects, and even the same injectable can serve different purposes depending on the method of application. Therefore, it is essential to adapt techniques flexibly according to the patient's needs and to consider combination therapies for optimal results.

7.3.1 Hyaluronic Acid Fillers

Hyaluronic acid (HA) filler is the most user-friendly and accessible option. With a wide range of products available on the market, each with different properties, practitioners have considerable flexibility in selection. HA fillers provide immediate results and have the added advantage of reversibility through hyaluronidase, a potent enzyme that allows for prompt correction in cases of overcorrection, nodule formation, or patient discomfort.

While fillers can be categorized as monophasic or biphasic based on their manufacturing process, the distinction between these types has become less critical. It is now more reasonable to choose fillers based on their rheological properties, such as elastic modulus (G'), viscosity, and cohesivity. In the treatment of perioral wrinkles, the primary role of fillers is to replace atrophied dermal fat. The goal is to create a "thin and broad filler cushion" by injecting into the subcutaneous layer just beneath the dermis.

Since the upper lip is subject to significant shear and compression forces, using a very soft filler—such as those typically used for neck lines or thin infraorbital skin—tends to yield suboptimal or short-lived results. Fillers with an elastic modulus (G') of 150–220 Pa (measured at 0.1 Hz) are generally effective in producing satisfactory outcomes while minimizing patient discomfort.

To reduce procedural pain, a nerve block or topical anesthesia is recommended. Using a 23-gauge cannula to access the area from the mouth corner toward the center with a fanning technique allows for more uniform wrinkle correction. However, care must be taken, as blunt trauma to the dermis or inadvertent vessel injury can lead to bruising. A 25G cannula is not recommended due to its lack of rigidity, which limits its ability to advance.

When using a needle, the injection can be performed retrogradely along lines from the vermilion border or via tiny serial punctures with a short needle. The serial puncture technique has the added benefit of providing a microneedling effect. On average, about 1 cc of filler is used per session, though the volume should be adjusted based on individual patient needs (Fig. 7.9).

In the case of mouth corners and marionette lines, stronger compression forces are at play, and the skin in these areas tends to be thicker. Therefore, using a relatively firmer filler is generally more effective. Fillers with an elastic modulus (G') of 250–350 Pa (at 0.1 Hz) are known to provide longer-lasting results. However, some patients may report discomfort, so selecting a softer filler based on the patient's preference is also acceptable.

Since wrinkles in these areas are typically firmly attached to both the dermis and underlying facial expression muscles, subdermal release using a cannula should be performed prior to injection. Care should be taken not to inject large volumes of filler outside the wrinkle line, as this may increase tissue heaviness and worsen sagging. For mouth corner wrinkles, 0.2–0.4 cc per side is generally sufficient, while 0.5–1 cc may be used for marionette lines (Fig. 7.10).

7.3.2 Biostimulatory Fillers (Poly-L-Lactic Acid, PDLLA, Calcium, PCL, etc.)

Biostimulatory fillers are a type of filler composed of biocompatible biomaterial particles that are injected into the body to induce a controlled foreign body reaction. This reaction stimulates fibroblasts to generate new collagen. Compared to HA fillers, biostimulators do not remain in the

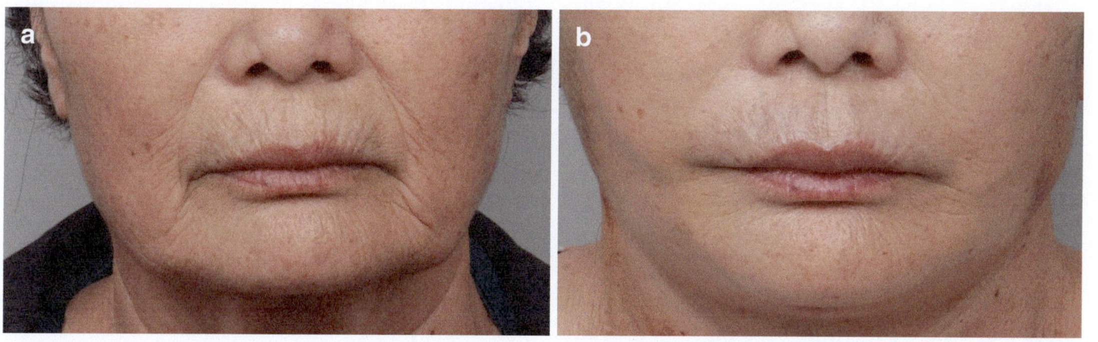

Fig. 7.9 67-year-old female patient. No improvement was observed in upper lip wrinkles after facelift surgery, so an additional filler treatment was performed. Two-week follow-up after using the serial puncture technique. (**a**) Before treatment. (**b**) Two weeks after treatment

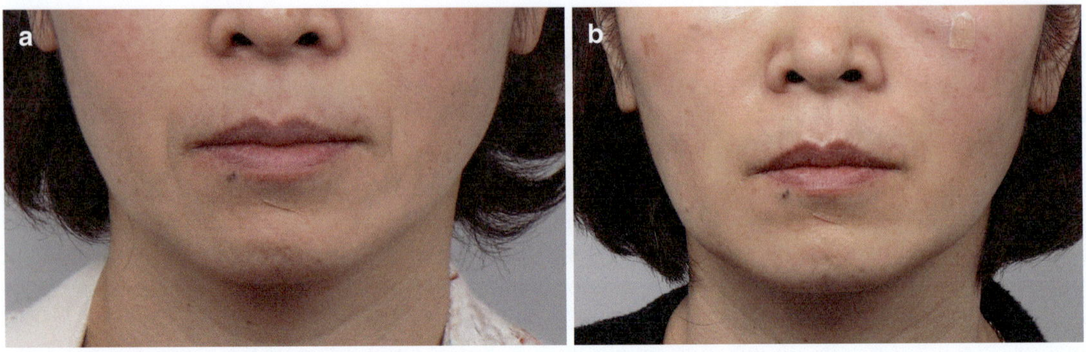

Fig. 7.10 52-year-old female patient. Visited for improvement of perioral wrinkles. 0.3 cc of filler was injected on each side. One-year follow-up. (**a**) Before treatment. (**b**) One year after treatment

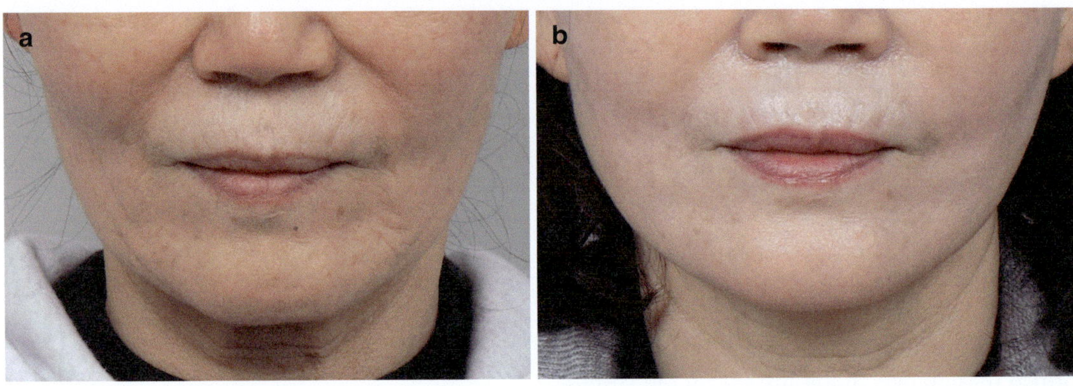

Fig. 7.11 69-year-old female patient. PLLA was diluted with 6 cc of sterile water and injected at the mouth corner using a cannula with a fanning technique. (**a**) Before treatment. (**b**) Six-month follow-up after two sessions at 6-week intervals

body permanently; instead, the particles dissolve over time, while the newly formed endogenous collagen provides long-lasting effects.

However, collagen synthesis typically begins 1.5–2 months after injection, during which visible effects are minimal. To compensate for this delay, many biostimulatory products incorporate carboxymethyl cellulose (CMC) to provide initial volume.

The mechanism of action for biostimulators is based entirely on dermal-level responses. Therefore, if injected into the subcutaneous layer, like HA fillers, they may not trigger the desired biological effect. Biostimulators must be injected within or very close to the dermis to achieve dermal volumization, which expands the skin and prevents sharp wrinkle lines from being pinched by reinforcing the area with newly formed, firm collagen fibers.

Poly-L-lactic acid (PLLA) was one of the first biostimulatory agents used and has demonstrated strong volumizing effects. However, it also carries one of the highest risks of nodule formation. Recently, newer formulations have emerged with improved particle shapes to reduce complications, along with safer reconstitution techniques. While using 5 cc of reconstituted solution can maximize collagen production, it is generally recommended to dilute to 6–7 cc when injecting around the perioral area to lower the risk of nodules (Fig. 7.11).

In addition to PLLA, other commonly used biostimulatory fillers include PDLLA, calcium hydroxylapatite (Ca-HA), and polycaprolactone

(PCL). These all work through a similar mechanism of collagen stimulation, although their duration of effect and specific handling techniques may vary depending on their individual properties.

A common procedural guideline is to perform agitation immediately before injection to ensure even distribution of particles within the reconstituted solution. After the procedure, manual massage should be performed for 2–3 days to minimize the risk of nodule formation caused by particle aggregation.

7.3.3 Neuromodulators (Botulinum Toxin)

Botox is essential for improving perioral wrinkles because the force generated by facial expression muscles is quite substantial. Reducing the folding energy exerted on the skin takes priority over other contributing factors (Fig. 7.12).

For upper lip wrinkles, botulinum toxin is injected targeting the orbicularis oris muscle (OOM). Injections are administered along a line 5 mm above the vermilion border at 8–10 points, with 1–1.5 units per point, totaling approximately 12 ± 4 units. This approach minimizes discomfort while providing effective results.

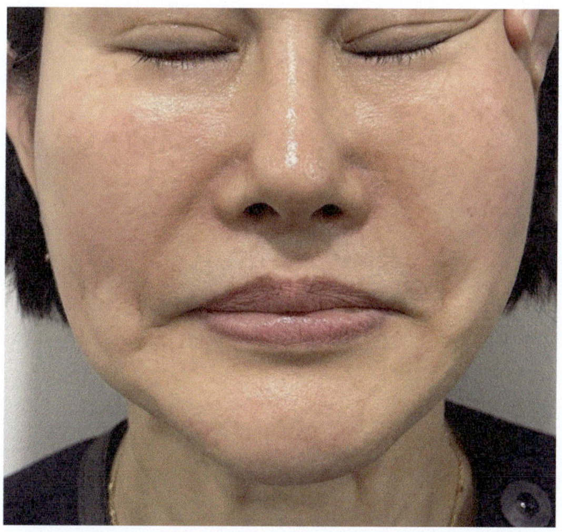

Fig. 7.12 The force exerted by the depressor anguli oris (DAO), which pulls tissues downward, is quite strong. When this muscle is activated, even manual lifting from the temple area results in limited movement

Mouth corner wrinkles require careful application, as improper injection or excessive dosage may affect the zygomaticus major or minor muscles, potentially causing facial asymmetry. Therefore, it is recommended to inject in a dermatoxin-like manner, targeting the deep dermis with 0.5 units at 2–3 points per side. Rather than using botulinum toxin alone, it is advisable to combine it with other treatments for optimal outcomes.

For marionette lines, the target is the depressor anguli oris (DAO). Inject 2–3 units at a point located 1 cm lateral and 1 cm inferior to the mouth corner. Alternatively, injections can be made 0.5 cm lateral to the marionette line. In all cases, the injection should be delivered on the surface of the DAO. Care should be taken to avoid injecting too medially, as this may impair the function of the depressor labii inferioris (DLI).

The mentalis muscle, which is also innervated by the marginal mandibular branch like the DAO, is believed to undergo simultaneous contraction through muscular interplay, particularly when expressing specific emotions. This often results in a cobblestone appearance in patients with static marionette lines. Therefore, the author also injects botulinum toxin into the mentalis muscle as part of marionette line correction (Fig. 7.13).

7.3.4 Skin Boosters and Mesotherapy (PN, HA, Peptides, Growth Factors, etc.)

Procedures aimed at improving skin quality affected by aging are essential for wrinkle correction, but when used alone, their effectiveness is limited. Therefore, combining them with other injectables to create a synergistic effect is more effective. The primary goal is to increase the reduced collagen levels caused by aging, restore the thickness of the thinned dermis, and improve skin elasticity.

There are two main approaches to achieve this:

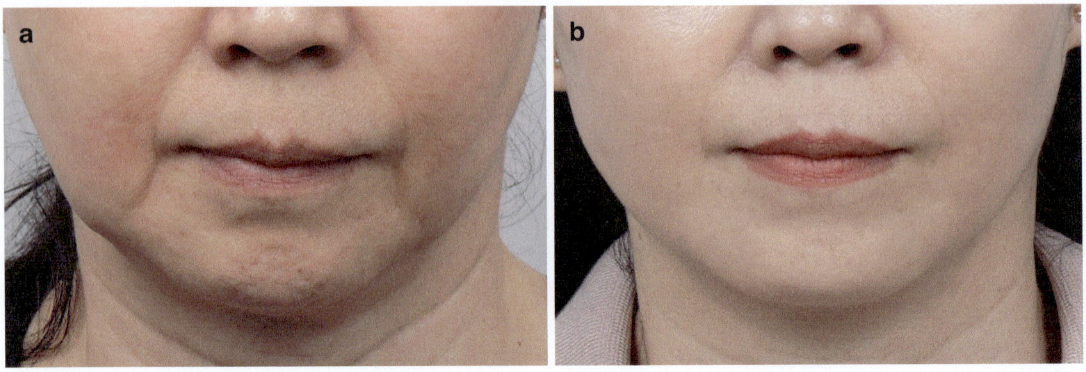

Fig. 7.13 56-year-old female patient. Both the DAO and mentalis muscles were simultaneously hyperactivated, although the patient was unaware of the muscle overactivity. (**a**) Before treatment. (**b**) Two weeks after botox injection

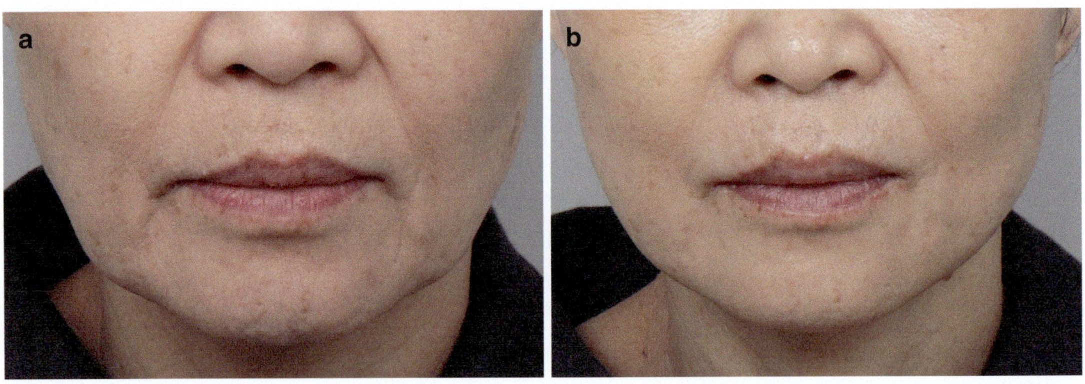

Fig. 7.14 65-year-old female patient. (**a**) Before treatment. (**b**) Two-month follow-up after two collagen injections administered at 2-week intervals

1. Using PN (polynucleotide) injections or applying skin boosters containing amino acids, peptides, and growth factors to directly or indirectly stimulate fibroblasts and induce neocollagenesis.
2. Directly supplementing the diminished extracellular matrix (ECM) by injecting hyaluronic acid or animal-derived collagen.

For ECM supplementation, performing 3–4 sessions at 2-week intervals is recommended to achieve longer-lasting results (Fig. 7.14).

7.4 Advanced Combination Strategies

While using a single injectable mentioned above may yield good results in younger patients, a combination strategy tends to produce more satisfying outcomes in patients over their 40s. Based on the treatment goals for perioral wrinkle correction, the author employs a "layering technique" that combines three components—filler, neuromodulator, and skin booster. This approach reduces muscle movement to lessen folding

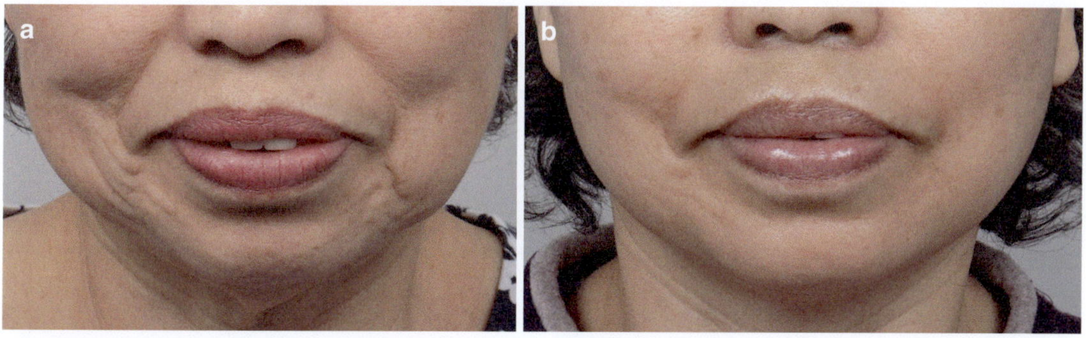

Fig. 7.15 68-year-old female patient. (**a**) Before treatment. (**b**) Two-month follow-up after mini lifting, 0.6 cc HA filler injection into the mouth corner wrinkles, 1.2 cc into the marionette lines, collagen injection into the upper lip, and simultaneous botox injection into the DAO, mentalis, and upper lip orbicularis oris muscle (OOM)

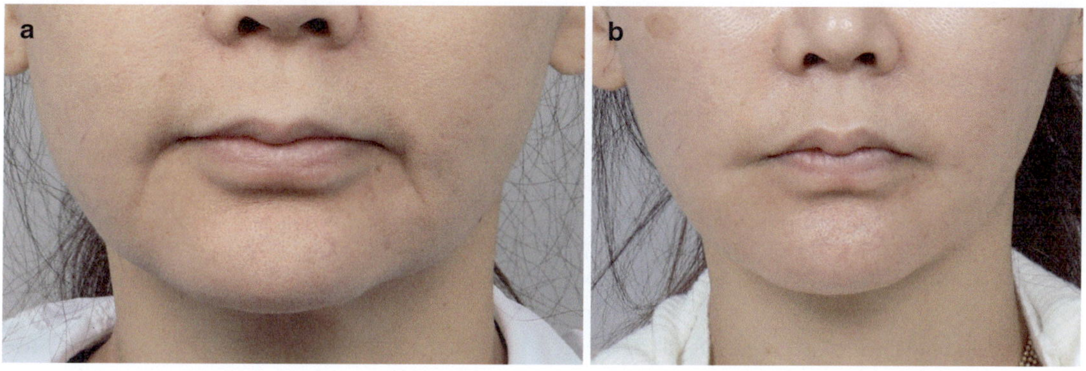

Fig. 7.16 49-year-old female patient. (**a**) Before treatment. (**b**) One-month follow-up after thread lifting, 0.8 cc HA filler injection into the marionette lines, and botox injection into the DAO and mentalis muscles

force, uses filler as a cushion to prevent the dermis from being sharply pinched, and strengthens the dermis with a skin booster to neutralize the energy that reaches deeper layers (Figs. 7.15 and 7.16).

Performing lip augmentation in parallel can enhance the improvement of upper lip wrinkles. In the case of marionette lines, the extent of buccal fat volume, the condition of superficial fat compartments, and skin laxity all influence the result. Therefore, for optimal outcomes, buccal fat removal, liposuction, or lifting procedures may be performed in combination (Fig. 7.17).

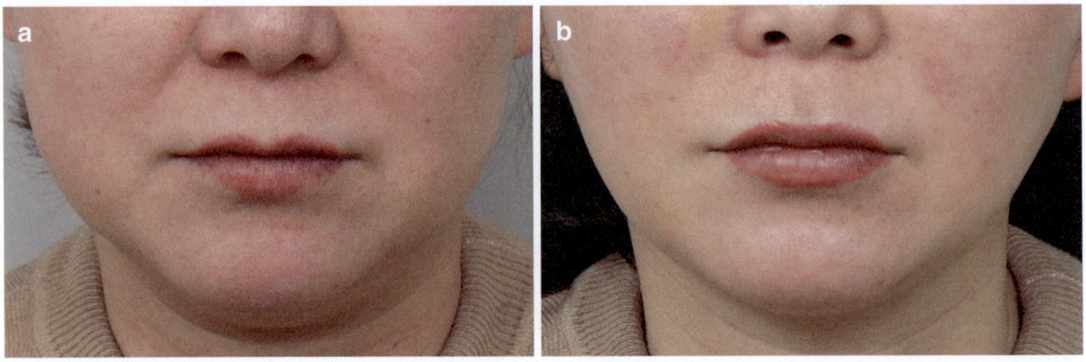

Fig. 7.17 51-year-old female patient. (**a**) Before treatment. (**b**) Combining HA filler-based lip augmentation with botox treatment for the upper lip and marionette lines provides enhanced results

7.5 Complications

The most common complications encountered during perioral wrinkle rejuvenation are bruising and swelling. This is particularly true when using a cannula, as the injectable target layer is typically the deep dermis or subcutaneous layer. Due to fat atrophy, there is an increased risk of trauma to the dermal plexus located just beneath the deep dermis. Therefore, in patients requiring more aggressive wrinkle correction, the potential for swelling and bruising must be clearly explained prior to the procedure (Fig. 7.18).

The superior labial artery, which supplies blood to the upper lip, is located between the mucosa and the orbicularis oris muscle (OOM), making it anatomically separate from the target injection layer. Similarly, the marionette line lies medial to the facial artery, resulting in a relatively low risk of vascular occlusion. Although the mouth corner wrinkles are closer to the course of the facial artery, the artery runs in a deeper plane than the zygomaticus major muscle. Therefore, as long as the injection is carefully administered just below the deep dermis, the risk of complications is minimal.

However, because these techniques involve injecting near the dermis, there is a risk of nodule formation. In the case of HA fillers, such nodules can be easily resolved using hyaluronidase. In contrast, nodules caused by biostimulators are more challenging to manage. A common solution involves injecting non-cross-linked HA around the nodule to promote particle hydrolysis, combined with the application of radiofrequency to induce thermal degradation. Nevertheless, this method is not typically resolved in a single session and may require multiple repeated treatments.

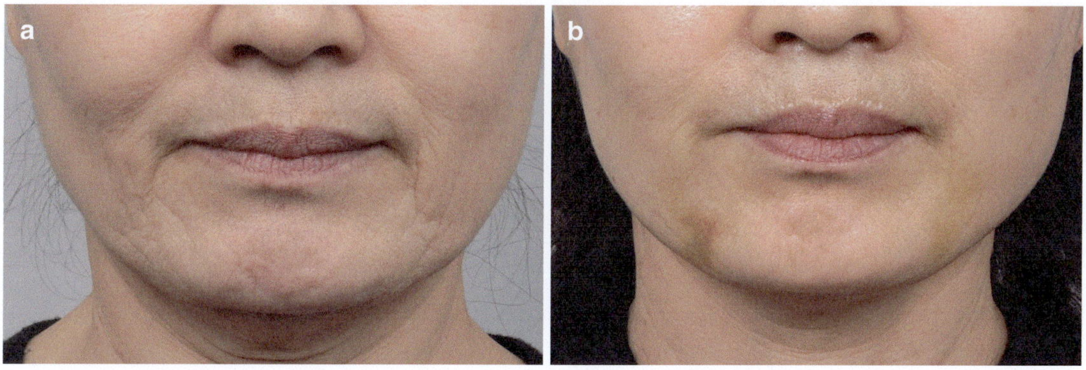

Fig. 7.18 60-year-old female patient. (**a**) Before treatment. (**b**) Case of fine wrinkle improvement around the mouth using PLLA. The patient reported bruising around the mouth at the 2-week follow-up

7.6 Conclusion

Before treatment, it is important to assess the patient's skin condition and degree of volume loss and to identify the primary contributing factors. Prioritizing the appropriate treatment sequence based on these findings leads to higher patient satisfaction. Additionally, habitual facial muscle use and occupational factors may influence outcomes, so it is essential to explain to patients that a single treatment session may not provide complete correction and that repeated sessions may be needed for both improvement and prevention.

From the practitioner's perspective, among the many available treatment options, it is important to choose the methods they are most skilled with and that best match the patient's needs. Since the causes of perioral wrinkles are multifactorial and the mouth area is one of the most noticeable and concerning regions for patients, a combination of different treatments is often the most appropriate strategy for achieving meaningful improvement.

References

1. Fujimura T, Hotta M. The preliminary study of the relationship between facial movements and wrinkle formation. Skin Res Technol. 2012;18(2):219–24. https://doi.org/10.1111/j.1600-0846.2011.00557.x. Epub 25 Aug 2011.
2. Cannarozzo G, Fazia G, Bennardo L, Tamburi F, Amoruso GF, Del Duca E, Nisticò SP. A new 675 nm laser device in the treatment of facial aging: a prospective observational study. Photobiomod Photomed Laser Surg. 2021;39(2):118–22. https://doi.org/10.1089/photob.2020.4908. Epub 15 Jan 2021.
3. Varani J, Dame MK, Rittie L, Fligiel SE, Kang S, Fisher GJ, Voorhees JJ. Decreased collagen production in chronologically aged skin: roles of age-dependent alteration in fibroblast function and defective mechanical stimulation. Am J Pathol. 2006;168(6):1861–8. https://doi.org/10.2353/ajpath.2006.051302.
4. Lee DH, Oh JH, Chung JH. Glycosaminoglycan and proteoglycan in skin aging. J Dermatol Sci. 2016;83(3):174–81. https://doi.org/10.1016/j.jdermsci.2016.05.016. Epub 27 May 2016.
5. Kuwazuru O, Miyamoto K, Yoshikawa N, Imayama S. Skin wrinkling morphology changes suddenly in the early 30s. Skin Res Technol. 2012;18(4):495–503. https://doi.org/10.1111/j.1600-0846.2011.00598.x. Epub 11 Jan 2012.
6. Chien AL, Qi J, Cheng N, Do TT, Mesfin M, Egbers R, Xie W, Chow C, Chubb H, Sachs D, Voorhees J, Kang S. Perioral wrinkles are associated with female gender, aging, and smoking: development of a gender-specific photonumeric scale. J Am Acad Dermatol. 2016;74(5):924–30. https://doi.org/10.1016/j.jaad.2015.11.042. Epub 20 Jan 2016.
7. Paes EC, Teepen HJ, Koop WA, Kon M. Perioral wrinkles: histologic differences between men and women. Aesthet Surg J. 2009;29(6):467–72. https://doi.org/10.1016/j.asj.2009.08.018.
8. Choi YJ, Kim JS, Gil YC, Phetudom T, Kim HJ, Tansatit T, Hu KS. Anatomical considerations regarding the location and boundary of the depressor anguli oris muscle with reference to botulinum toxin injection. Plast Reconstr Surg. 2014;134(5):917–21. https://doi.org/10.1097/PRS.0000000000000589.
9. Hong GW, Wong S, Yoon SE, Wan J, Yi KH. Anatomical-based diagnosis and filler injection techniques: marionette line (static labiomandibular fold). J Dermatolog Treat. 2025;36(1):2452954. https://doi.org/10.1080/09546634.2025.2452954. Epub 2 Feb 2025.

8 New Techniques for Ultrasound-Guided Hyaluronic Acid Filler Injection

Benjamin Ascher, Audrey Melin, and Won Lee

8.1 Introduction

The introduction of hyaluronic acid (HA) filler injections has significantly transformed modern aesthetic medicine, offering a minimally invasive alternative to traditional cosmetic surgery. This injectable therapy, capable of restoring skin texture, volume, and contouring facial structures within minutes, ranks among the most widely performed aesthetic treatments, alongside botulinum toxin injections [1]. A key advantage of HA fillers is their reversibility, as they can be enzymatically degraded by hyaluronidase, making them a safer option compared to other fillers. However, despite their safety profile, HA fillers are not without risks. Severe complications can arise if the filler is inadvertently injected into blood vessels, potentially leading to vascular occlusion and tissue necrosis and blindness [2].

To minimize these risks, a thorough understanding of facial anatomy, particularly the vascular network, is essential. However, due to individual anatomical variations, it is nearly impossible to completely avoid all vascular structures during injection. Consequently, real-time visualization of internal facial structures has become an indispensable tool in filler procedures.

Among available imaging techniques, ultrasound has emerged as the most effective tool for real-time vascular assessment. While other imaging modalities, such as computed tomography (CT) or magnetic resonance imaging (MRI), can provide valuable anatomical insights, they lack the dynamic, real-time capability necessary for guided injections. In contrast, Doppler ultrasound is widely utilized for vascular mapping, allowing practitioners to identify critical blood vessels and enhance procedural safety [3].

Beyond pre-procedural assessment, ultrasound also plays a vital role in the detection and management of vascular complications. In cases of vascular compromise, ultrasound enables the precise, targeted administration of hyaluronidase, facilitating rapid filler dissolution in high-risk areas [4].

However, despite its advantages, real-time ultrasound guidance during filler injections traditionally requires an additional practitioner, leading to various practical constraints. However, recent technological advancements have led to the development of an innovative device that integrates an ultrasound probe with a finger attachment, allowing single-operator use during filler injection. This breakthrough enhances procedural efficiency and safety, making

B. Ascher
Think-In Tech, Paris, France

A. Melin
CHU Henri Mondor, Paris, France

W. Lee (✉)
Yonsei E1 Plastic Surgery Clinic, Anyang, Kyonggi-do, Korea (Republic of)

W. Lee (ed.), *Innovative Injectable Techniques in Minimally Invasive Aesthetics*,
https://doi.org/10.1007/978-981-95-2161-6_8

ultrasound-guided injections more accessible in everyday aesthetic practice.

This chapter aims to explore the existing ultrasound techniques in aesthetic medicine, strategies for identifying key vascular structures and layers, as well as the latest innovations in real-time ultrasound-guided filler procedures.

8.2 Practical Application of Ultrasound in Aesthetic Medicine

8.2.1 Forehead and Glabellar Filler Injection

Achieving aesthetically pleasing and safe results in forehead augmentation requires precise and even distribution of hyaluronic acid fillers. However, due to the vascular complexity of this region, thorough anatomical knowledge and careful injection planning are essential. The forehead and glabellar region contain critical arteries that must be carefully identified before injection: the supratrochlear artery, the supraorbital artery, and the frontal branch of the superficial temporal artery.

Among these, the supratrochlear artery (Fig. 8.1) is of particular concern, as it has a direct connection to the ophthalmic artery. This anatomical feature makes the glabellar region highly vulnerable to vascular complications, including retrograde embolization, which can lead to severe adverse effects such as blindness [5].

To minimize risks, vascular mapping using ultrasound is highly recommended before forehead filler procedures (Fig. 8.2). Doppler ultrasound allows practitioners to visualize and assess the location and depth of critical vascular structures. After confirming the vascular locations, the safest technique involves creating an entry point above the eyebrow, allowing for precise filler placement while avoiding major blood vessels [6].

8.2.2 Nose Filler Injection

Injecting hyaluronic acid filler in the nasal area is a commonly performed non-surgical rhinoplasty procedure.

While minimally invasive, it carries a significant risk of vascular complications, particularly ocular complications, due to the dorsal nasal artery. This artery is of high clinical relevance as it connects directly to the ophthalmic artery, increasing the potential for vascular occlusion and blindness [7].

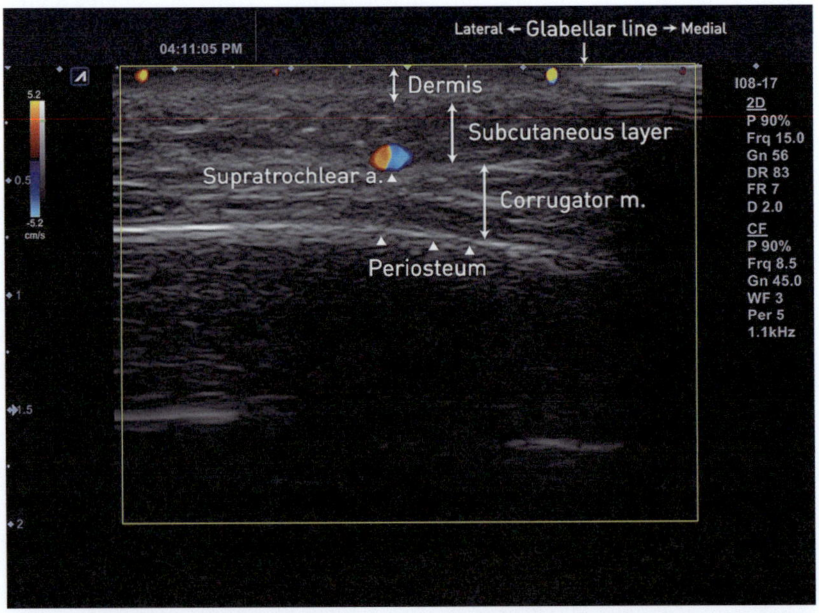

Fig. 8.1 Supratrochlear artery located in the subcutaneous fat layer

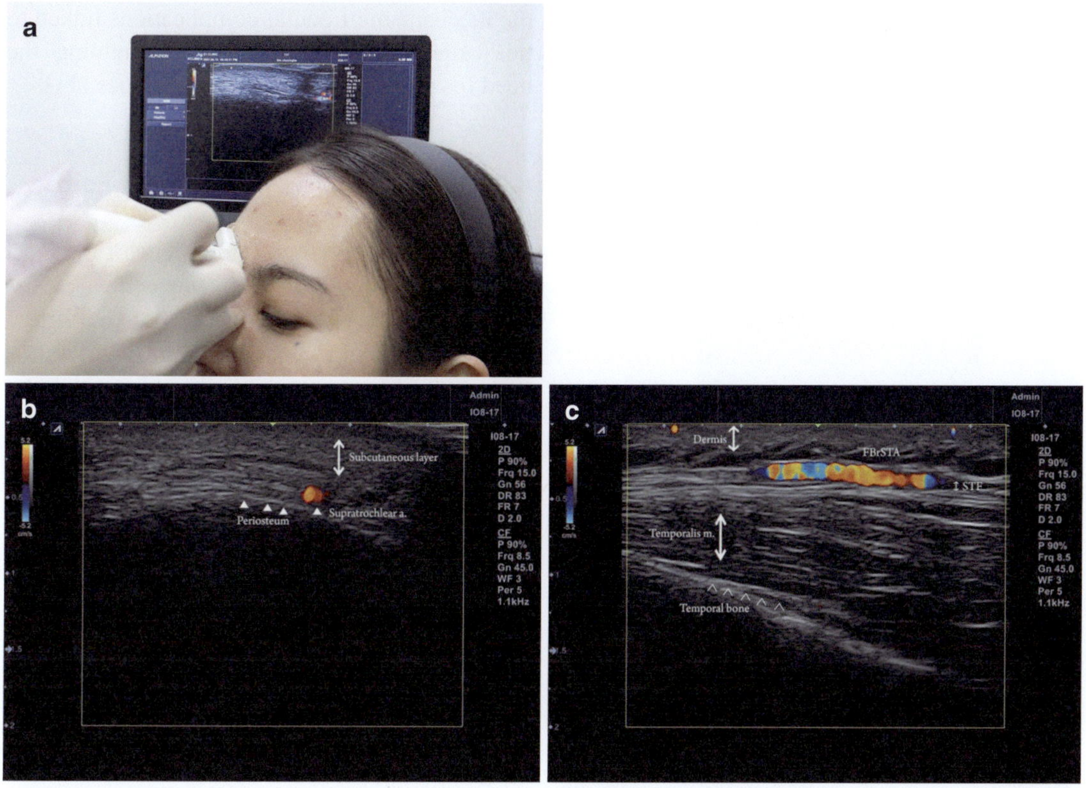

Fig. 8.2 Ultrasound-Guided Assessment Before Forehead Treatment. (**a**) Ultrasound imaging in Doppler mode at medial forehead. (**b**) Supratrochlear artery. (**c**) Identification of the superficial temporal artery at lateral forehead

To mitigate these risks and enhance procedural safety, ultrasound-guided vascular mapping should be a standard practice prior to injection. This pre-procedural assessment allows practitioners to identify the precise course of the dorsal nasal artery and other critical vessels, reducing the risk of intravascular injection and subsequent complications (Fig. 8.3) [8].

8.2.3 Temples Filler Injection

The temple region consists of multiple anatomical layers, making ultrasound guidance a valuable tool for precise filler placement (Fig. 8.4).

Hyaluronic acid (HA) fillers can be injected at different depths, including the following:

- The subcutaneous fat layer
- The interfascial space (between the superficial temporal fascia (STF) and deep temporal fascia (DTF)) [9]
- The deep periosteal layer (injections placed directly onto the bone)

For temple injections, a medium-viscosity hyaluronic acid filler is typically used, as shown in Table 8.1, Lorient No. 4 is preferred for this procedure.

By identifying anatomical layers, ultrasound guidance considerably improves injection safety and precision in this particular area.

While the deep-layer injection technique (advancing a needle until it contacts bone) is widely used, it poses a significant risk of vascular complications. The deep temporal artery, a branch of the maxillary artery, runs within this region, making intravascular injection a potential hazard [10]. Recent studies have also investigated the mechanism of ocular complications linked to this arterial pathway, further highlighting the need for meticulous injection techniques [11].

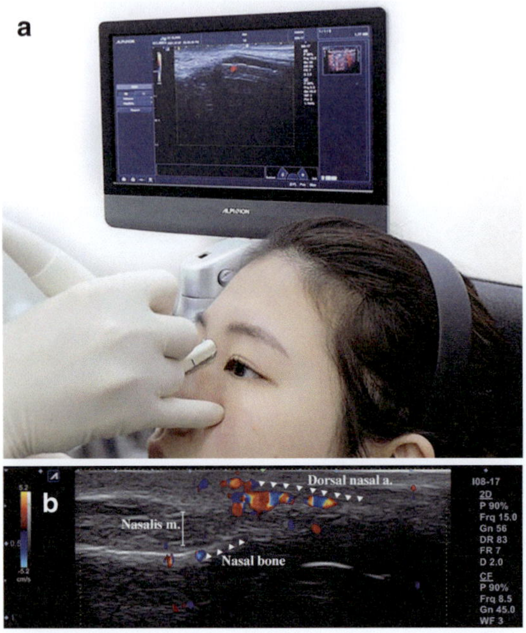

Fig. 8.3 Ultrasound-guided nose filler injection. (**a**) Ultrasound assessment performed prior to a nose filler injection. (**b**) Ultrasound visualization of the dorsal nasal artery, highlighting its course in relation to the nasal bone and surrounding soft tissues

8.2.4 Correction of Nasolabial Folds

Correction of nasolabial folds is one of the most commonly performed filler procedures across both Eastern and Western practices. The formation of nasolabial folds is linked to multiple factors such as sagging of the nasolabial fat compartments, loss of deep medial cheek fat (DMCF) leading to pseudoptosis, and decreased dermal elasticity due to aging [12, 13]. Furthermore, it is noted that lip elevators attach to the dermal layer around the nasolabial folds, and repeated muscle movements contribute to the formation of nasolabial folds [14].

A key anatomical feature in this region is Ristow's space, located between the DMCF and the periosteum. Injecting HA filler into this space is a critical step in achieving natural and effective NLF correction.

One of the primary safety concerns in this area is the facial artery, which often courses within the subcutaneous layer. Given its relatively large diameter and variable location, ultrasound guidance is highly recommended to reduce the risk of

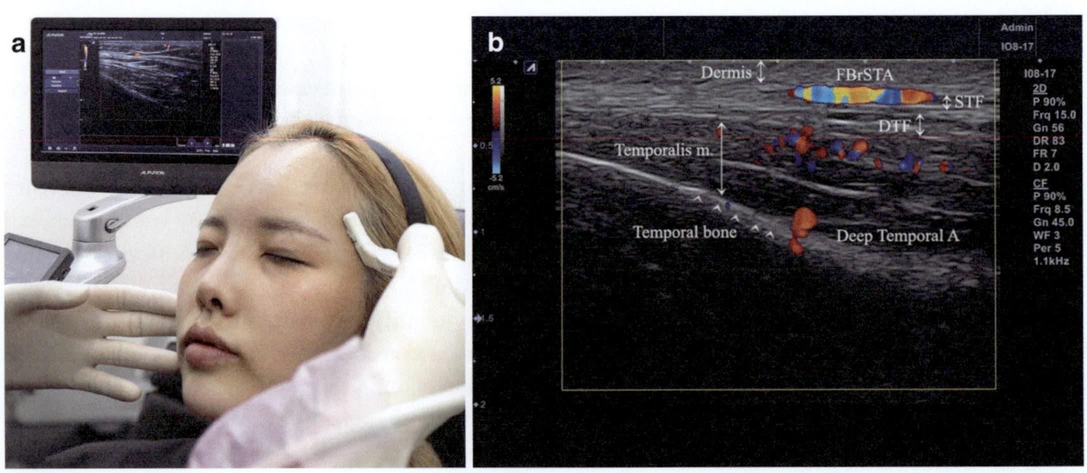

Fig. 8.4 Ultrasound imaging of the temporal region. (**a**) Pre-procedural ultrasound assessment of the temple area before filler injection, illustrating the use of real-time imaging for anatomical visualization. (**b**) Ultrasound findings highlighting key anatomical structures, including the superficial and deep temporal arteries, temporalis muscle, and temporal bone, providing critical guidance for safe and precise injection placement

Table 8.1 Rheological results of Lorient filler. The author used No. 4 in the temple area

Product	G′ (Pa)	G″ (Pa)	Complex viscosity (μ)	Tan delta	Cohesiveness (*N*)
Lorient No 2	203	41	1,673,007	0.20	0.4401
Lorient No 4	338	95	2,795,776	0.28	0.4237
Lorient No 6	413	121	3,423,232	0.29	0.4454

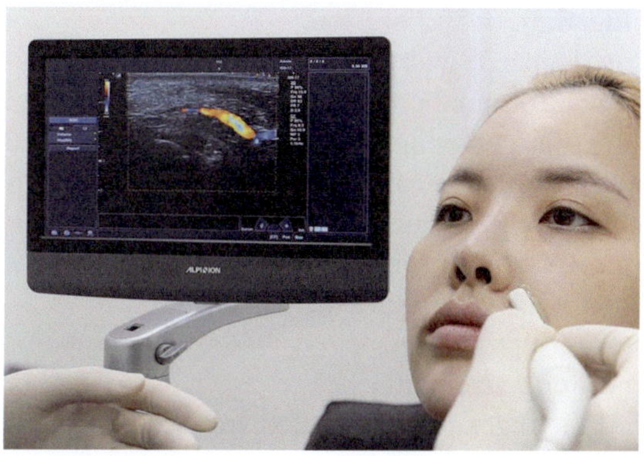

Fig. 8.5 Ultrasound findings of the facial artery around the nasolabial folds

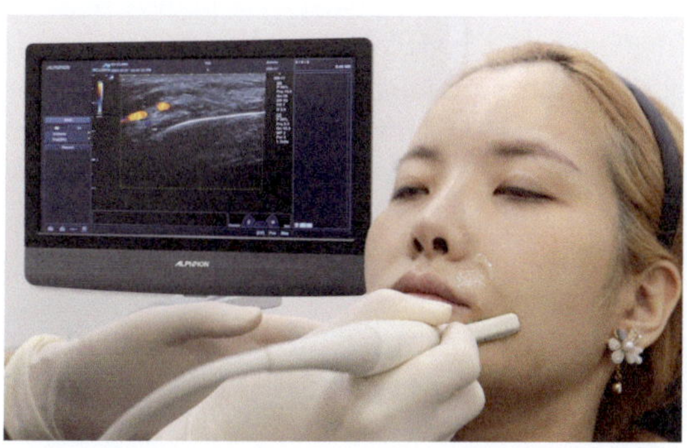

Fig. 8.6 Ultrasound findings of the inferior labial artery

vascular occlusion [15] (Fig. 8.5). By providing real-time visualization, ultrasound enables precise localization of the facial artery and allows practitioners to tailor their injection technique accordingly. This facilitates the choice between a cannula or a needle injection against the bone, enhancing both safety and precision while minimizing vascular complications.

Ultrasound imaging reveals the course of the facial artery within the subcutaneous tissue around the nasolabial folds. Its superficial location allows for both cannula-based and needle injections, with ultrasound guidance enhancing precision and minimizing the risk of vascular complications.

8.2.5 Lip Augmentation

As a result of aging process, the lip border loses definition, leading to structural loss and a less youthful appearance. Hyaluronic acid (HA) fillers can restore lip contour and enhance volume, with an ideal lip ratio of 1:1.5 (upper to lower lip) for natural aesthetics. The procedure should be performed with the patient in an upright position for optimal results.

A key safety consideration in lip augmentation is vascular anatomy, as the superior labial artery (SLA) and inferior labial artery (ILA) supply the lips. These arteries exhibit significant anatomical variability, making ultrasound mapping essential to reduce the risk of vascular occlusion (Fig. 8.6).

8.2.6 Midface Augmentation

Midface filler procedures often involve the simultaneous correction of several areas, including treating the tear trough, the anterior malar, and lateral cheek fat compartments.

Generally, an entry point is created vertically at the lateral canthus level, and the filler is injected into the desired area using a cannula.

Several key vascular structures must be identified before midface augmentation, such as the angular artery, which frequently passes through the tear trough area, the infraorbital artery, and the zygomaticofacial artery.

Due to their variable course and close proximity to injection sites, ultrasound-guided vascular mapping is strongly recommended. This minimizes the risk of inadvertent intravascular injection and enhances procedural safety (Fig. 8.7).

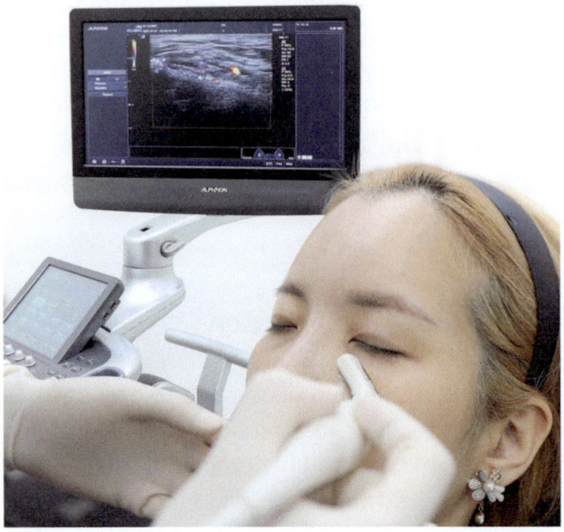

Fig. 8.7 Ultrasound findings of the angular artery in the tear trough area

8.2.7 Conclusion

The transformative impact of ultrasound-guided injection in aesthetic medicine ultrasound is becoming a cornerstone technology in aesthetic medicine, significantly improving the safety and precision of dermal filler injections. By providing real-time vascular mapping, it enables practitioners to identify key vascular structures, optimize filler placement, and minimize the risk of vascular complications.

8.3 The Birth of Finger-Held Ultrasound: SIBUS-In™ Technology

8.3.1 Introduction

Vascular complications are the most severe risks of dermal fillers, making Doppler ultrasound-guided injection a crucial safety measure [16].

However, conventional ultrasound devices typically require two or more practitioners—one to operate the ultrasound probe and the other to perform the injection—making real-time ultrasound-assisted filler procedures challenging with existing equipment.

A groundbreaking innovation, SIBUS-IN™ (Safe Injection By UltraSound), has transformed this approach by integrating an ultrasound probe into a compact, finger-held device. This technological advancement allows practitioners to use their non-dominant hand for ultrasound imaging while simultaneously performing filler injections with their dominant hand, ensuring greater precision and safety. By eliminating the need for a secondary operator, SIBUS technology streamlines procedures while enhancing accuracy and control (Fig. 8.8).

Compared with traditional linear and hockey-stick ultrasound probes, the SIBUS device offers superior ergonomics, enabling two-handed maneuverability and improved workflow efficiency. What's more, SIBUS technology minimizes the use of gel, improving both procedure accuracy and patient experience.

For optimal maneuverability, the probe is most effectively attached to either the second or fourth finger. Once secured, ultrasound gel is applied to ensure proper imaging transmission, and a sterile glove is worn to maintain aseptic conditions. The ultrasound screen, connected to the probe, is then adjusted to a high-resolution frequency of 15 MHz. Depending on the procedure, it can be configured to visualize vascular structures in Doppler mode or assess facial layers in B-mode, allowing for precise and real-time guidance (Fig. 8.9).

8.3.2 Ultrasound-Guided Temporal Injection with SIBUS

For temporal augmentation, several injection techniques can be used as follows:

- Needle injection directly onto the bone
- Cannula injection into the subcutaneous fat
- Cannula injection into the interfascial space (between the superficial temporal fascia and the deep temporal fascia) (Figs. 8.10 and 8.11)

When injecting directly onto the bone, the deep temporal artery (DTA) may sometimes be in direct contact with the periosteum at the injection

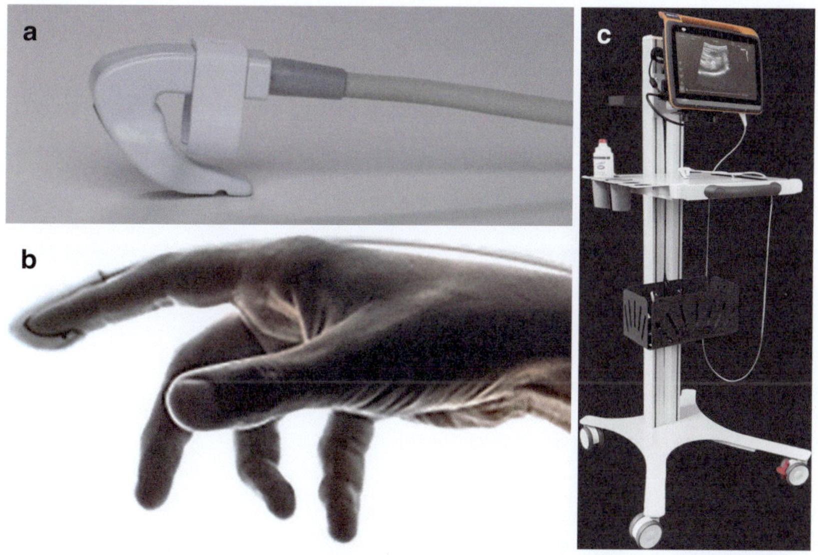

Fig. 8.8 SIBUS-IN™ (Safe Injection By UltraSound) Finger Probe Ultrasound. (**a**) SIBUS-IN Probe. (**b**) Finger-held device in practice. (**c**) Proposed device design

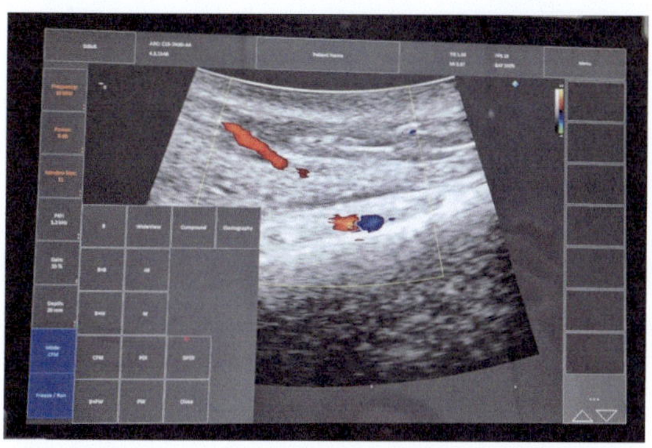

Fig. 8.9 Doppler ultrasound setting screen high-resolution 15 MHz display. The interface includes various imaging settings, such as vascular/Doppler (CFM) and B-mode, allowing for real-time assessment of blood flow dynamics. SIBUS-IN™ Technology

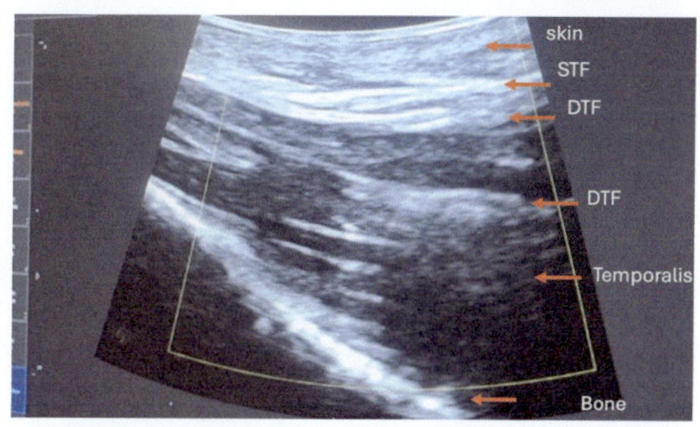

Fig. 8.10 Visualization of the anatomical planes of the temporal fossa: skin, subcutaneous fat, superficial temporal fascia (STF), deep temporal fascia (DTF) housing superficial temporal fat, temporalis muscle, and temporal bone

site, making this technique inherently risky. Even with careful aspiration before injecting, accidental intravascular injection remains a concern. The use of SIBUS technology allows real-time visualization of the deep temporal artery, enabling the practitioner to precisely adjust the injection site or modify the technique to enhance safety.

When injecting into the interfascial space, maintaining the correct anatomical plane can be challenging. The cannula may inadvertently shift into the subcutaneous fat layer or the superficial temporal fat pad (located between the two layers of the deep temporal fascia). Within the superficial temporal fat pad, practitioners must also be mindful of the middle temporal artery (MTA), which can pose additional risks.

By utilizing ultrasound guidance with SIBUS probe, practitioners can precisely confirm the cannula's or needle's position within the desired anatomical plane, ensuring safe and effective filler placement while minimizing vascular complications (Figs. 8.10, 8.11, 8.12, 8.13, and 8.14).

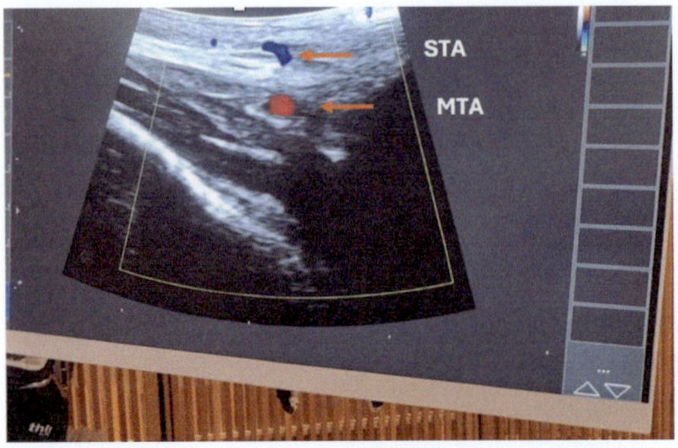

Fig. 8.11 Doppler visualization of the superficial temporal artery (STA) in subcutaneous fat and the middle temporal artery (MTA) in superficial temporal fat

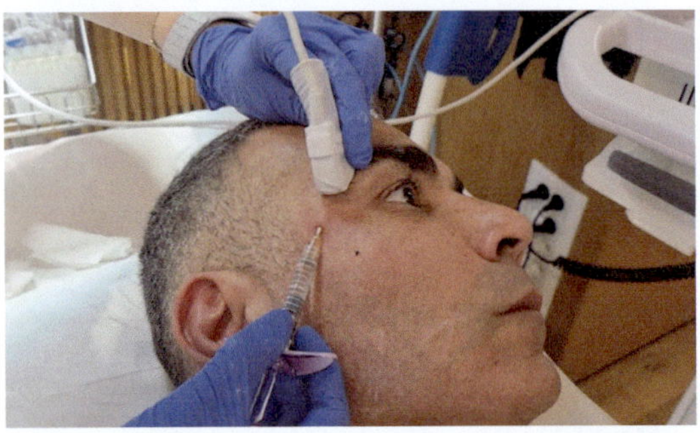

Fig. 8.12 Ultrasound-guided hyaluronic acid filler injection in the temple using SIBUS-IN™

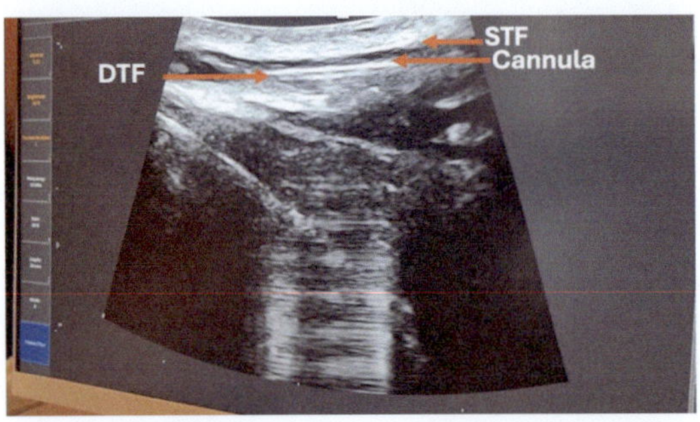

Fig. 8.13 Example of cannula injection in the interfascial space, between the superficial temporal fascia (STF) and the deep temporal fascia (DTP) using SIBUS-IN™

8.3.3 Ultrasound-Guided Nasolabial Fold Injection with SIBUS

SIBUS technology is particularly beneficial for nasolabial fold injections, where the facial artery typically courses through the subcutaneous fat layer but may also be in direct contact with the

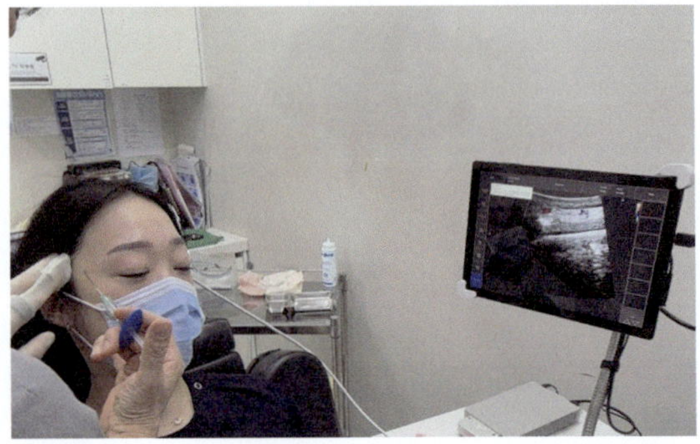

Fig. 8.14 Ultrasound-guided temporal filler injection *using SIBUS-IN™*

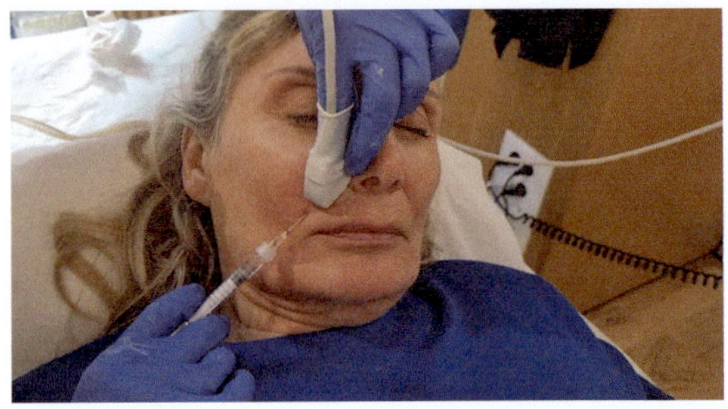

Fig. 8.15 Ultrasound-guided hyaluronic acid filler injection

bone. In the latter scenario, performing needle injections poses a significant risk of vascular complications, as inadvertent intravascular injection can occur.

Since the course of the facial artery differs not only among individuals but also between the two sides of the same face, pre-procedural vascular mapping is crucial.

Identifying the artery's precise location helps the practitioner determine the most appropriate injection technique, whether using a cannula for a safer, more controlled placement or a needle when appropriate precautions are taken [15] (Figs. 8.15, 8.16, and 8.17).

8.3.4 Ultrasound-Guided Nasal Injection with SIBUS

When performing non-surgical rhinoplasty, ultrasound can confirm the position of the dorsal nasal artery, reducing the risk of vascular occlusion. The

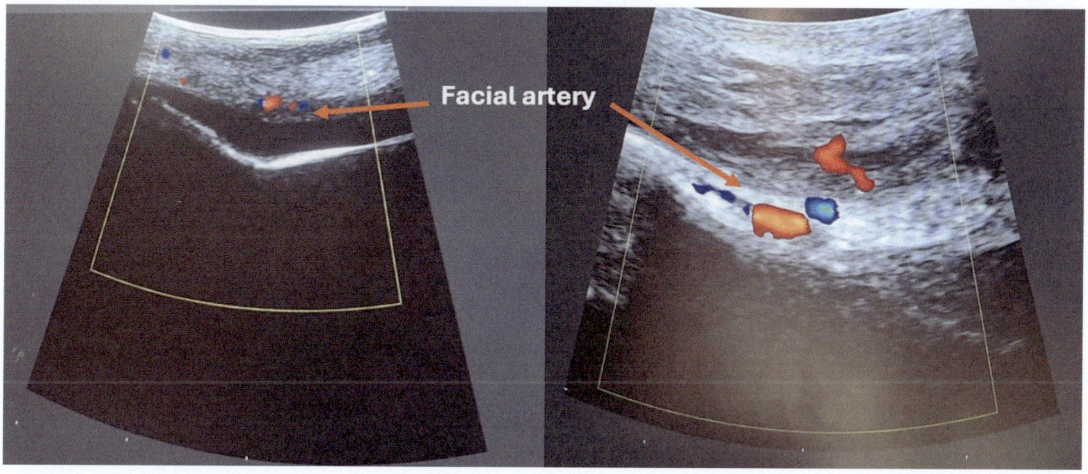

Fig. 8.16 Visualization of the facial artery running subcutaneously (on the left) and in direct contact with the bone (on the right), using SIBUS-IN™

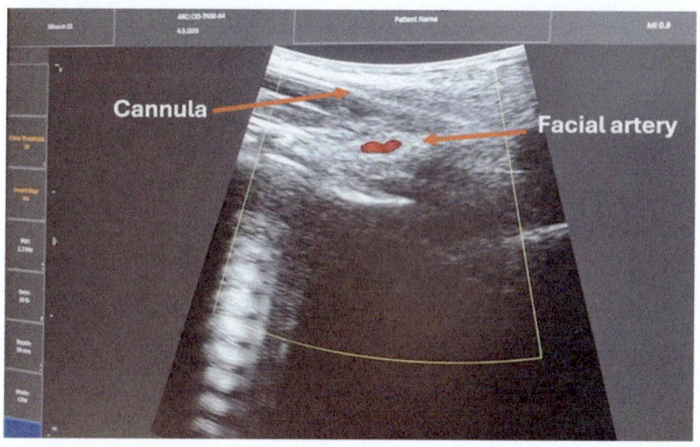

Fig. 8.17 Real-time nasolabial fold hyaluronic acid filler injection using a cannula

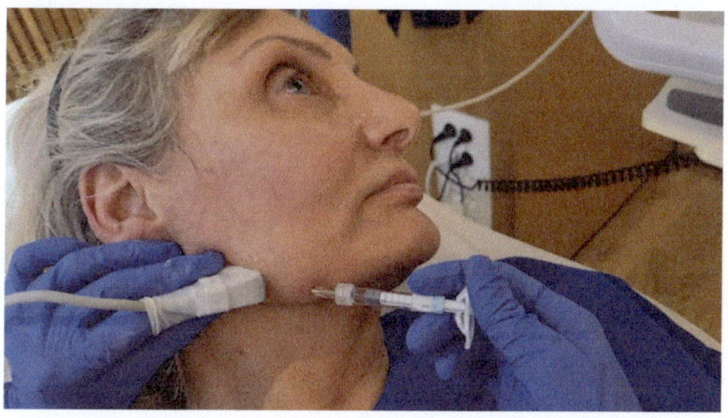

Fig. 8.18 Real-time monitoring of jawline filler injection—cannula placement of hyaluronic acid into subcutaneous fat for jawline contouring

cannula's movement can be monitored during filler placement, and the height of the nose can be precisely adjusted using the hand holding the ultrasound probe, ensuring accurate and safe filler deposition.

8.3.5 Ultrasound-Guided Jawline Injection with SIBUS

For jawline contouring, filler injections can be performed using the following:

- Needle injections (onto the mandibular angle, within masseter fibers)
- Cannula injections (into the subcutaneous fat layer)

During cannula injections, there is a risk of inadvertent displacement into the parotid gland, particularly when the cannula shifts planes. This misplacement can result in the unintended deposition of hyaluronic acid (HA) fillers or collagen stimulators within the parotid, potentially leading to ineffective clinical outcomes, unnatural aesthetic results, localized pain, and an increased risk of secondary infections or inflammatory nodes and nodules.

By utilizing SIBUS technology, practitioners can visualize the cannula's precise location in real-time, ensuring accurate, safe, and optimal placement of the injected product, thereby minimizing complications and enhancing treatment efficacy (Figs. 8.18, 8.19, and 8.20).

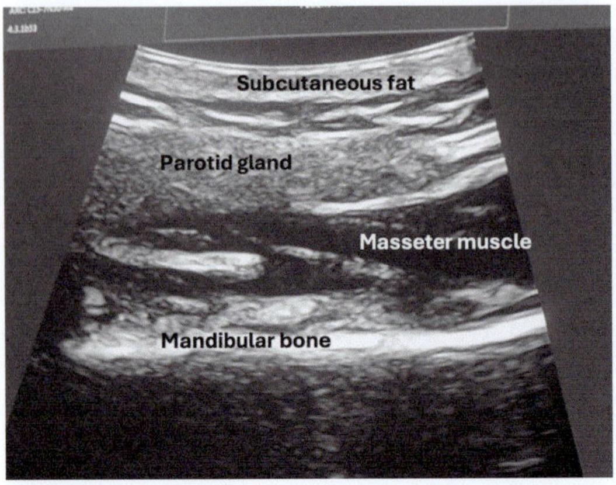

Fig. 8.19 B-mode visualization: subcutaneous fat, parotid gland, masseter muscle, and mandibular bone

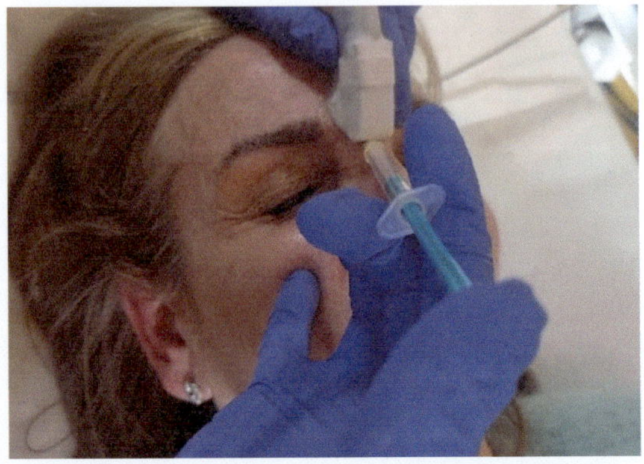

Fig. 8.21 Ultrasound-guided injection of botulinum toxin in the procerus muscle, using SIBUS-IN™

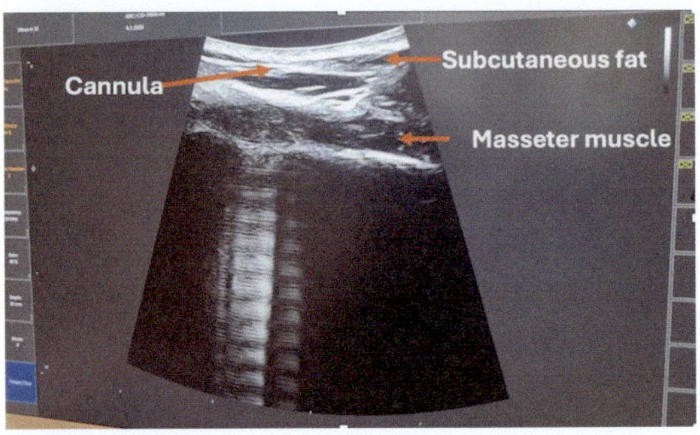

Fig. 8.20 Cannula injection of HA into subcutaneous fat for jaw contour enhancement

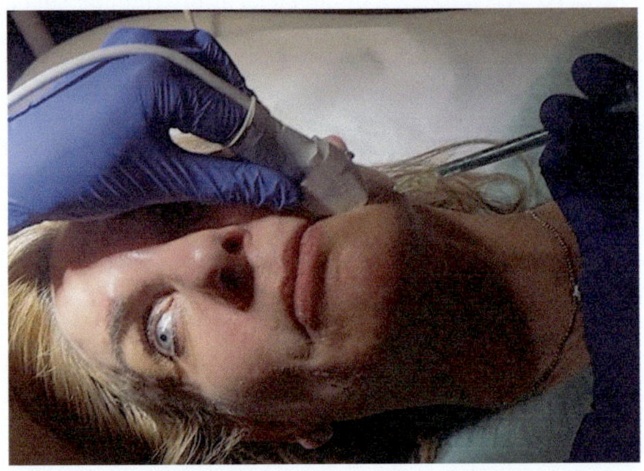

Fig. 8.22 Ultrasound-guided injection of botulinum toxin in the DAO muscle, using SIBUS-IN™

8.3.6 SIBUS Ultrasound Technology for Botulinum Toxin Injections

Beyond filler procedures, SIBUS ultrasound technology has emerged as an invaluable tool for botulinum toxin injections, significantly enhancing precision and safety. By utilizing B-mode ultrasound imaging, practitioners can directly visualize muscle layers, allowing for a more targeted and controlled injection of botulinum toxin while minimizing complications.

This technique is particularly beneficial for the following muscle groups:

- Frontalis muscle: Ensures precise placement to smooth forehead wrinkles while avoiding excessive diffusion that could lead to brow ptosis.
- Corrugator and procerus muscles: Facilitates accurate injections for glabellar line correction, reducing the risk of asymmetry or unwanted diffusion to adjacent structures (Fig. 8.21).
- Orbicularis oculi muscle: Enhances control over periorbital (crow's feet) injections.
- Depressor anguli oris (DAO) muscle: Enables more precise targeting to improve marionette lines and downturned mouth corners while minimizing toxin migration to surrounding facial muscles (depressor labii inferioris, DLI) (Fig. 8.22).
- Masseter muscle: Provides superior guidance for jawline slimming procedures, ensuring the toxin is deposited at the correct depth and within the appropriate portion of the masseter,

reducing the risk of excessive weakening or unintended effects on mastication.

By integrating ultrasound guidance, practitioners can optimize treatment precision, reduce the risk of unwanted toxin diffusion, and achieve more predictable and refined aesthetic outcome.

8.3.7 Conclusion: The transformative Impact of SIBUS-IN™ in Aesthetic Medicine

By integrating real-time ultrasound guidance into routine procedures, SIBUS-IN™ represents a technological breakthrough in aesthetic medicine.

One of the key benefits of SIBUS technology is the real-time visualization of critical structures, enabling practitioners to precisely map vascular pathways and adjust injection techniques accordingly. This minimizes the risk of intravascular injection, which can lead to vascular occlusion, tissue necrosis, and even blindness.

Beyond safety, SIBUS optimizes the placement of fillers, ensuring symmetrical, natural-looking results. Whether used for nasolabial folds, temple augmentation, midface enhancement, jaw contouring, or non-surgical rhinoplasty, this system offers an excellent precision. Its use for botulinum toxin injections also ensures targeted delivery, reducing inadvertent diffusion and maximizing treatment efficacy.

By enabling the use of a single operator, the system eliminates the need for an additional practitioner, streamlining workflow efficiency and making ultrasound-guided injections more accessible in everyday practice.

As non-surgical facial rejuvenation continues to evolve, the SIBUS-IN™ system sets a new standard of care by bridging the gap between advanced imaging and precision injections. This innovation marks a paradigm shift, enabling safer, better-controlled, and highly effective aesthetic treatments.

8.4 Conclusion

Ultrasound technology has revolutionized the safety of injectable treatments, particularly hyaluronic acid fillers. The introduction of finger-mounted ultrasound technology (SIBUS-IN™) represents a major breakthrough in aesthetic medicine, providing real-time visualization, enhanced safety, and greater procedural precision. Unlike conventional ultrasound systems, this innovation allows practitioners to inject with both hands, eliminating the need for an additional operator or the inconvenience of holding a probe. Additionally, it optimizes product use by reducing the required quantity of filler, ensuring more efficient and controlled injections. By seamlessly integrating ultrasound guidance into routine filler and toxin procedures, injectors can achieve safer, more precise, and aesthetically superior results, while streamlining the overall treatment process.

References

1. Aesthetic Plastic Surgery National Databank Statistics 2020–2021. Aesthet Surg J. 2022;42(Suppl 1):1–18.
2. DeLorenzi C. Complications of injectable fillers, Part 2: Vascular complications. Aesthet Surg J. 2014;34(4):584–600.
3. Schelke LW, Decates TS, Velthuis PJ. Ultrasound to improve the safety of hyaluronic acid filler treatments. J Cosmet Dermatol. 2018;17(6):1019–24.
4. Schelke LW, Velthuis PJ, Decates T, Kadouch J, Alfertshofer M, Frank K, Cotofana S. Ultrasound-guided targeted vs regional flooding: a comparative study for improving the clinical outcome in soft tissue filler vascular adverse event management. Aesthet Surg J. 2023;43(1):86–96. https://doi.org/10.1093/asj/sjac227.
5. Lee W, Moon HJ, Kim JS, Yang EJ. Safe glabellar wrinkle correction with soft tissue filler using Doppler ultrasound. Aesthet Surg J. 2021;41(9):1081–9. https://doi.org/10.1093/asj/sjaa197.
6. Lee W, Kim TH, Yang EJ. Mapping high-risk arteries using Doppler ultrasound for forehead contouring in Korean patients. Dermatol Surg. 2024;50(11):1029–33. https://doi.org/10.1097/DSS.0000000000004292.
7. Lee W, Koh IS, Oh W, et al. Ocular complications of soft tissue filler injections: a review of literature. 2020;19(4):772–81.

8. Lee W, Kim JS, Oh W, Koh IS, Yang EJ. Nasal dorsum augmentation using soft tissue filler injection. J Cosmet Dermatol. 2019;
9. Lee W, Park JW, Yang EJ. Temple augmentation by injecting a hyaluronic acid filler between the superficial and deep temporal fasciae. J Cosmet Dermatol. 2022;
10. Lee W, Moon HJ, Kim MS, Cheon GW, Yang EJ. Pre-injection ultrasound scanning for treating temporal hollowing. J Cosmet Dermatol. 2022;21(6):2420–5.
11. Sheth NT, Hauck EF, Bibawy JM, Lee IT, Dermarkarian CR, Saadat D, Woodward JA. Risk of blindness from temple filler injections: investigating vascular anastomoses between the deep temporal and ophthalmic arteries. Ophthalmic Plast Reconstr Surg. 2025; https://doi.org/10.1097/IOP.0000000000002897.
12. Ezure T, Amano S. Involvement of upper cheek sagging in nasolabial fold formation. Skin Res Technol. 2012;18(3):259–64. https://doi.org/10.1111/j.1600-0846.2011.00567.x.
13. Rohrich RJ, Pessa JE, Ristow B. The youthful cheek and the deep medial fat compartment. Plast Reconstr Surg. 2008;121(6):2107–12. https://doi.org/10.1097/PRS.0b013e31817123c6.
14. Beer GM, Manestar M, Mihic-Probst D. The causes of the nasolabial crease: a histomorphological study. Clin Anat. 2013;26(2):196–203. https://doi.org/10.1002/ca.22100.
15. Lee W, Kim JS, Moon HJ, Yang EJ. A safe Doppler ultrasound-guided method for nasolabial fold correction with hyaluronic acid filler. Aesthet Surg J. 2021;41(6):NP486–92.
16. Lee W. Hyaluronic acid filler injection guided by Doppler ultrasound. Arch Plast Surg. 2023;50(4):348–53. https://doi.org/10.1055/s-0043-1770078.

9 Artificial Intelligence and Injectables in Cosmetic Dermatology

Diala Haykal and Won Lee

9.1 Introduction

Artificial intelligence (AI) is revolutionizing medicine, with the global healthcare AI market projected to reach $45 billion by 2026 [1]. This unprecedented growth is transforming cosmetic dermatology, offering unparalleled precision, efficiency, and personalization in injectable treatments. The potential for AI to revolutionize injectables spans from data-driven decision-making to groundbreaking research applications, enabling a new era of innovation in aesthetic medicine [2, 3]. This chapter explores the intersection of AI and injectables, focusing on personalized care, precision diagnostics, streamlined treatment processes, post-treatment monitoring, and ethical frameworks to ensure safe and effective adoption in clinical practice. Injectables have long been a cornerstone of cosmetic dermatology, with demand growing exponentially over the past decade. This demand, coupled with the increasing complexity of aesthetic procedures, has necessitated the adoption of advanced tools and methodologies to optimize results [4]. AI has emerged as a game changer in this regard, offering the ability to analyze vast datasets, predict outcomes with remarkable accuracy, and guide clinicians with real-time feedback. Beyond its technical capabilities, AI also holds the promise of democratizing access to high-quality aesthetic care, reducing variability in outcomes, and fostering a more patient-centric approach [2].

The role of AI in cosmetic dermatology is multifaceted (Table 9.1). From assisting in initial consultations to predicting long-term outcomes, AI has the potential to touch every aspect of the patient journey [5]. By combining the expertise of clinicians with the analytical power of AI, the field is poised to achieve unprecedented levels of precision, safety, and efficiency. However, this integration is not without its challenges. Issues such as data privacy, algorithmic bias, and the need for comprehensive regulatory frameworks must be addressed to fully realize the benefits of AI in injectables (Figs. 9.1 and 9.2 illustrate the key areas of AI influence and the workflow process, respectively) [6].

D. Haykal
Centre Médical Laser Palaiseau, Palaiseau, France

W. Lee (✉)
Yonsei E1 Plastic Surgery Clinic,
Anyang, Kyonggi-do, Korea (Republic of)

W. Lee (ed.), *Innovative Injectable Techniques in Minimally Invasive Aesthetics*,
https://doi.org/10.1007/978-981-95-2161-6_9

Table 9.1 Examples of AI technologies in aesthetic dermatology

Company	Device	Software	Measurements	AI
Canfield	Vectra H2, Visia Skin Analysis	Face reveal, RBX technology	Spots, wrinkles, texture, pore	Simulate 3D
QuantifiCare	LifeViz Mini Face	Facial shape, pore, oiliness	Facial angles,	Automatic image organization
Miravex	Antera 3D	Full 3D image	Wrinkle, texture, pore, volume	Analysis of aesthetic treatments
FotoFinder	ATBM Master	Automated detection	Hair and scalp analysis	Automated analysis
Aram Huvis	AI Scalp Grader	Automated hair analysis	Scalp assessment	Scalp photo

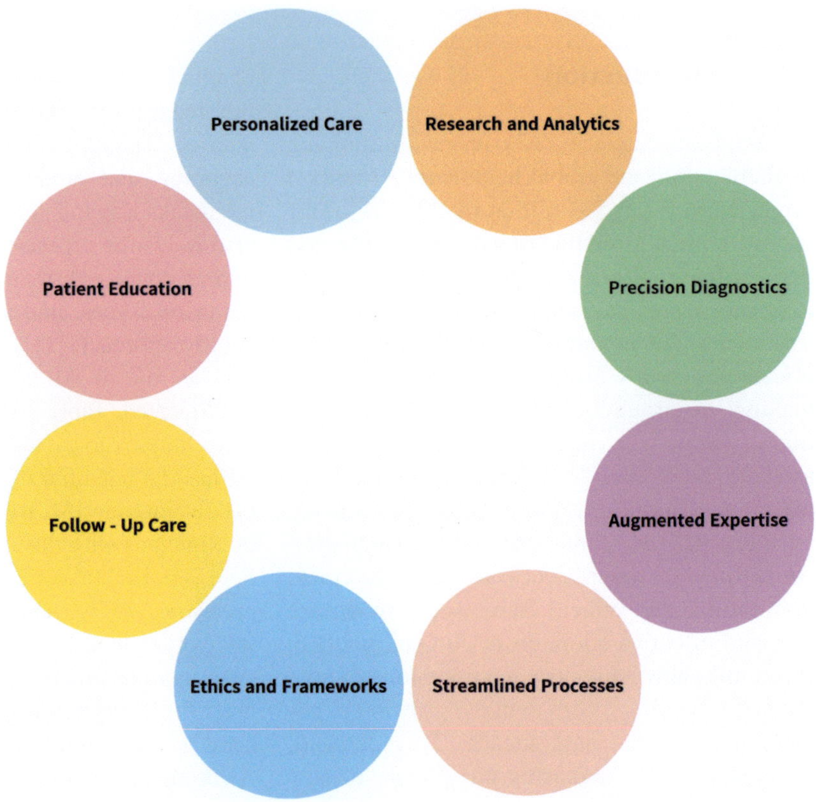

Fig. 9.1 Key areas of AI influence

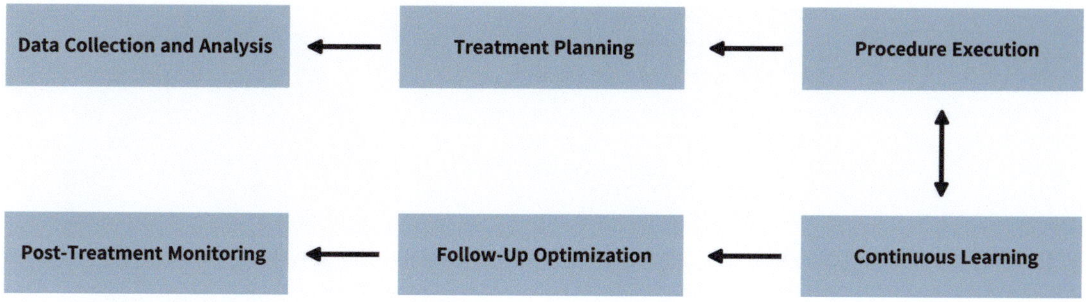

Fig. 9.2 Workflow process

9.2 Historical Context and Evolution

The use of injectables in cosmetic dermatology dates back several decades, initially focused on addressing facial wrinkles and volume loss. Early techniques relied heavily on manual precision and clinician expertise, with limited tools available for advanced diagnostics or personalized planning [7]. Over time, advancements in imaging, 3D modeling, and algorithmic analysis laid the groundwork for the integration of AI into aesthetic medicine. The evolution from simple dermal fillers to sophisticated injectable formulations designed for specific anatomical and dynamic needs reflects the growing complexity of the field. AI represents the next frontier, enabling clinicians to move beyond intuition and anecdotal experience to data-driven decision-making [8].

9.3 Personalized Care: Enhancing Individual Outcomes

One of the most profound impacts of AI in cosmetic dermatology lies in its ability to provide hyper-personalized care. By utilizing algorithms trained on extensive datasets, AI can analyze patient-specific factors such as skin type and texture, anatomical structure derived from 3D imaging, and genetic predispositions affecting treatment response [9]. For instance, AI systems can analyze 3D scans of a patient's face to predict the ideal filler type, volume, and precise injection sites to achieve natural results tailored to the patient's unique facial anatomy. These systems take into account dynamic facial expressions, offering a holistic approach to volumetric restoration [10, 11].

Furthermore, AI-powered visualization tools now allow patients to see projected results before undergoing treatment, bridging the communication gap between patient expectations and achievable outcomes (Figs. 9.3, 9.4, 9.5, 9.6, 9.7, and 9.8). Such tools also empower clinicians by providing a simulated roadmap for treatment, reducing the likelihood of errors and ensuring higher satisfaction rates among patients [12, 13].

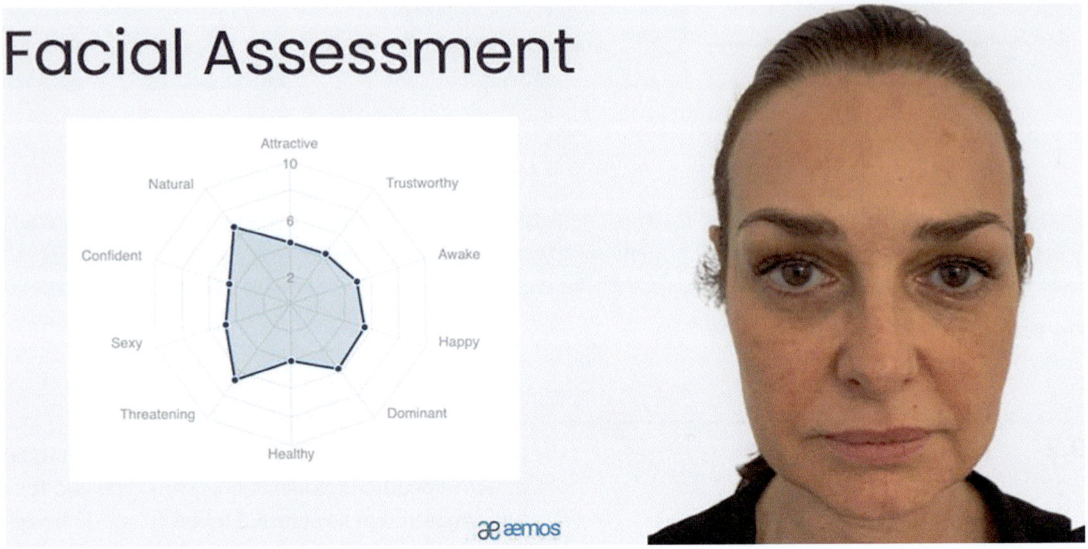

Fig. 9.3 Facial analysis by AI program. (Provided Aemos GmbH)

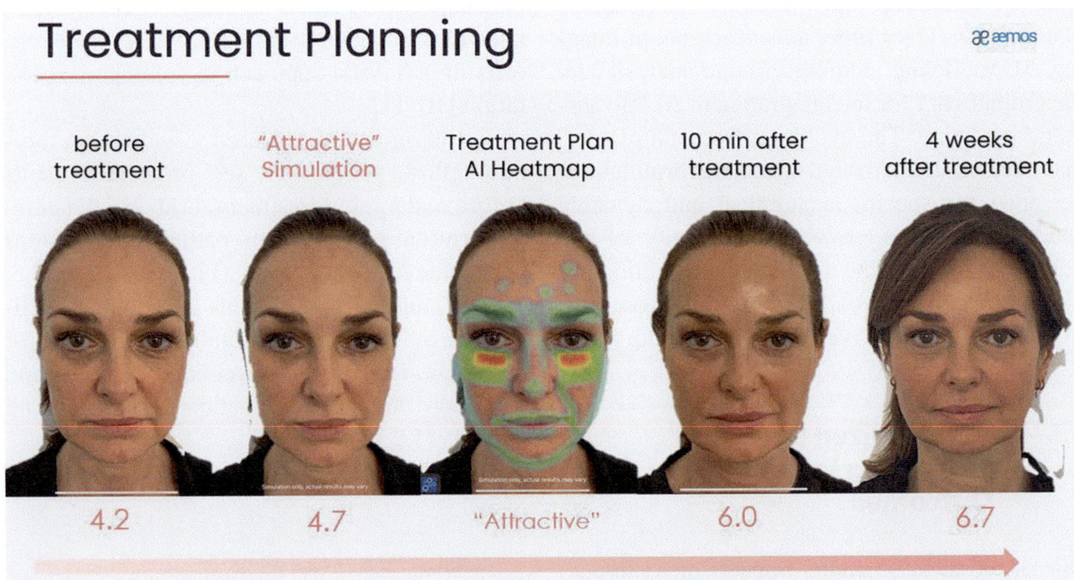

Fig. 9.4 Before and after the injection of 5 mL of hyaluronic acid and botulinum toxin injection into the forehead and around the mouth according to the AI's proposal. The attractive score reached 6.0 immediately after the procedure, up from 4.2. (Provided Aemos GmbH)

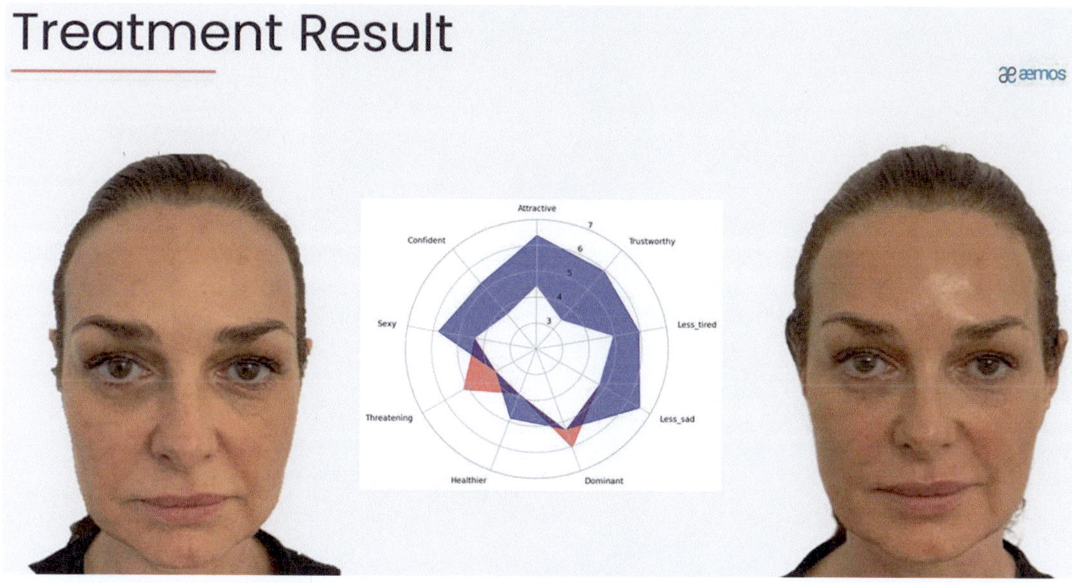

Fig. 9.5 Assessment after injection. (Provided Aemos GmbH)

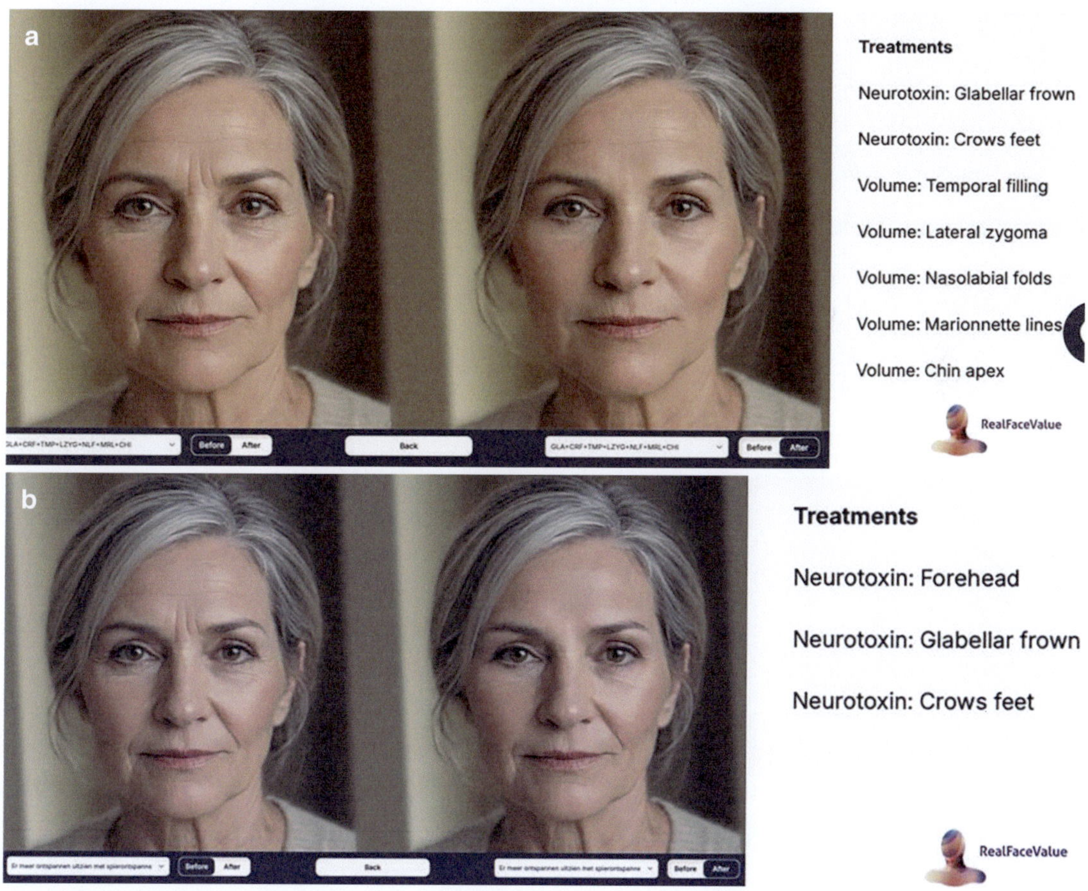

Fig. 9.6 AI simulation images. (**a**) Botulinum toxin and filler injection. (**b**) Botulinum toxin injection. (Provided RealFaceValue B.V.)

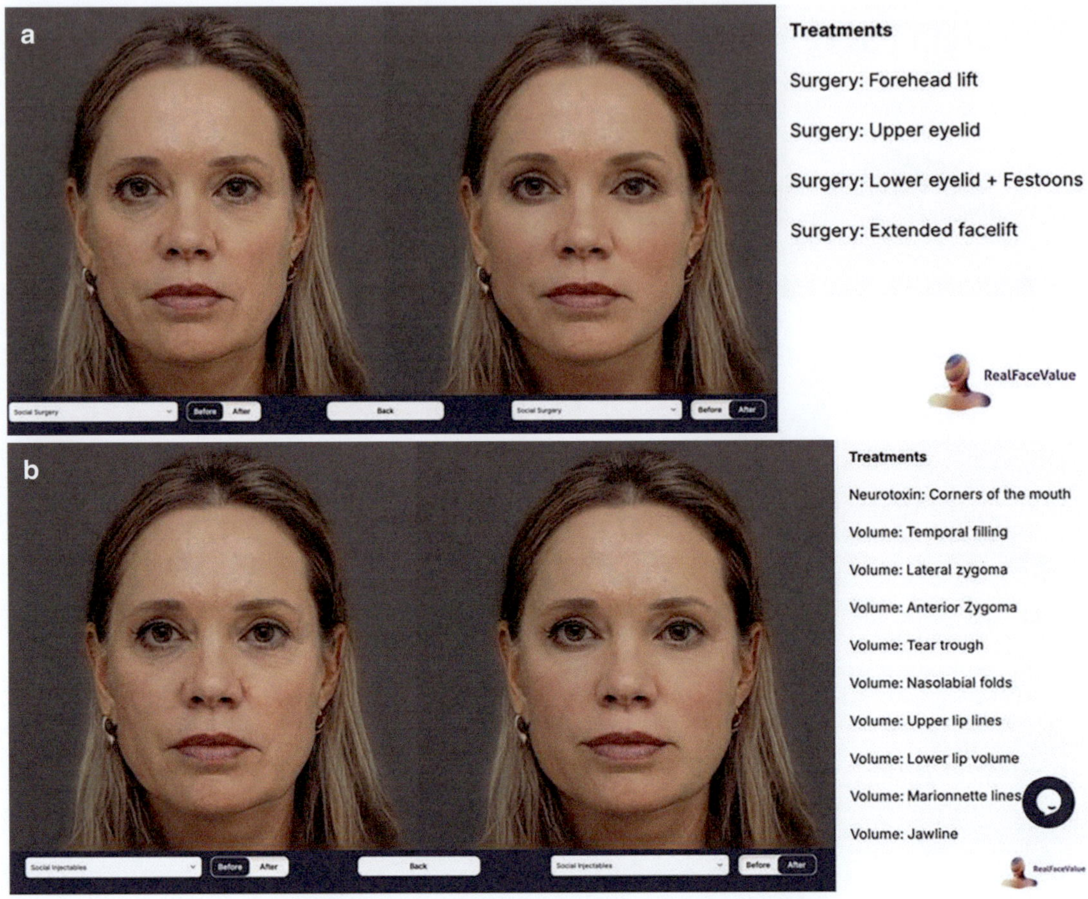

Fig. 9.7 AI simulation images. (**a**) Plastic surgery. (**b**) Injection. (Provided RealFaceValue B.V.)

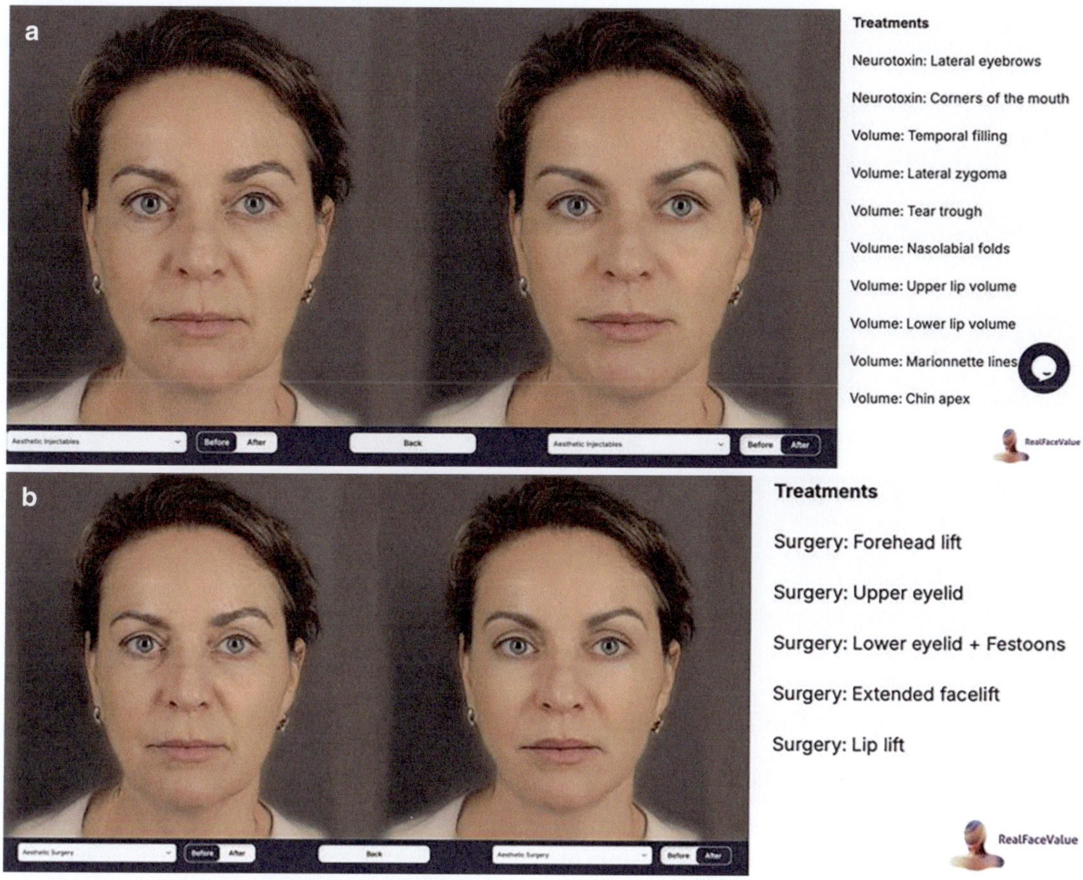

Fig. 9.8 AI simulation images. (**a**) Injection. (**b**) Plastic surgery. (Provided RealFaceValue B.V.)

9.4 Precision in Diagnostics

Accurate diagnostics are at the core of effective injectable treatments. AI enhances this precision by leveraging advanced imaging technologies and machine learning algorithms. For example, facial mapping technologies can identify subtle asymmetries or volume deficits that may not be apparent during a manual assessment (Fig. 9.9). High-resolution imaging, combined with AI analytics, enables clinicians to develop highly customized treatment plans [14].

Additionally, AI can aid in detecting underlying anatomical challenges, such as vascular networks, ensuring safer procedures. Real-time feedback from AI-enabled devices during injections minimizes risks such as vascular occlusion and overfilling. This combination of diagnostic precision and real-time guidance represents a paradigm shift in how injectables are administered, offering unprecedented levels of accuracy and safety [15].

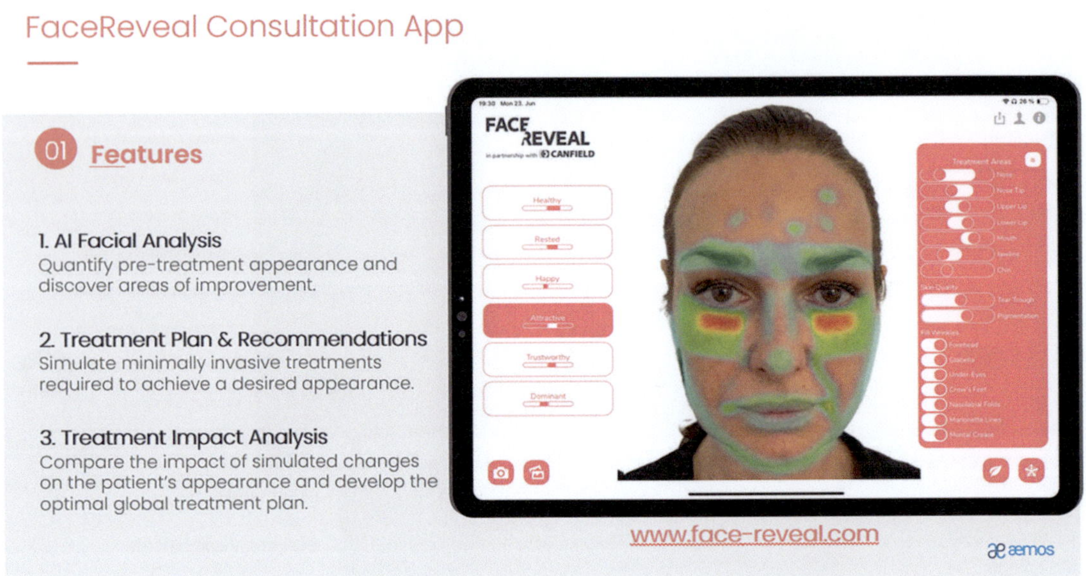

Fig. 9.9 Facial analysis AI program. (Provided Aemos GmbH)

9.5 Streamlining the Treatment Process

AI has the potential to streamline the entire injectable treatment process, from consultation to follow-up care. In the consultation phase, AI-powered platforms can analyze patient data to provide clinicians with detailed treatment recommendations. These platforms integrate medical history, facial analysis, and even patient-reported goals to propose an optimized treatment plan (Fig. 9.10) [16].

During the procedure, AI-guided robotic systems for injectable treatments would be a promise for the future. These systems aim to ensure consistent depth and placement, potentially leading to improved patient satisfaction. They use advanced algorithms to ensure consistent depth, volume, and placement of injectables. By minimizing human error, robotic-assisted systems enhance both safety and aesthetic outcomes [17, 18].

After the procedure, AI-driven monitoring tools can track patient recovery through apps or

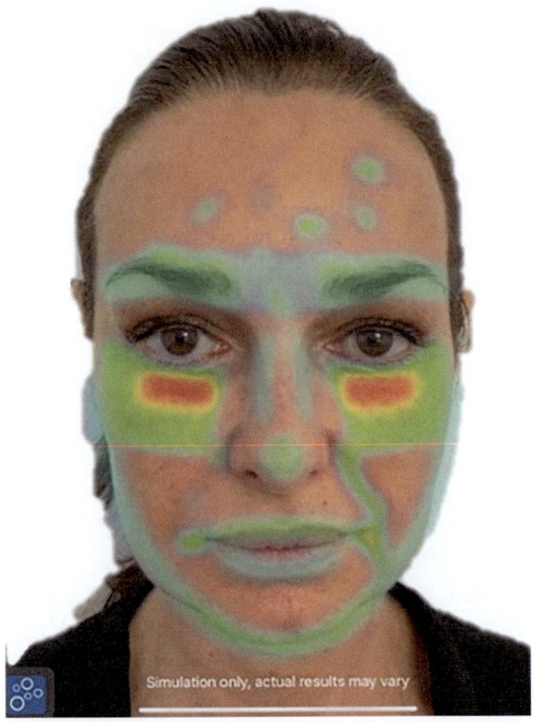

Fig. 9.10 AI recommended changes to facial features to create a certain appearance. (Provided Aemos GmbH)

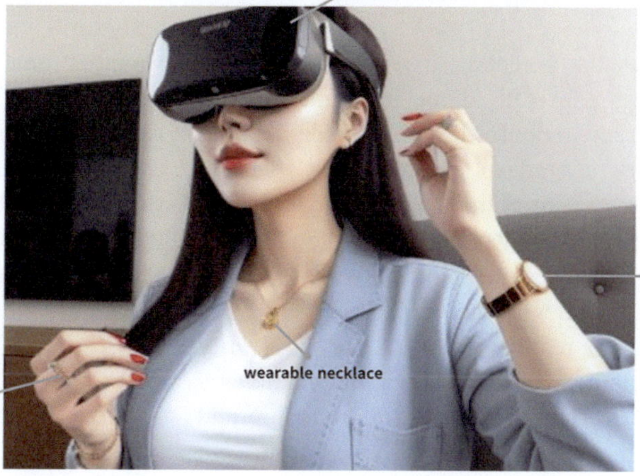

Fig. 9.11 Wearable device monitoring of AI made virtual patient (AI image)

wearable devices (Fig. 9.11). These tools can identify early signs of complications, such as swelling, infection, or filler migration, allowing for timely interventions. They also provide patients with tailored aftercare instructions, improving adherence and overall satisfaction [19, 20].

9.6 Follow-Up and Long-Term Care

AI's capabilities extend beyond the treatment itself, revolutionizing follow-up care and long-term maintenance. Sensors and biosensors are emerging as critical tools in this domain, offering real-time monitoring of physiological parameters and treatment effects. Embedded biosensors can measure biomarkers such as skin hydration, inflammation, or pH levels, providing clinicians with valuable data to assess treatment efficacy and detect complications early [19]. These devices can transmit information directly to AI systems, enabling dynamic adjustments to post-treatment protocols and ensuring a personalized approach to recovery. Predictive analytics, powered by machine learning, can forecast when a patient may require a touch-up or additional treatment, allowing clinicians to schedule follow-ups proactively and ensuring optimal results over time [21]. Telemedicine platforms integrated with AI further enhance post-treatment care. These platforms enable virtual consultations, during which patients can share real-time images of treated areas for evaluation. This approach reduces the need for in-person visits, making follow-up care more accessible and efficient [22].

9.7 Enhancing Patient Education

AI also has the potential to revolutionize how patients are educated about injectable procedures. Interactive platforms can provide detailed information tailored to an individual's needs, including treatment options, risks, and expected outcomes [23]. AI-powered chatbots can address frequently asked questions, offering 24/7 support and helping to alleviate patient anxiety [24].

Augmented reality (AR) and virtual reality (VR) simulations further enhance education by allowing patients to visualize the procedure and its effects in a realistic, immersive environment. These tools can increase patient understanding and confidence, leading to better overall experiences [25].

9.8 Augmented Reality and Virtual Reality in Cosmetic Dermatology

AR and VR are emerging as powerful tools in cosmetic dermatology, revolutionizing how procedures are planned, communicated, and executed. AR overlays digital information onto the real-world environment, enabling clinicians to visualize anatomical structures, injection sites, and projected outcomes directly on the patient's face. This enhances precision during treatments and provides a dynamic, interactive approach to patient consultations. For instance, AR can simulate the effects of dermal fillers, allowing patients to preview results and make more informed decisions [25]. This also can be used for plastic surgery (Fig. 9.12).

VR, on the other hand, offers immersive training experiences for clinicians, recreating real-life scenarios to refine techniques and enhance skillsets. By simulating complex procedures in a risk-free environment, VR enables practitioners to gain confidence and proficiency in performing advanced injectable treatments. Additionally, VR can serve as a patient education tool, helping individuals understand the procedure steps and expected outcomes through engaging, 3D visualizations. Together, AR and VR are reshaping the landscape of cosmetic dermatology by bridging the gap between patient expectations and clinical capabilities, ultimately fostering greater trust and satisfaction [26, 27].

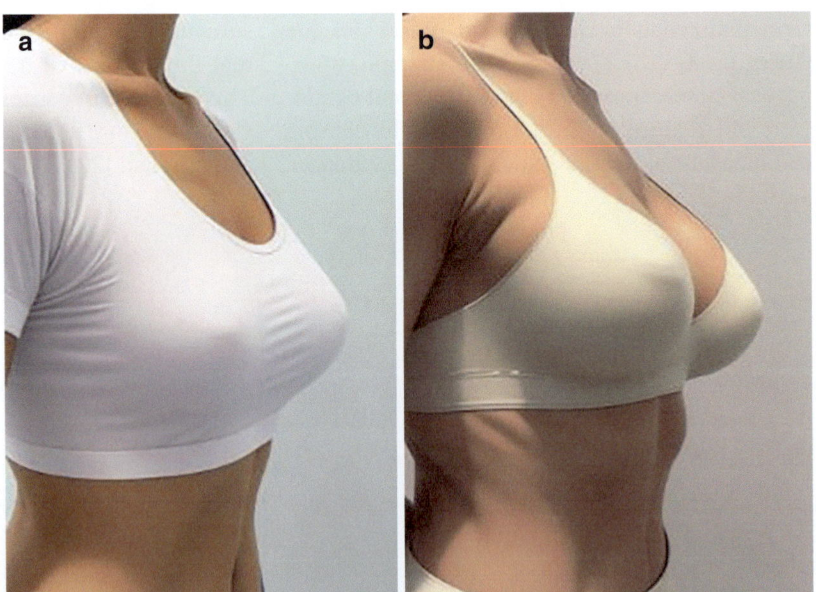

Fig. 9.12 Virtual augmentation mammoplasty preoperative (**a**) and postoperative (**b**) images made by AI program (AI images)

9.9 AI and Ultrasound-Guided Injections

The combination of AI and ultrasound technology (US) is revolutionizing the precision and safety of injectable procedures. US-guided injections allow clinicians to visualize the underlying anatomy in real time, providing critical insights into vascular structures, tissue layers, and the precise location of injectable products (Figs. 9.13 and 9.14).

When integrated with AI, this approach is elevated further, as machine learning algorithms can analyze US images to identify key anatomical landmarks, predict potential complications, and recommend optimal injection sites. AI-powered US systems enhance the safety profile of injectable treatments by minimizing the risk of vascular occlusion and ensuring even product distribution. For example, these systems can highlight high-risk areas, such as arteries and veins, reducing the likelihood of accidental intravascular injection. Additionally, AI algorithms can adapt in real time to dynamic changes in tissue anatomy during the procedure, offering clinicians actionable feedback to refine their techniques. This combination also plays a significant role in training and education. AI-integrated US platforms can simulate various anatomical scenarios, enabling practitioners to gain hands-on experience in a controlled environment. These tools help clinicians develop a deeper understanding of individual variations in anatomy, ultimately improving the consistency and quality of injectable procedures [28].

The adoption of AI and US-guided injections represents a breakthrough in cosmetic dermatology, merging technology with clinical expertise to achieve unparalleled levels of precision, safety, and patient satisfaction. This synergy not only enhances procedural outcomes but also builds trust among patients by demonstrating a commitment to evidence-based care [29, 30].

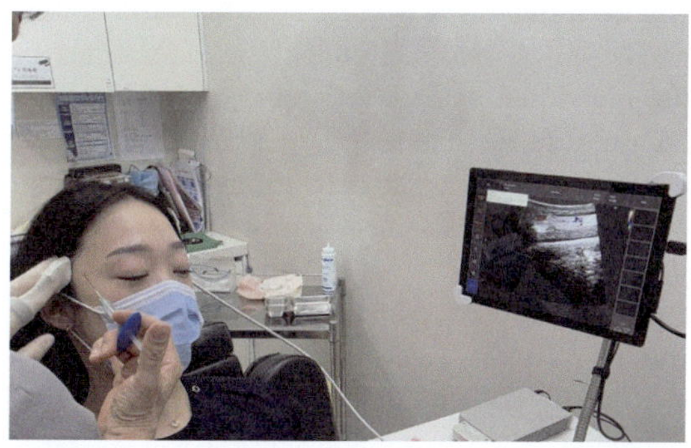

Fig. 9.14 Finger-held probe of SIBUS technology. Doppler ultrasound-guided injection

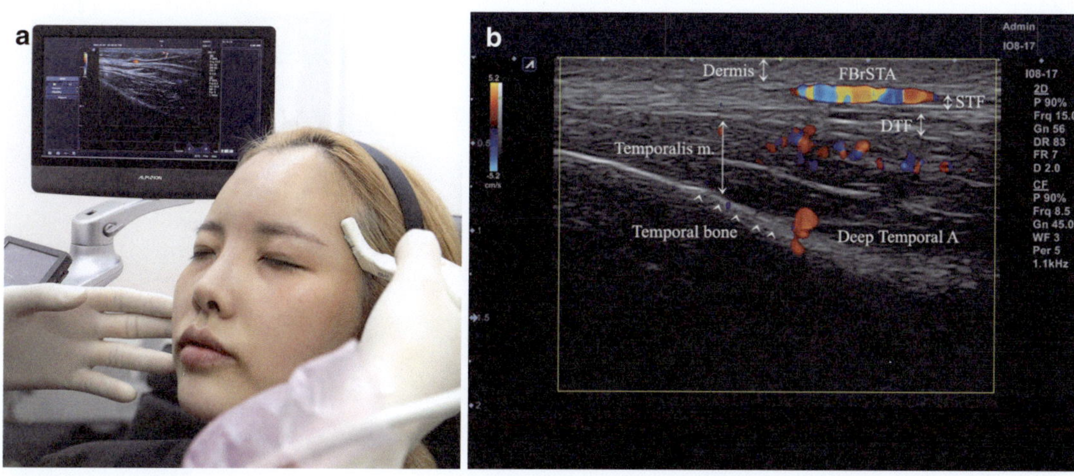

Fig. 9.13 Facial detection by Doppler ultrasound. (**a**) Temple area detection. (**b**) Frontal branch of superficial temporal artery and deep temporal artery

9.10 AI in Coordinating Multimodal Treatment Strategies

AI is not limited to isolated applications but can play a significant role in coordinating multimodal treatment strategies. For patients requiring combined approaches, such as injectables, lasers, and other energy-based devices, AI can serve as a central hub for treatment planning and monitoring [31]. By integrating data from various modalities, AI ensures that treatments are complementary, avoiding overlaps or contraindications [32]. This holistic approach optimizes patient outcomes and enhances the overall treatment experience. Ultimately, this integration underscores the importance of personalization, and each treatment plan is tailored to the unique needs, goals, and anatomical considerations of the individual patient. AI's ability to synthesize complex datasets and provide actionable insights empowers clinicians to deliver results that are not only effective but also harmonious with the patient's natural aesthetics [33, 34]. Personalization, facilitated by AI, transforms the traditional "one-size-fits-all" approach into a dynamic, patient-centric process, fostering greater satisfaction and long-term trust.

9.11 Ethics and Regulatory Frameworks

While AI offers numerous benefits, its integration into cosmetic dermatology raises important ethical and regulatory considerations. Data privacy is a significant concern, as AI relies heavily on patient-specific information. The history of AI shows that it has been developed since the 1950s, but with the advent of machine learning and deep learning, we are now witnessing the era of OpenAI, characterized by vast amounts of information and recent advancements (Fig. 9.15 [8]).

Therefore, vast amounts of data are essential. Compliance with regulations such as the General Data Protection Regulation (GDPR) is essential to protect patient confidentiality and build trust [35]. Bias in AI algorithms is another critical issue. If training datasets are not diverse, AI systems may produce biased recommendations that do not account for variations in skin tone, facial anatomy, or cultural preferences. To address this, developers must ensure that datasets are representative of all demographics and that algorithms are rigorously tested for fairness [36, 37]. Accountability is another concern. As AI systems become more autonomous, clear guidelines must delineate the responsibilities of clinicians versus

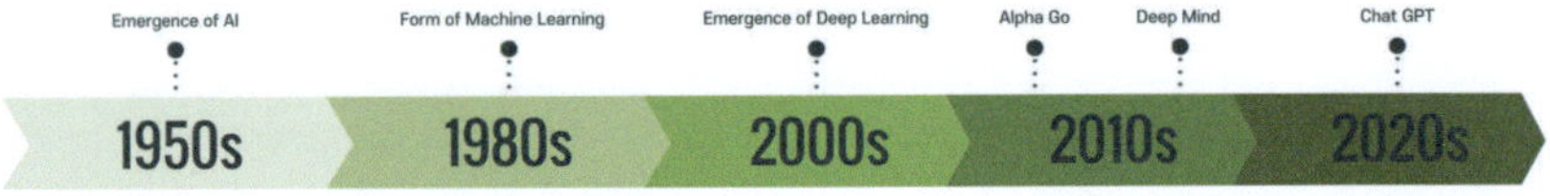

Fig. 9.15 The history of AI

AI tools. For example, in the event of an adverse outcome, it must be clear whether the clinician or the AI system is accountable. Establishing robust frameworks for accountability will be crucial as AI adoption increases [38].

9.12 Frameworks for Safe Implementation

To ensure the safe and ethical integration of AI in cosmetic dermatology, several frameworks must be established. Standardized protocols should guide the use of AI tools, from patient data collection to treatment planning and execution. Continuous monitoring and periodic audits of AI systems are necessary to assess their performance and safety [39, 40]. Clinician training is equally important. Practitioners must be equipped with the knowledge and skills to interpret AI-generated insights and incorporate them into their clinical decision-making. Certification programs focusing on AI applications in aesthetic medicine would help bridge this knowledge gap. Collaboration between clinicians, AI developers, and regulatory bodies is essential to create a unified approach to AI integration. Such collaboration can also foster innovation, ensuring that AI tools are designed with both clinical efficacy and patient safety in mind [6].

9.13 AI-Driven Research and Data Analytics

AI is enabling groundbreaking research in the field of injectables by analyzing large datasets to identify trends, optimize techniques, and predict outcomes. Machine learning models can uncover previously unnoticed correlations between treatment parameters and patient satisfaction, leading to data-driven improvements in clinical practice [41]. By identifying patterns across diverse datasets, AI also enhances the development of new treatment protocols, ensuring they are backed by robust evidence. AI-powered data analytics can assist in designing clinical trials by identifying suitable candidates and predicting potential complications. For example, algorithms can screen patient profiles to determine eligibility, streamlining the recruitment process and reducing dropout rates. Predictive modeling can also simulate trial outcomes under various conditions, allowing researchers to refine methodologies before implementation [42]. Additionally, AI supports post-market surveillance by monitoring the long-term effects of injectables across large patient populations. Real-time analysis of adverse event reports and patient feedback ensures continuous improvement in product safety and efficacy [43]. This dynamic approach to research accelerates innovation, enabling clinicians and manufacturers to respond rapidly to emerging trends and challenges. AI-driven insights are not limited to clinical applications; they also inform business strategies within the cosmetic dermatology industry. By analyzing market trends and consumer preferences, AI enables companies to tailor product development and marketing campaigns to meet evolving patient needs [2].

9.14 Collaborative AI and Augmented Expertise

AI should not replace human expertise but rather augment it. Collaborative AI systems provide real-time suggestions and data-driven insights while allowing clinicians to exercise their judgment [44]. This partnership ensures that the clinician remains at the center of the decision-making process, with AI serving as a supportive tool [45]. For example, during complex procedures like non-surgical rhinoplasty, AI can offer guidance on injection depth and filler distribution while the clinician adjusts techniques based on patient feedback and anatomical nuances (Fig. 9.16).

While AI provides critical insights, the clinician's expertise in adapting to subtle anatomical variations and dynamic patient responses ensures a bespoke approach to each procedure. Additionally, AI tools can analyze patient feedback in real time, allowing for intra-procedure adjustments that further refine outcomes [46].

This blend of human expertise and machine precision creates an ideal environment for achiev-

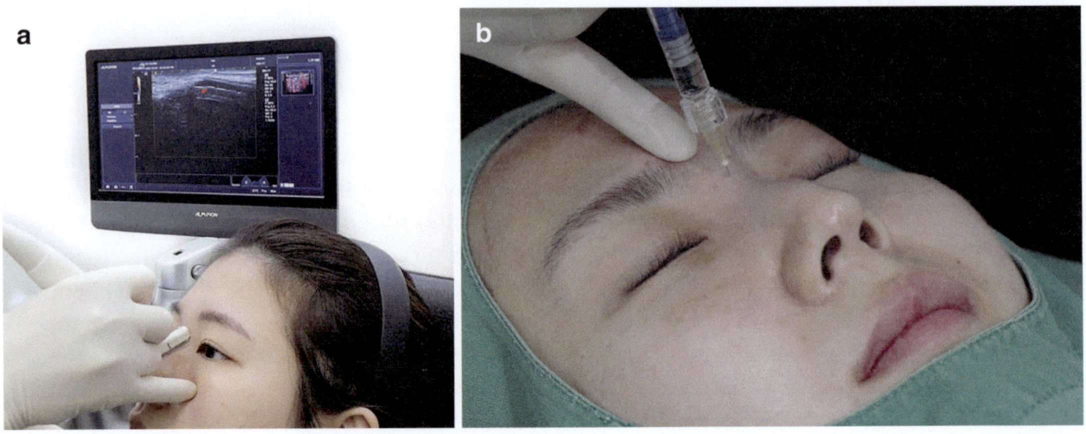

Fig. 9.16 AI technology can provide more detailed ultrasound images and injection depth for safer injection. (**a**) Prescanning ultrasound. (**b**) Injection rhinoplasty

ing superior outcomes. The collaboration between AI and clinicians represents a turning point, where the strengths of both are synergized to elevate the standard of care [47]. This approach not only optimizes procedural results but also builds patient trust by maintaining the essential human touch in aesthetic treatments.

9.15 Global Implications

The adoption of AI is reshaping aesthetic practices worldwide, but regional disparities remain a significant challenge [48]. High-resource settings benefit from access to cutting-edge AI tools and training programs, enabling rapid adoption and innovation. In contrast, low-resource settings face barriers such as high costs, lack of infrastructure, and limited clinician training [49]. Addressing these disparities requires a concerted effort to develop cost-effective AI solutions and educational initiatives tailored to diverse healthcare environments. AI also holds the potential to democratize access to aesthetic care by enabling remote consultations and telemedicine-based treatment planning [50].

9.16 Patient Perspectives

Understanding patient perceptions of AI-driven treatments is critical for successful adoption. Many patients appreciate the enhanced precision and transparency offered by AI, particularly when tools such as outcome simulation and facial mapping are used during consultations [17]. However, concerns about data privacy and the potential loss of the "human touch" in aesthetic care persist [51]. Educating patients about the role of AI as a supportive tool rather than a replacement for clinician expertise can help alleviate these concerns and build trust. Surveys and focus groups indicate that patients value a balanced approach, where AI complements but does not overshadow the clinician's role [52].

9.17 Future-Proofing Practices

To thrive in an AI-driven landscape, clinics and practitioners must adopt strategies for continuous adaptation. Investing in clinician training programs focused on AI applications, creating multidisciplinary teams to integrate AI tools into workflows, and collaborating with technology developers are essential steps [53]. Clinics can also benefit from adopting flexible business models that allow for the incremental adoption of AI tools, reducing financial and operational risks [54]. Moreover, engaging in collaborative research initiatives and contributing to the development of ethical and regulatory frameworks will position practitioners as leaders in the evolving field of aesthetic medicine [55].

9.18 The Role of Stakeholders in Establishing Fair, Responsible, and Ethical AI for Injectables in Cosmetic Dermatology

The successful integration of AI in injectables hinges on the collaboration and contributions of various stakeholders, including doctors, industry leaders, payers, and data analysts [56]. Clinicians are at the forefront of this transformation, using their expertise to implement AI tools effectively, interpret data, and ensure patient-centered care. Industry leaders play a pivotal role in driving innovation, funding research, and fostering partnerships between academia and technology developers to create cutting-edge solutions [57]. Payers, including insurance companies and healthcare organizations, are instrumental in establishing reimbursement models and frameworks that support the accessibility and sustainability of AI advancements in aesthetic medicine. Meanwhile, data analysts and AI developers are responsible for designing, testing, and refining algorithms to enhance precision, safety, and unbiased outcomes in clinical practice [58]. Regulatory bodies and policymakers ensure a supportive and ethical environment, addressing critical concerns such as data privacy, patient safety, and equitable access [37, 59]. By working together, these stakeholders create a cohesive ecosystem that leverages the transformative potential of AI to enhance both clinical outcomes and patient satisfaction. This taxonomy of stakeholders highlights their critical roles in fostering innovation, ensuring ethical implementation, and advancing patient care. Clinicians provide the expertise needed to apply AI tools effectively, industry leaders drive innovation and collaborations, payers establish reimbursement models for accessibility, and data analysts refine algorithms for precision and safety [60]. Regulatory bodies, meanwhile, ensure ethical frameworks and patient safety, creating a supportive environment for AI-driven advancements. Their combined efforts are essential to unlocking the full potential of AI in injectables [61].

9.19 Future Directions

The future of AI in injectables is promising but requires ongoing research and development. Expanding datasets to include diverse populations will enhance the accuracy and applicability of AI algorithms, ensuring that AI tools can deliver equitable and effective care for patients of all backgrounds [62]. Beyond expanding datasets, efforts should focus on refining algorithmic precision to accommodate variations in anatomy, skin types, and cultural aesthetics. Seamless integration of AI tools into existing clinical workflows remains a critical goal. AI must be designed to complement, rather than disrupt, the natural flow of consultations and treatments [63].

Interoperability between AI systems and clinical management platforms will play a significant role in achieving this balance, enabling practitioners to access insights in real time without technological hindrances [64].

Emerging technologies, such as AR and VR, are poised to further complement AI in injectables. AR tools can overlay advanced facial mapping data onto a patient's face during consultations, providing real-time guidance for injection planning while visualizing potential outcomes. This capability enhances communication between clinicians and patients, ensuring that treatment plans align closely with patient expectations. Mixed reality (MR) also can be applied using hologram (Fig. 9.17).

VR platforms, meanwhile, will continue to evolve as critical training tools, offering immersive simulations of complex procedures (Fig. 9.18).

These environments can replicate diverse scenarios, enabling clinicians to refine their techniques in a controlled and risk-free setting. In addition, the use of AI for predictive modeling holds vast potential. By analyzing longitudinal patient data, AI can predict the durability of injectable treatments and suggest optimal timelines for maintenance sessions. Such advancements will empower both clinicians and patients to adopt a proactive approach to aesthetic care, enhancing long-term satisfaction and treatment efficiency [25].

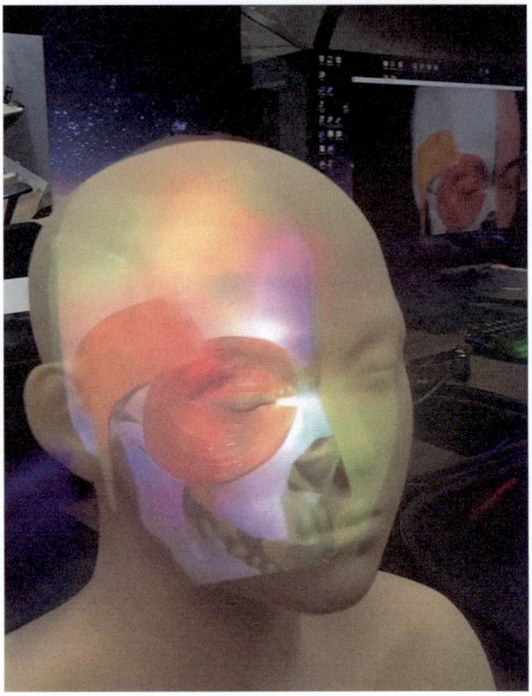

Fig. 9.17 Mixed reality applied to dummy using HoloLens 2

Finally, ethical considerations and regulatory frameworks must keep pace with technological innovation. Ensuring data privacy, addressing algorithmic bias, and maintaining transparency in AI-driven decisions are essential to fostering trust and accountability [65].

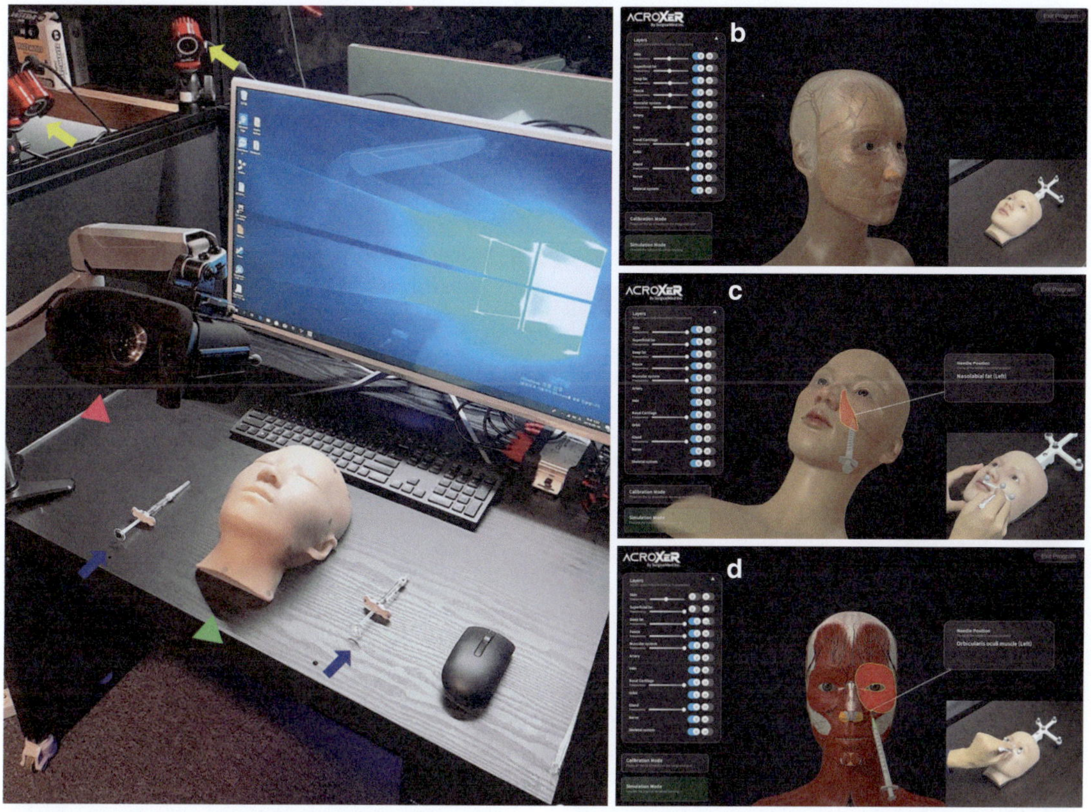

Fig. 9.18 Filler injection education program by virtual reality (SurgicalMind Co.). (**a**) Hardware of VR, optical motion tracking system (yellow arrow), dummy (green arrowhead), motion syringe (blue arrow), and VR headset (red arrowhead). (**b**) VR simulation. (**c**) Nasolabial fold filler injection simulation. (**d**) Orbicularis oculi muscle location simulation

9.20 Conclusion

The integration of AI into the realm of injectables represents a transformative leap in cosmetic dermatology, promising to redefine the standards of precision, personalization, and patient satisfaction. Through the collaborative efforts of stakeholders such as clinicians, industry leaders, policymakers, and data scientists, AI has the potential to address some of the most pressing challenges in aesthetic medicine, including variability in outcomes, safety concerns, and accessibility barriers. By leveraging AI-driven tools, clinicians can achieve unparalleled levels of accuracy and efficiency, enhancing both procedural outcomes and long-term patient care. The journey toward ethical and effective AI integration is far from over. Ensuring data privacy, mitigating algorithmic bias, and fostering equitable access remain pivotal challenges that demand ongoing attention and innovation. Moreover, the role of education and training cannot be overstated, as practitioners must adapt to this rapidly evolving technological landscape to maximize the benefits of AI tools. Stakeholders must prioritize transparency, collaboration, and continuous improvement to create a robust ecosystem where AI serves as an enabler of progress rather than a source of disparity.

As we look to the future, the intersection of AI and injectables holds immense potential to drive innovation across aesthetic medicine. With a focus on developing advanced applications, promoting interdisciplinary research, and addressing ethical concerns, AI can become a cornerstone of a more inclusive and patient-focused approach to cosmetic dermatology. By embracing this transformative technology responsibly, the field can unlock new possibilities, ultimately enhancing the quality of care and outcomes for patients worldwide.

References

1. Statista. AI healthcare market by application worldwide 2026. https://www.statista.com/statistics/938819/global-healthcare-artificial-intelligence-market-value-by-application/. Accessed 19 Jan 2025.
2. Haykal D. Emerging and pioneering AI technologies in aesthetic dermatology: sketching a path toward personalized, predictive, and proactive care. Cosmetics. 2024;11(6):206. https://doi.org/10.3390/cosmetics11060206.
3. Frank K, Day D, Few J, et al. AI assistance in aesthetic medicine-A consensus on objective medical standards. J Cosmet Dermatol. 2024;23(12):4110–5. https://doi.org/10.1111/jocd.16481.
4. BCG Global. Medical aesthetics is resilient, growing, and attracting investors. 8 May 2023. https://www.bcg.com/publications/2023/medical-aesthetics-industry-growth-attracting-investors. Accessed 19 Jan 2025.
5. Elder A, Ring C, Heitmiller K, Gabriel Z, Saedi N. The role of artificial intelligence in cosmetic dermatology-current, upcoming, and future trends. J Cosmet Dermatol. 2021;20(1):48–52. https://doi.org/10.1111/jocd.13797.
6. Haykal D, Cartier H, du Crest D, Galadari H, Landau M, Haddad A. What happens when simulations get real and cosmetic dermatology goes virtual? J Cosmet Dermatol. 2023;22:2682–4. https://doi.org/10.1111/jocd.15888.
7. Vatiwutipong P, Vachmanus S, Noraset T, Tuarob S. Artificial intelligence in cosmetic dermatology: a systematic literature review. IEEE Access. 2023;11:71407–25. https://doi.org/10.1109/ACCESS.2023.3295001.
8. Li Z, Koban KC, Schenck TL, Giunta RE, Li Q, Sun Y. Artificial intelligence in dermatology image analysis: current developments and future trends. J Clin Med. 2022;11(22):6826. https://doi.org/10.3390/jcm11226826.
9. Haykal D. The suitability of AI in dermatology for enhanced skin care. J Aesthet Nurs. 2024;13(5):240–51. https://doi.org/10.12968/joan.2024.0006.
10. du Crest D, Madhumita M, Enbiale W, et al. Skin and digital – the 2024 narrative. Mayo Clin Proc Digit Health. 2024;2(3):322–30. https://doi.org/10.1016/j.mcpdig.2024.05.008.
11. Duong TV, Vy VPT, Hung TNK. Artificial intelligence in plastic surgery: advancements, applications, and future. Cosmetics. 2024;11(4):109. https://doi.org/10.3390/cosmetics11040109.
12. Alowais SA, Alghamdi SS, Alsuhebany N, et al. Revolutionizing healthcare: the role of artificial intelligence in clinical practice. BMC Med Educ. 2023;23:689. https://doi.org/10.1186/s12909-023-04698-z.
13. Maleki Varnosfaderani S, Forouzanfar M. The role of AI in hospitals and clinics: transforming healthcare in the 21st century. Bioengineering. 2024;11(4):337. https://doi.org/10.3390/bioengineering11040337.
14. Pinto-Coelho L. How artificial intelligence is shaping medical imaging technology: a survey of innovations and applications. Bioengineering. 2023;10(12):1435. https://doi.org/10.3390/bioengineering10121435.
15. Hong G-W, et al. Adverse effects associated with dermal filler treatments: part II vascular complication. Diagnostics. 2024;14:1555. https://www.mdpi.com/2075-4418/14/14/1555. Accessed 19 Jan 2025.
16. Al Kuwaiti A, Nazer K, Al-Reedy A, et al. A review of the role of artificial intelligence in healthcare. J Pers Med. 2023;13(6):951. https://doi.org/10.3390/jpm13060951.
17. Johnson KB, Wei W, Weeraratne D, et al. Precision medicine, AI, and the future of personalized health care. Clin Transl Sci. 2021;14(1):86–93. https://doi.org/10.1111/cts.12884.
18. Bekbolatova M, Mayer J, Ong CW, Toma M. Transformative potential of AI in healthcare: definitions, applications, and navigating the ethical landscape and public perspectives. Healthcare. 2024;12(2):125. https://doi.org/10.3390/healthcare12020125.
19. Haykal D. Unleashing the power of biosensors and AI in dermatology. Aesthet Surg J Open Forum. 2024;6:ojae030. https://doi.org/10.1093/asjof/ojae030.
20. Shajari S, Kuruvinashetti K, Komeili A, Sundararaj U. The emergence of AI-based wearable sensors for digital health technology: a review. Sensors. 2023;23(23):9498. https://doi.org/10.3390/s23239498.
21. Dixon D, Sattar H, Moros N, et al. Unveiling the influence of AI predictive analytics on patient outcomes: a comprehensive narrative review. Cureus. 2024;16(5):e59954. https://doi.org/10.7759/cureus.59954.
22. Haykal D, Garibyan L, Flament F, Cartier H. Hybrid cosmetic dermatology: AI generated horizon. Skin Res Technol. 2024;30(5):e13721. https://doi.org/10.1111/srt.13721.
23. Ngo B, Nguyen D, vanSonnenberg E. Artificial intelligence: has its time come for inclusion in medical school education? Maybe…maybe not. MedEdPublish. 2021;10:131. https://doi.org/10.15694/mep.2021.000131.2.

24. Chen R, Zhang Y, Choi S, Nguyen D, Levin NA. The chatbots are coming: risks and benefits of consumer-facing artificial intelligence in clinical dermatology. J Am Acad Dermatol. 2023;89(4):872–4. https://doi.org/10.1016/j.jaad.2023.05.088.
25. Haykal D, Cartier H, Flament F. A psychosocial exploration of augmented reality and virtual reality apps in cosmetic procedures. J Cosmet Dermatol. 2024;23(12):3863–70. https://doi.org/10.1111/jocd.16612.
26. An S, Chen J, Zhu Z, et al. ARCosmetics: a real-time augmented reality cosmetics try-on system. Front Comput Sci. 2022;17(4):174706. https://doi.org/10.1007/s11704-022-2059-8.
27. Bonmarin M, Läuchli S, Navarini A. Augmented and virtual reality in dermatology—where do we stand and what comes next? Dermato. 2022;2(1):1–7. https://doi.org/10.3390/dermato2010001.
28. Cavallieri FA, Balassiano LKDA, Munhoz G, Tembra MF, Wortsman X. Ultrasound in aesthetics: filler and non-filler applications. Semin Ultrasound CT MR. 2024;45(3):251–63. https://doi.org/10.1053/j.sult.2023.11.005.
29. Haykal D, Cartier H, Benzaquen M, Damiani G, Habib SM. The growing importance of ultrasonography in cosmetic dermatology: an update after the 23rd IMCAS Annual World Congress (2022). J Cosmet Dermatol. 2023;22(1):222–5. https://doi.org/10.1111/jocd.15503.
30. Haykal D, Cartier H, Yi K, Wortsman X. The transformative potential of AI in ultrasound for facial aesthetics. J Cosmet Dermatol. 2025;24:e16691. https://doi.org/10.1111/jocd.16691.
31. Haykal D. Harnessing AI in laser aesthetic treatments: revolutionizing precision, safety, and personalization. J Cosmet Dermatol. 2025;24:e16704. https://doi.org/10.1111/jocd.16704.
32. Wang C, He T, Zhou H, Zhang Z, Lee C. Artificial intelligence enhanced sensors – enabling technologies to next-generation healthcare and biomedical platform. Bioelectron Med. 2023;9(1):17. https://doi.org/10.1186/s42234-023-00118-1.
33. Alzeer J. Integrating medicine with lifestyle for personalized and holistic healthcare. J Public Health Emerg. 2023;7:33. https://doi.org/10.21037/jphe-23-71.
34. Haykal D, Treacy P, Lim T, et al. Cross-cultural perspectives on patient expectations in cosmetic dermatology: a comparative analysis across countries and ethnicities. J Cosmet Dermatol. 2023;22(12):3237–40. https://doi.org/10.1111/jocd.16023.
35. Carmi L, Zohar M, Riva GM. The European General Data Protection Regulation (GDPR) in mHealth: theoretical and practical aspects for practitioners' use. Med Sci Law. 2023;63(1):61–8. https://doi.org/10.1177/00258024221118411.
36. Elston DM. Availability bias and artificial intelligence. J Am Acad Dermatol. 2023;89(1):29–30. https://doi.org/10.1016/j.jaad.2019.07.051.
37. Sangers TE, Kittler H, Blum A, et al. Position statement of the EADV Artificial Intelligence (AI) Task Force on AI-assisted smartphone apps and web-based services for skin disease. J Eur Acad Dermatol Venereol. 2024;38:22–30. https://doi.org/10.1111/jdv.19521.
38. Daneshjou R, Kittler H. Empowering the next generation of artificial intelligence in dermatology: the datasets and benchmarks track of the Journal of Investigative Dermatology. J Invest Dermatol. 2024;144(3):437–8. https://doi.org/10.1016/j.jid.2023.11.011.
39. Goktas P, Grzybowski A. Assessing the impact of ChatGPT in dermatology: a comprehensive rapid review. J Clin Med. 2024;13(19):5909. https://doi.org/10.3390/jcm13195909.
40. Haykal D, Ascher B, Cartier H, Gold M. Exploring the landscape of AI adoption in cosmetic medicine and surgery: insights from the 25th IMCAS Congress (International Master Course in Aging Science). J Cosmet Dermatol. 2024;23(8):2673–5. https://doi.org/10.1111/jocd.16316.
41. Rehman AU, Li M, Wu B, et al. Role of artificial intelligence in revolutionizing drug discovery. Fundam Res. 2025;5:1273–87. https://doi.org/10.1016/j.fmre.2024.04.021.
42. Saady M, Eissa M, Yacoub AS, Hamed AB, Azzazy HMES. Implementation of artificial intelligence approaches in oncology clinical trials: a systematic review. Artif Intell Med. 2025;161:103066. https://doi.org/10.1016/j.artmed.2025.103066.
43. Huanbutta K, Burapapadh K, Kraisit P, et al. Artificial intelligence-driven pharmaceutical industry: a paradigm shift in drug discovery, formulation development, manufacturing, quality control, and post-market surveillance. Eur J Pharm Sci. 2024;203:106938. https://doi.org/10.1016/j.ejps.2024.106938.
44. Göndöcs D, Dörfler V. AI in medical diagnosis: AI prediction & human judgment. Artif Intell Med. 2024;149:102769. https://doi.org/10.1016/j.artmed.2024.102769.
45. Alves M, Seringa J, Silvestre T, Magalhães T. Use of artificial intelligence tools in supporting decision-making in hospital management. BMC Health Serv Res. 2024;24(1):1282. https://doi.org/10.1186/s12913-024-11602-y.
46. Gala D, Behl H, Shah M, Makaryus AN. The role of artificial intelligence in improving patient outcomes and future of healthcare delivery in cardiology: a narrative review of the literature. Healthcare. 2024;12(4):481. https://doi.org/10.3390/healthcare12040481.
47. Yelne S, Chaudhary M, Dod K, Sayyad A, Sharma R. Harnessing the power of AI: a comprehensive review of its impact and challenges in nursing science and healthcare. Cureus. 2023;15(11):e49252. https://doi.org/10.7759/cureus.49252.
48. Khogali HO, Mekid S. The blended future of automation and AI: examining some long-term societal and

ethical impact features. Technol Soc. 2023;73:102232. https://doi.org/10.1016/j.techsoc.2023.102232.
49. Olawade DB, Wada OJ, David-Olawade AC, Kunonga E, Abaire O, Ling J. Using artificial intelligence to improve public health: a narrative review. Front Public Health. 2023;11:1196397. https://doi.org/10.3389/fpubh.2023.1196397.
50. Nwankwo E, Emeihe E, Ajegbile M, Olaboye J, Maha C. Telemedicine and AI to improve healthcare access in rural settings. Int J Life Sci Res Arch. 2024;7:59–077. https://doi.org/10.53771/ijlsra.2024.7.1.0061.
51. Esmaeilzadeh P, Mirzaei T, Dharanikota S. Patients' perceptions toward human–artificial intelligence interaction in health care: experimental study. J Med Internet Res. 2021;23(11):e25856. https://doi.org/10.2196/25856.
52. Asan O, Bayrak AE, Choudhury A. Artificial intelligence and human trust in healthcare: focus on clinicians. J Med Internet Res. 2020;22(6):e15154. https://doi.org/10.2196/15154.
53. Carini C, Seyhan AA. Tribulations and future opportunities for artificial intelligence in precision medicine. J Transl Med. 2024;22:411. https://doi.org/10.1186/s12967-024-05067-0.
54. Jorzik P, Klein SP, Kanbach DK, Kraus S. AI-driven business model innovation: a systematic review and research agenda. J Bus Res. 2024;182:114764. https://doi.org/10.1016/j.jbusres.2024.114764.
55. Ramirez S, Cullen C, Ahdoot R, Scherz G. The primacy of ethics in aesthetic medicine: a review. Plast Reconstr Surg Glob Open. 2024;12(6):e5935. https://doi.org/10.1097/GOX.0000000000005935.
56. Sadeghi Z, Alizadehsani R, Cifci MA, et al. A review of explainable artificial intelligence in healthcare. Comput Electr Eng. 2024;118:109370. https://doi.org/10.1016/j.compeleceng.2024.109370.
57. Schubert T, Oosterlinck T, Stevens RD, Maxwell PH, van der Schaar M. AI education for clinicians. eClinicalMedicine. 2025;79:102968. https://doi.org/10.1016/j.eclinm.2024.102968.
58. Siala H, Wang Y. SHIFTing artificial intelligence to be responsible in healthcare: a systematic review. Soc Sci Med. 2022;296:114782. https://doi.org/10.1016/j.socscimed.2022.114782.
59. European Commission. The European AI Alliance | Shaping Europe's digital future. 24 Mar 2023. https://digital-strategy.ec.europa.eu/en/policies/european-ai-alliance. Accessed 1 May 2023.
60. Hogg HDJ, Al-Zubaidy M, Talks J, et al. Stakeholder perspectives of clinical artificial intelligence implementation: systematic review of qualitative evidence. J Med Internet Res. 2023;25:e39742. https://doi.org/10.2196/39742.
61. González-Gonzalo C, Thee EF, Klaver CCW, et al. Trustworthy AI: closing the gap between development and integration of AI systems in ophthalmic practice. Prog Retin Eye Res. 2022;90:101034. https://doi.org/10.1016/j.preteyeres.2021.101034.
62. Singh S, Gupta H, Sharma P, Sahi S. Advances in artificial intelligence (AI)-assisted approaches in drug screening. Artif Intell Chem. 2024;2(1):100039. https://doi.org/10.1016/j.aichem.2023.100039.
63. Mennella C, Maniscalco U, De Pietro G, Esposito M. Ethical and regulatory challenges of AI technologies in healthcare: a narrative review. Heliyon. 2024;10(4):e26297. https://doi.org/10.1016/j.heliyon.2024.e26297.
64. Ahmed MI, Spooner B, Isherwood J, Lane M, Orrock E, Dennison A. A systematic review of the barriers to the implementation of artificial intelligence in healthcare. Cureus. 2023;15(10):e46454. https://doi.org/10.7759/cureus.46454.
65. Hanna M, Pantanowitz L, Jackson B, et al. Ethical and bias considerations in artificial intelligence (AI)/machine learning. Mod Pathol. 2025;38:100686. https://doi.org/10.1016/j.modpat.2024.100686.

10 Superficial Injections to Enhance the Infraorbital Area: When Deep and When Superficial

Marina Landau and Won Lee

10.1 Introduction

The infraorbital region plays an essential role in the perception of facial aging. Recently, a clinical study using eye-tracking technology revealed that the periorbital region is the second most crucial area in terms of aging perception [1]. Infraorbital area changes affect a wide range of ages, both sexes, and all races, and many patients seek treatments specifically for this area, with the most common complaint being a "tired look" or "infraorbital dark circles" [2–4].

10.2 Infraorbital Pathology Classification

Despite the prevalence of this condition, there is considerable confusion regarding the contributing anatomical and biological mechanisms. The lower eyelid area has been, for years, a victim of a "one size fits all" approach, and only a few publications are making a systematic classification of the pathological processes in this area, to assist in the selection of clinical correction options [5, 6]. Factors contributing to a "tired look" or "dark circles" include periorbital melanosis, visibility of infraorbital veins, wrinkling of the skin, visibility of previously injected filler, and shadowing due to tear troughs and infra-orbital fat herniation, with the last two being probably the most prevalent.

Hollows or Bulges? (Fig. 10.1)

Most of the publications discussing the enhancement of the infraorbital area by injectables refer to tear trough deformities, while looking at the cases included in the publications, some of them actually demonstrate bulging due to infraorbital fat herniation [7, 8]. Even some of the statistically validated scales targeting to assess the infraorbital hollowing objectively contain cases of infraorbital fat herniation [9]. Our long-lasting experience, as well as that of others, shows that the pre-treatment differentiation between the "hollow" and the "bulging" is crucial for the treatment success, as different pathologies require different therapeutic approaches [10]. "Hills" and "Valleys" approach was suggested to simplify the assessment of the lower eyelid area to ease the diagnosis and treatment method [5].

M. Landau
Arena Dermatology, Herzliya, Israel

W. Lee (✉)
Yonsei E1 Plastic Surgery Clinic,
Anyang, Kyonggi-do, Korea (Republic of)

W. Lee (ed.), *Innovative Injectable Techniques in Minimally Invasive Aesthetics*,
https://doi.org/10.1007/978-981-95-2161-6_10

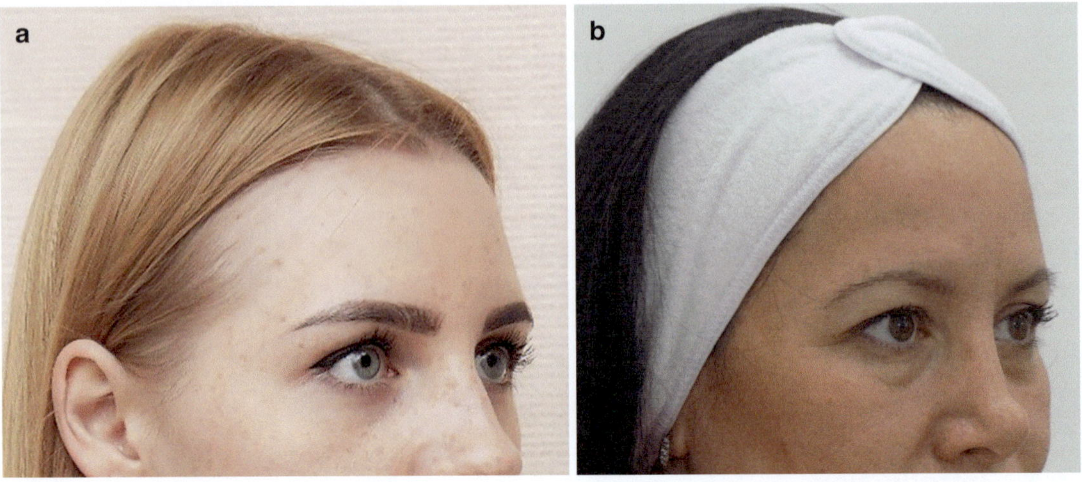

Fig. 10.1 Infraorbital deformity. (**a**) Hollow (tear trough deformity). (**b**) Bulging (infraorbital fat herniation)

10.3 Infraorbital Hollows (Tear Trough Deformity)

The infraorbital groove can be differentiated into nasojugal groove (or fold), tear trough deformity, and palpebromalar groove; these conditions are caused by atrophy of the skin and subcutaneous fat, contraction of the orbital part of orbicular oculi muscle or squinting, and malar bone resorption [11]. The most common method described for the correction of the infraorbital groove is placement of the hyaluronic-based filler deeply on the periosteum between the orbicularis oculi muscle and the inferior orbital rim, using the inferior orbital rim or nasojugal groove as an injection point landmark, either by using a blunt cannula or a sharp needle [12, 13].

10.4 Bulges

A significant number of the patients present to aesthetic clinics not with an infraorbital groove, but rather with infraorbital bags. They arise from a complex aging process following a progressive laxity of the eyelid support apparatus (Lockwood suspensory ligament and lateral canthal tendon), which allows the eyeball to descend posteriorly, displacing the post-septal fat anteriorly, causing the appearance of a bulge or pseudo-herniation across the orbital septum [14, 15].

Infraorbital fat bags can be treated either surgically or non-surgically. When using a non-surgical approach, the injection technique should be completely different from this, applied for tear-trough deformity correction. According to Kato et al. in Japanese patients, infraorbital pathology (called in the publication incorrectly again "tear trough deformities") can be classified into three types according to the presence or absence of a "negative vector" based on retrusion of the maxilla relative to the anterior corneal surface, with or without eye-bag protrusion when smiling. Type 1 patients (infraorbital hollowness without the negative vector) can be treated by filling the depression in the tear trough and the palpebromalar groove region. Type 2 patients (hollowness with a negative vector and no eye-bag protrusion on smiling) require in addition volume restoration in the mid-cheek Type 3 patients (with a negative vector and eye-bag protrusion on smiling) require in addition superficial placing of a filler in front of the eye bags [16].

10.5 My Method to Treat Infraorbital Bulges

To conceal infraorbital fat herniation, I use hyaluronic acid-based "soft filler" with relatively low G prime. Since all the HA-based fillers are hydrophilic, attract water, and swell after the injection, I prefer to use the same product for all my patients to master the nuances of its "in vivo" behavior. Before the injection, I ask a patient to look upward and mark a line corresponding to the lower border of the herniated fat.

For the injection, I rarely use the original 1.0 ml syringes, but prefer to transfer 0.2 ml of the original filler to 0.3 ml "baby insulin" syringes with a 6 mm × 25 mm (31G) needle (Fig. 10.2).

I inject small aliquots of the filler in the subdermal plane along the palpebral-malar transition, pulling the skin up away from the bone throughout all the entire injection process. I usually start the injection from the most medial part, with the first entry point about 4 to 6 mm away from the medial border of the herniation. The needle insertion is superficial to the point of being seen through transparency (Fig. 10.3). A delicate massage is done in regions with a punctual accumulation of product. The lateral part of the transition line can be injected deeper to the bone. I use 0.6–1.0 ml of the product for both eyes' correction.

I aspire to achieve no more than 80% correction. The patient is scheduled for a follow-up visit after 8 weeks (Fig. 10.4). I rarely agree to see patients earlier than two months, since in most cases this is the time required for the complete product "saturation" with the in-tissue water. If, after a 2-month period, there is still a remaining defect, I carefully touch the patient up, injecting usually not more than 0.2 ml.

Infraorbital injection of cross-linked HA-based products usually provides long-lasting (more than 12 months) correction (Figs. 10.5, 10.6, 10.7, 10.8, and 10.9).

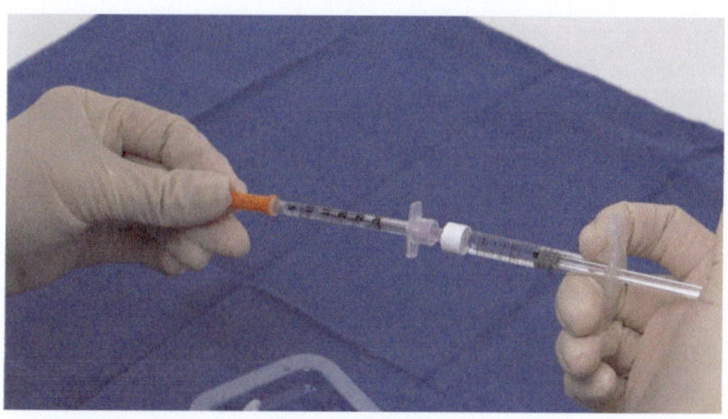

Fig. 10.2 Partition of HA filler

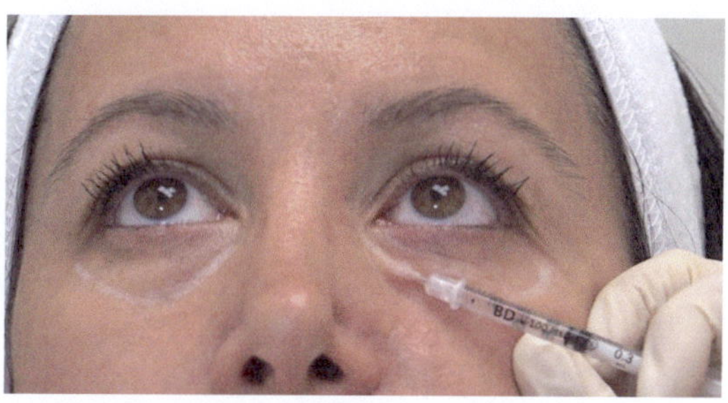

Fig. 10.3 Injection technique

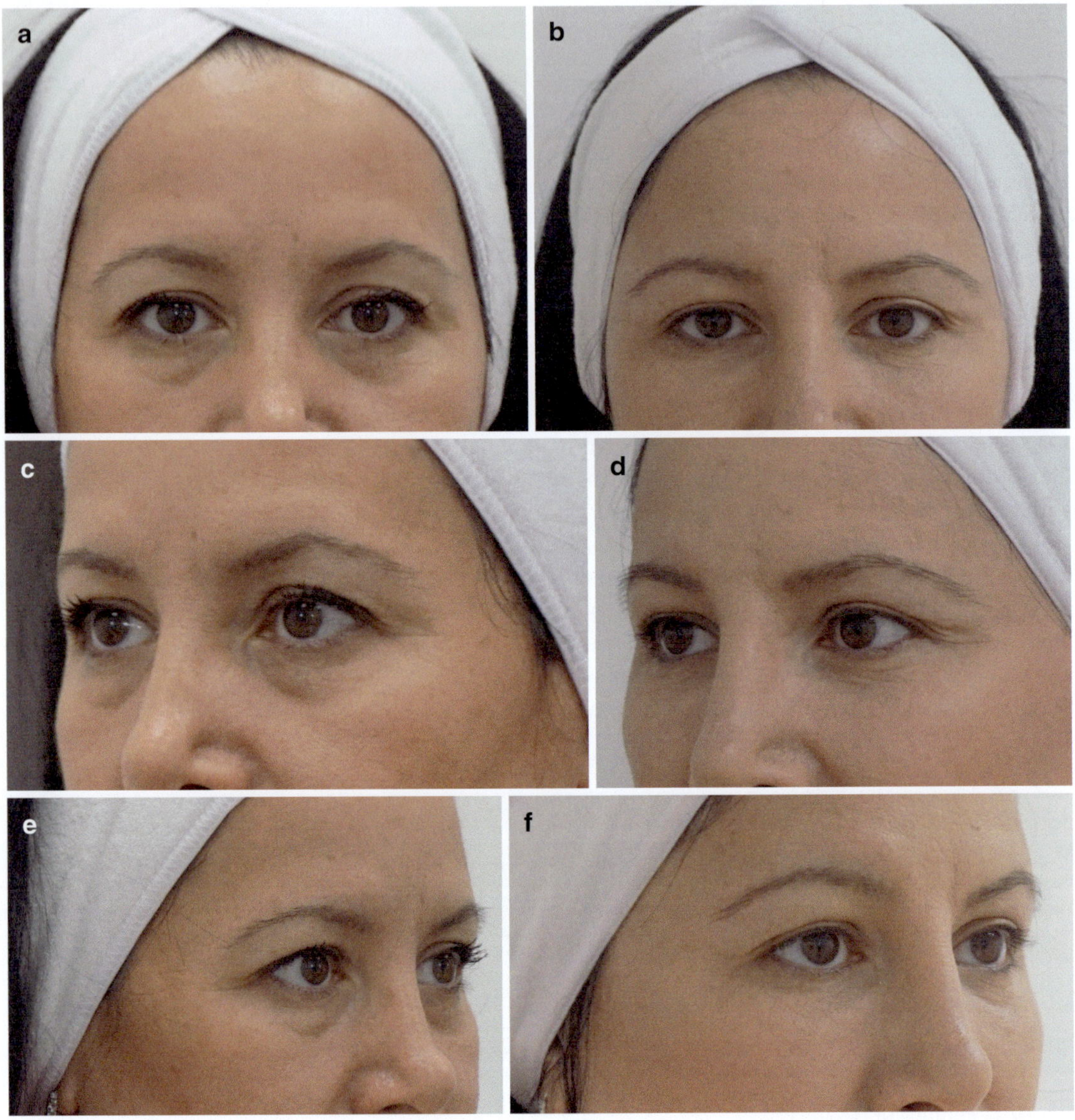

Fig. 10.4 Infraorbital HA filler injection. (**a**) Preoperative frontal view. (**b**) Postoperative 8 weeks frontal view. (**c**) Preoperative three quarter view. (**d**) Postoperative 8 weeks three quarter view. (**e**) Preoperative three quarter view. (**f**) Postoperative 8 weeks three quarter view

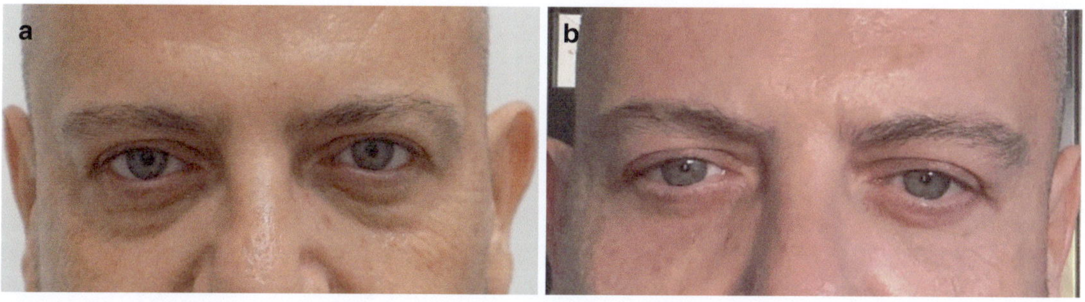

Fig. 10.5 Infraorbital HA filler injection. (**a**) Preoperative frontal view. (**b**) Postoperative frontal view

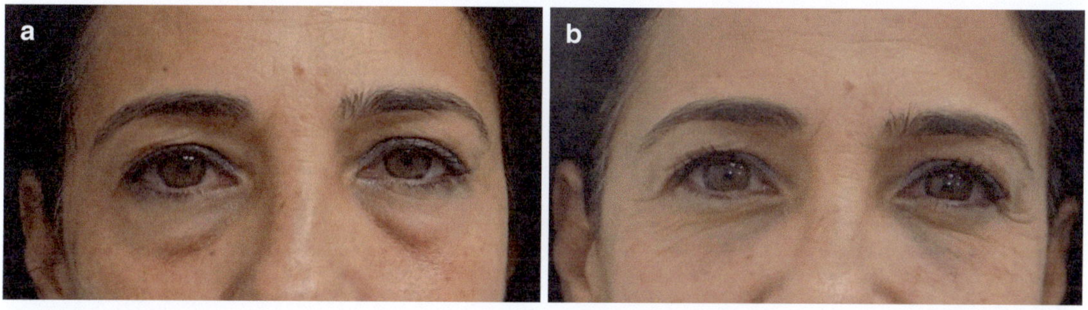

Fig. 10.6 Infraorbital HA filler injection. (**a**) Preoperative frontal view. (**b**) Postoperative frontal view after 2 months

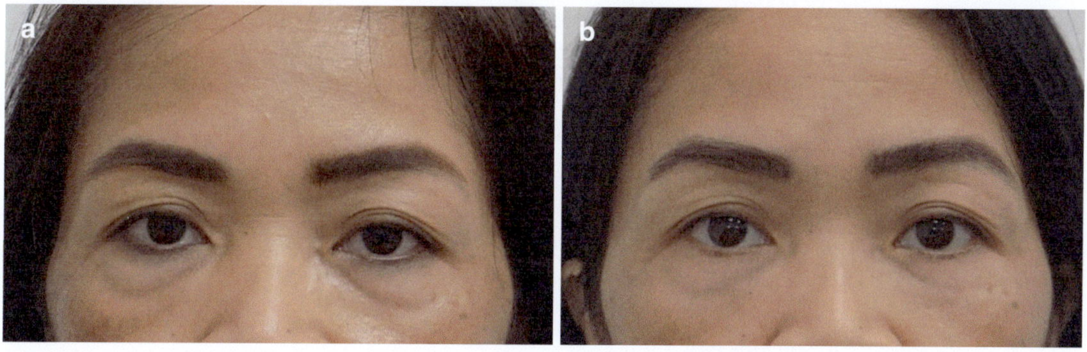

Fig. 10.7 Infraorbital HA filler injection. (**a**) Preoperative frontal view. (**b**) Postoperative frontal view

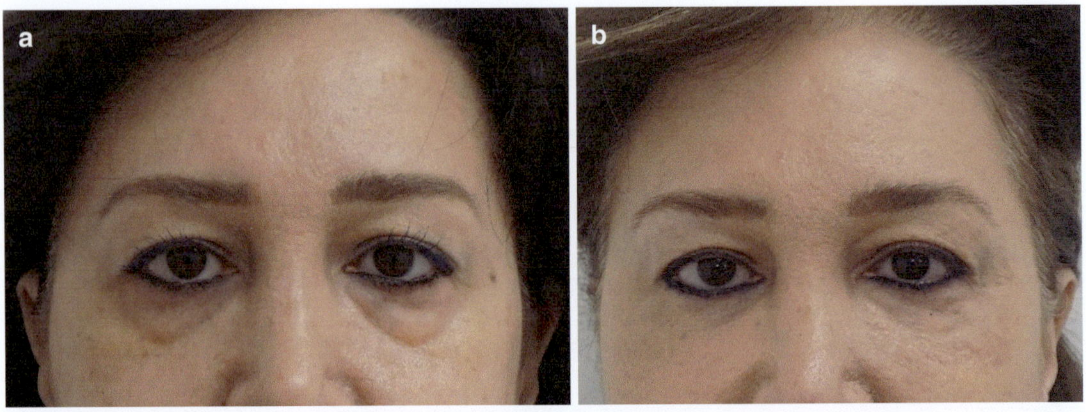

Fig. 10.8 Infraorbital HA filler injection. (**a**) Preoperative frontal view. (**b**) Postoperative frontal view

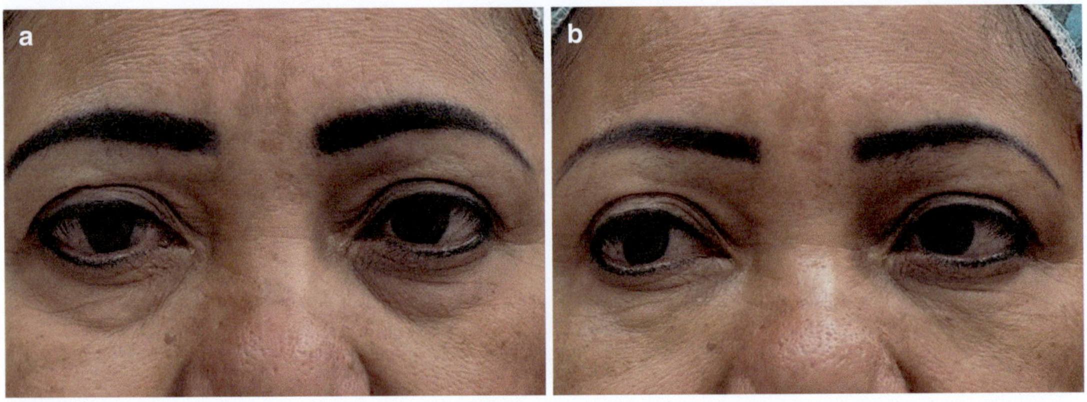

Fig. 10.9 Infraorbital HA filler injection. (**a**) Preoperative frontal view. (**b**) Postoperative frontal view

10.6 Safety of the Procedure

In spite of the potential of injury to the artery in the infraorbital area, due to abundance of the arteries in this area, severe vascular complications are only rarely reported [17, 18]. Since infraorbital neurovascular bundle is located deeply on the bone, superficial injections, while retracting the tissue away from the bone should be considered relatively safe.

10.7 Complications

The most common complications include bruising, transient irregularity, and insufficient correction. Overcorrection and Tyndall effect are extremely rare as long as one respects the "rule" of 80% correction during the first session.

In addition, I instruct all the patients treated for infraorbital pathology to avoid using swimming goggles, as those can push the product up, causing secondary product dislocation.

References

1. Frank K, Ehrl D, Bernardini F, Walbrun A, Moellhoff N, Alfertshofer M, et al. How we look at mature faces – an eye-tracking investigation into the perception of age. Aesthetic Surg J. 2023;43:115–22. https://doi.org/10.1093/asj/sjac251.
2. Nkengne A, Bertin C, Stamatas GN, Giron A, Rossi A, Issachar N, et al. Influence of facial skin attributes on the perceived age of Caucasian women. J Eur Acad Dermatol Venereol. 2008;22:982–91.
3. Camp MC, Wong WW, Filip Z, Carter CS, Gupta SC. A quantitative analysis of periorbital aging with three dimensional surface imaging. J Plast Reconstr Aesthet Surg. 2011;64:148–54.

4. Mayes AE, Murray PG, Gunn DA, Tomlin CC, Catt SD, Wen YB, et al. Ageing appearance in China: biophysical profile of facial skin and its relationship to perceived age. J Eur Acad Dermatol Venereol. 2010;24:341–8.
5. Naik MN. Hills and valleys: understanding the under-eye. J Cutan Aesthet Surg. 2016;9(2):61–4. https://doi.org/10.4103/0974-2077.184048.
6. Park KY, Kwon HJ, Youn CS, Seo SJ, Kim MN. Treatments of infra-orbital dark circles by various etiologies. Ann Dermatol. 2018;30(5):522–8. https://doi.org/10.5021/ad.2018.30.5.522.
7. Woodward J, Cox SE, Kato K, Urdiales-Galvez F, Boyd C, Ashourian N. Infraorbital hollow rejuvenation: considerations, complications, and the contributions of midface volumization. Aesthet Surg J Open Forum. 2023;5:ojad016. https://doi.org/10.1093/asjof/ojad016.
8. Hong GW, Choi W, Yoon SE, Wan J, Yi KH. Anatomical-based filler injection diagnosis to treatment techniques: infraorbital groove and hollowness. Life (Basel). 2025;15(2):237. https://doi.org/10.3390/life15020237.
9. Lorenc ZP, Smith S, Bass LS, Bank D, Weiss R, Canfield D, D'Alessandro BM, Cramer LM. Validating the reliability and clinical relevance of an infraorbital hollow photonumeric scale. Aesthet Surg J Open Forum. 2023;5:ojad052. https://doi.org/10.1093/asjof/ojad052.
10. Siperstein R. Infraorbital hyaluronic acid filler: common aesthetic side effects with treatment and prevention options. Aesthet Surg J Open Forum. 2022;4:ojac001. https://doi.org/10.1093/asjof/ojac001.
11. Lee JH, Hong G. Definitions of groove and hollowness of the infraorbital region and clinical treatment using soft-tissue filler. Arch Plast Surg. 2018;45:214–21. https://doi.org/10.5999/aps.2017.01193.
12. Trinh LN, Grond SE, Gupta A. Dermal fillers for tear trough rejuvenation: a systematic review. Facial Plast Surg. 2022;38(3):228–39. https://doi.org/10.1055/s-0041-1731348.
13. Berros P, Atlan L, Hubschman S, Converset S, Enright KM, Nikolis A. Novel treatment protocol for combined tear trough ligament stretching and injection. Plast Reconstr Surg. 2023;152(5):808e–16e. https://doi.org/10.1097/PRS.0000000000010410.
14. Branham GH. Lower eyelid blepharoplasty. Facial Plast Surg Clin North Am. 2016;24:129–38. https://doi.org/10.1016/j.fsc.2015.12.004.115.
15. Pack S, Quereshy FA, Altay MA, Baur DA. Transconjunctival lower blepharoplasty. Atlas Oral Maxillofac Surg Clin. 2016;24:147–51. https://doi.org/10.1016/j.cxom.2016.05.011.
16. Kato K, Kajiwara T, Furuyama N, Liew S. Filler-based correction of tear trough depressions and eye bags in Japanese patients: a classification system and treatment algorithm. J Cosmet Dermatol. 2023;22(2):439–48. https://doi.org/10.1111/jocd.15449.
17. Jitaree B, Phumyoo T, Uruwan S, Sawatwong W, McCormick L, Tansatit T. The feasibility determination of risky severe complications of arterial vasculature regarding the filler injection sites at the tear trough. Plast Reconstr Surg. 2018;142(5):1153–63. https://doi.org/10.1097/PRS.0000000000004893.
18. Santiago Díaz A, Montes JR, Nieves MI. Injection-related visual compromise. Plast Reconstr Surg Glob Open. 2024;12(1):e5494. https://doi.org/10.1097/GOX.0000000000005494.

Facial Overfilled Syndrome (FOS): Pathophysiology, Diagnosis, and Management

11

Lim Tingsong and Won Lee

11.1 Introduction

Facial overfilled syndrome (FOS) is a progressively disfiguring complication arising from excessive or improperly administered dermal filler injections. While dermal fillers have revolutionized aesthetic medicine by addressing volume loss and aging, their misuse can result in unnatural facial contours, excessive fullness, and distortion of facial proportions. The widespread adoption of hyaluronic acid (HA) and non-HA fillers has significantly increased the prevalence of FOS, necessitating heightened clinical awareness [1, 2].

FOS manifests across a spectrum, ranging from overt puffiness (e.g., "sausage-like" lips) to subtler distortions such as midface heaviness, nasal broadening, and chin or jawline over corrections. A critical barrier to early diagnosis is visual adaptation, wherein practitioners and patients normalize overfilled features due to repeated exposure to exaggerated aesthetics prevalent in social media and filtered imagery. This perceptual phenomenon entrenches unrealistic ideals, obscuring objective assessment [3].

This chapter examines the pathophysiology, clinical presentation, diagnostic strategies, prevention, and evidence-based management of FOS, including emerging therapies such as collagenase for non-HA filler complications.

11.2 Pathophysiology of FOS

FOS is driven by a triad of factors: patient preferences, practitioner practices, and filler properties [2, 4].

1. Patient-Driven Factors
Patients often demand overcorrection of age-related volume loss, influenced by social media platforms and beauty filters that promote hyper-augmented facial ideals [5].

2. Physician-Driven Factors
Poor anatomical knowledge and improper injection techniques—such as superficial placement of volumizing fillers—lead to unnatural outcomes. Overcorrection driven by commercial incentives exacerbates tissue burden, while inadequate understanding of filler longevity delays diagnosis [6]. Visual adaptation further compounds this issue, as practitioners exposed to prevalent overfilled aesthetics may fail to recognize deviations from natural proportions [3].

L. Tingsong
Clique Clinic, Kuala Lumpur, Malaysia
e-mail: drlim@cliqueclinic.com

W. Lee (✉)
Yonsei E1 Plastic Surgery Clinic,
Anyang, Kyonggi-do, Korea (Republic of)

W. Lee (ed.), *Innovative Injectable Techniques in Minimally Invasive Aesthetics*,
https://doi.org/10.1007/978-981-95-2161-6_11

3. Misconceptions About Aging
The erroneous belief that aging is solely due to volume loss (rather than sagging or structural collagen decline) results in overreliance on fillers. This overlooks the role of skin-tightening procedures (e.g., radiofrequency) or regenerative therapies (e.g., polynucleotides) [7].

4. Filler Longevity and Integration
HA fillers, once assumed to degrade within 6–12 months, persist for years, as shown by MRI studies [8]. Non-HA fillers (e.g., poly-L-lactic acid [PLLA], calcium hydroxylapatite [CaHA]) induce biostimulation, creating permanent fibrotic collagen networks that complicate reversal [9].

11.3 Clinical Presentation and Diagnosis

The "See-Touch-Feel-Express" Diagnostic Framework (Figs. 11.1 and 11.2)

1. See: Puffy lips, overprojected forehead, drooping oral commissures, and loss of infraorbital topography. Visual adaptation may obscure these signs; practitioners must consciously compare findings to age-appropriate norms [3].
2. Touch: Firm, immobile deposits in overfilled areas; liquid-like consistency in thin-skinned regions (e.g., infraorbital hollows) (Fig. 11.3).

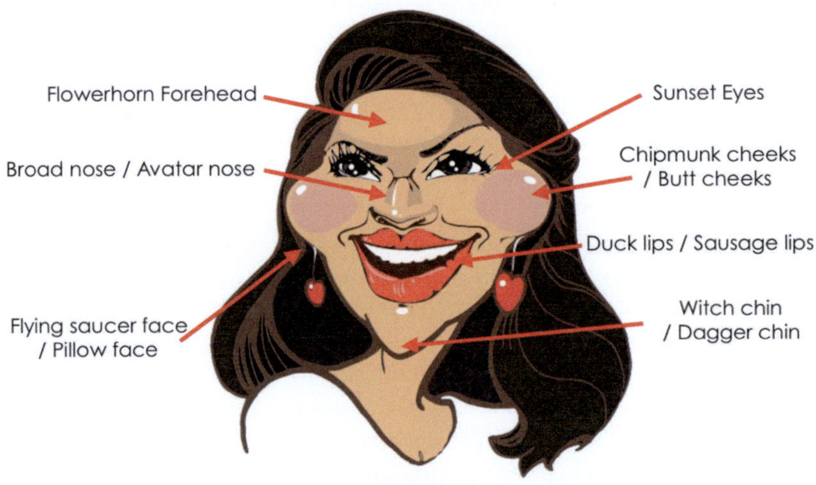

Fig. 11.1 Female patient facial overfilled syndrome

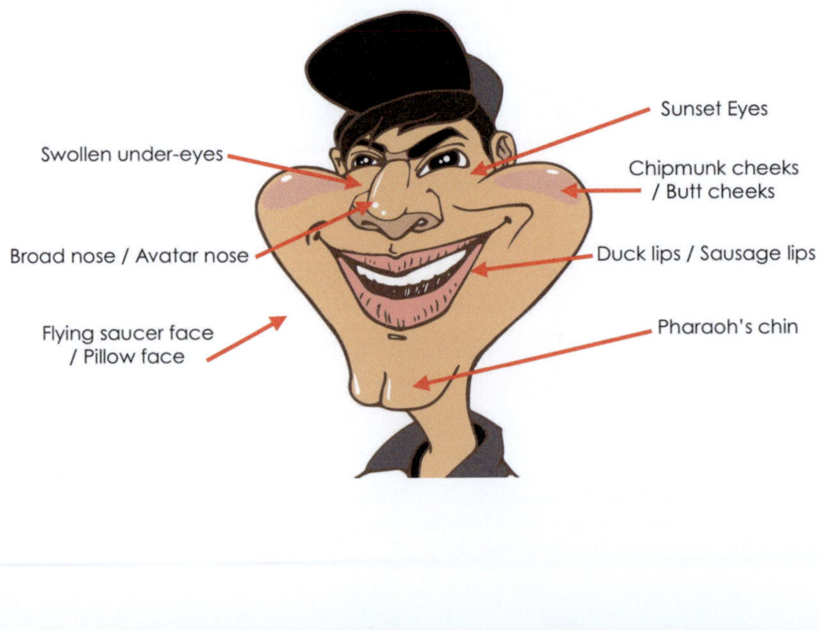

Fig. 11.2 Male patient facial overfilled syndrome

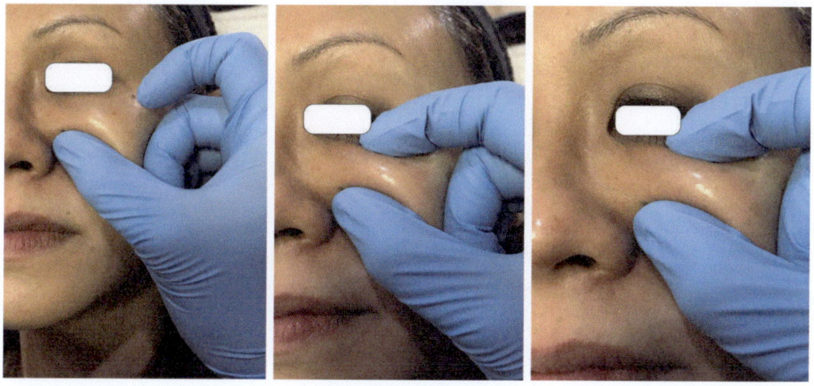

Fig. 11.3 Assessment of facial overfilled syndrome

3. Feel: Patient-reported tightness or palpable lumps.
4. Express: Dynamic facial movements reveal asymmetrical contours or filler migration.

11.4 Prevention Strategies

1. Filler Selection

Low-viscosity high cohesivity HA fillers are preferred for superficial regions to avoid visibility, while high projection capacity products suit deep volumizing [7].

2. Injection Techniques
   - Target-Specific Sandwich Technique (TSST): Layering fillers in deep (supraperiosteal) and superficial planes reduces migration [7].
   - Avoid high-volume injections in mobile areas (e.g., lips) to prevent "pillowing" [6].
3. Patient Education

Pre-treatment counseling using 3D imaging tools mitigates unrealistic expectations [5]. Addressing visual adaptation through side-by-side comparisons of natural versus hyper-augmented outcomes reinforces realistic goals [3].

11.5 Management of FOS

1. Mild FOS

Non-invasive modalities (e.g., microfocused ultrasound, radiofrequency) redistribute filler and stimulate collagen remodeling [10].

2. Moderate-Severe HA FOS
   - Hyaluronidase: 1500 IU diluted in lidocaine, injected via 30G needle; repeat sessions required for cross-linked HA [6, 11] (Figs. 11.4 and 11.5).
3. Non-HA FOS
   - Collagenase clostridium histolyticum (CCH): Degrades fibrotic collagen around PLLA/CaHA, though efficacy varies [9].
   - Surgical excision: Indicated for PMMA or refractory cases [12].
4. Post-treatment Recovery

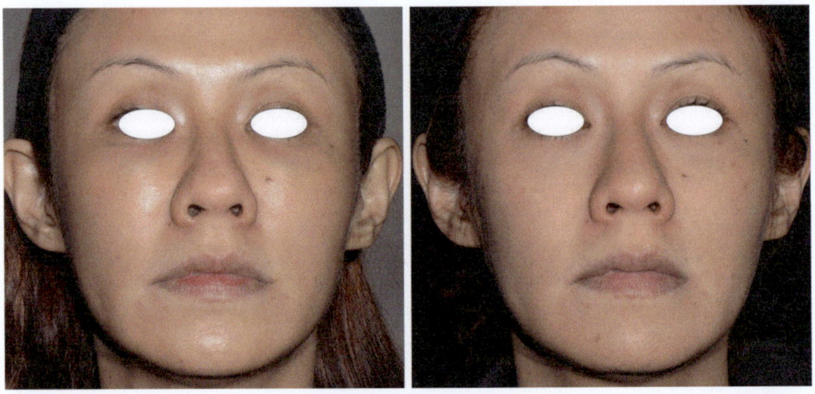

Fig. 11.4 Hyaluronidase injection of facial overfilled syndrome Before (Lt) and after (Rt)

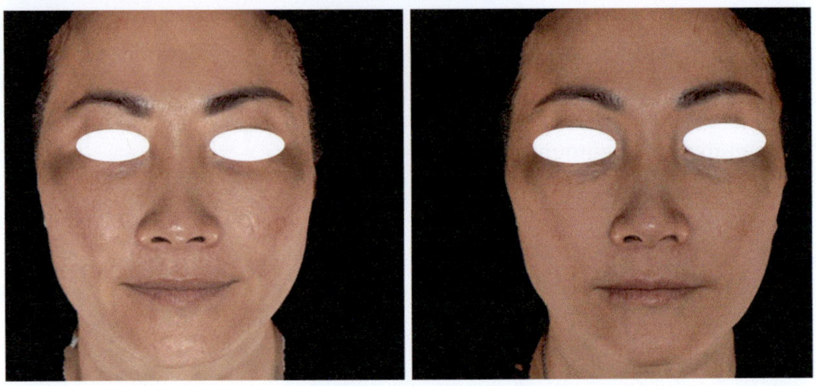

Fig. 11.5 Hyaluronidase injection of facial overfilled syndrome Before (Lt) and after (Rt)

Bioregenerative agents and fractional lasers restore skin integrity [7].

11.6 Conclusion

FOS underscores the need for ethical practices, anatomical expertise, and patient-centered care. Emerging therapies like collagenase and regenerative techniques offer hope, but prevention through education remains paramount. Combating visual adaptation requires continuous training and objective assessment tools to counteract normalized distortions.

Key Takeaways

1. Prevention: Prioritize low-volume, deep-plane injections and patient counseling [2].
2. Diagnosis: Combine clinical assessment with MRI/ultrasound; account for visual adaptation in practitioner judgment [3, 8, 12].
3. Treatment: Enzymatic dissolution for HA, collagenase trials for non-HA, and surgery for permanent fillers [6, 9, 12].
4. Recovery: Leverage bioregenerative agents to restore skin health [7].

References

1. De Boulle K, Heydenrych I. Patient factors influencing dermal filler complications: prevention, assessment, and treatment. Clin Cosmet Investig Dermatol. 2015;8:205–14. https://doi.org/10.2147/CCID.S80446.
2. Lim TS. Facial overfilled syndrome. Dermatol Clin. 2024;42(1):121–8. https://doi.org/10.1016/j.det.2023.06.007.
3. Goldie K, Cumming D, Voropai D, et al. Aesthetic delusions: an investigation into the role of rapid visual adaptation in aesthetic practice. Clin Cosmet Investig Dermatol. 2021;14:1079–87. https://doi.org/10.2147/CCID.S305976.
4. Lim TS, Wanitphakdeedecha R, Yi KH. Exploring facial overfilled syndrome from the perspective of anatomy and the mismatched delivery of fillers. J Cosmet Dermatol. 2024;23(6):1964–8. https://doi.org/10.1111/jocd.16244.
5. Buzzaccarini G, Degliuomini RS, Borin M. The impact of social media-driven fame in aesthetic medicine: when followers overshadow science. Aesthet Surg J. 2023;43(10):NP807–8. https://doi.org/10.1093/asj/sjad190.
6. DeLorenzi C. Complications of injectable fillers, Part I. Aesthet Surg J. 2013;33(4):561–75. https://doi.org/10.1177/1090820X13484492.
7. Lim TS, Frank K, Hadjab B. Target-specific sandwich technique: facial rejuvenation leveraging CPM technology. J Cosmet Dermatol. 2022;21(1):207–19. https://doi.org/10.1111/jocd.14342.
8. Master M, Azizeddin A, Master V. Hyaluronic acid filler longevity in the mid-face: a review of 33 magnetic resonance imaging studies. Plast Reconstr Surg Glob Open. 2024;12(7):e5934. https://doi.org/10.1097/GOX.0000000000005934.
9. Salles AG, Lotierzo PH, Gimenez RP. Management of complications from permanent and semipermanent fillers: recommendations for surgical excision. Plast Reconstr Surg. 2021;148(3):447e–56e. https://doi.org/10.1097/PRS.0000000000008244.
10. Alam M, Dover JS. Management of complications and sequelae with temporary injectable fillers. Plast Reconstr Surg. 2007;120(6 Suppl):98S–105S. https://doi.org/10.1097/01.prs.0000248859.14788.60.
11. Hong GW, Hu H, Chang K, et al. Review of the adverse effects associated with dermal filler treatments: Part I Nodules, granuloma, and migration. Diagnostics (Basel). 2024;14(15):1640. https://doi.org/10.3390/diagnostics14151640.
12. Schelke LW, Decates TS, Velthuis PJ. Ultrasound-guided hyaluronidase injection for filler complications: a standardized protocol. Dermatol Surg. 2020;46(11):1364–71. https://doi.org/10.1097/DSS.0000000000002367.

Injectables for Hair Loss Treatment

12

Jino Kim and Won Lee

12.1 Introduction

Alopecia is a common condition affecting a significant portion of the global population, manifesting in a variety of forms, including androgenetic alopecia (AGA), alopecia areata, and scarring alopecia. The spectrum ranges from male and female pattern hair loss to autoimmune-mediated conditions such as alopecia areata [1]. As hair loss progresses, it raises not only cosmetic concerns but also profoundly affects overall quality of life, leading to psychological distress and diminished social confidence.

Conventional treatments for alopecia include oral medications (finasteride, dutasteride), topical therapies (minoxidil), low-level laser therapy (LLLT), and hair transplantation [2]. Recently, injectable therapies have gained considerable attention as a method to deliver active substances directly into the scalp, thereby maximizing localized effects (Fig. 12.1). This approach offers significant advantages, such as minimizing systemic side effects and overcoming the limitations of skin barrier penetration, while enabling faster therapeutic action [3].

J. Kim
New Hair Plastic Surgery Clinic,
Seoul, Republic of Korea
e-mail: jinokim@newhairps.com

W. Lee (✉)
Yonsei E1 Plastic Surgery Clinic,
Anyang, Kyonggi-do, Korea (Republic of)

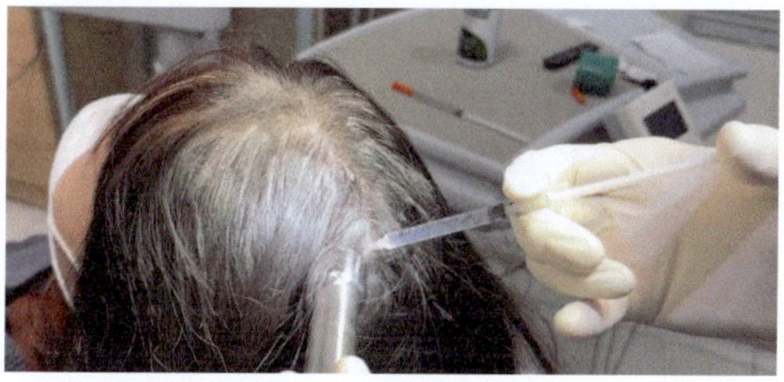

Fig. 12.1 Application of injectable therapies for the treatment of hair loss

In this chapter, we will systematically explore the mechanisms of action underlying injectable treatments for hair loss and examine the specific types currently utilized in clinical practice. Particular focus will be given to emerging therapies such as platelet-rich plasma (PRP), polydeoxyribonucleotide (PDRN)/polynucleotide (PN) solutions, polymer-based agents, botulinum toxin, and autologous micrografts, highlighting their clinical significance and limitations.

12.2 Pathophysiology of Hair Loss

12.2.1 Androgenetic Alopecia (AGA)

- Dihydrotestosterone (DHT) acts on genetically predisposed hair follicles, leading to progressive miniaturization and shortening of the

W. Lee (ed.), *Innovative Injectable Techniques in Minimally Invasive Aesthetics*,
https://doi.org/10.1007/978-981-95-2161-6_12

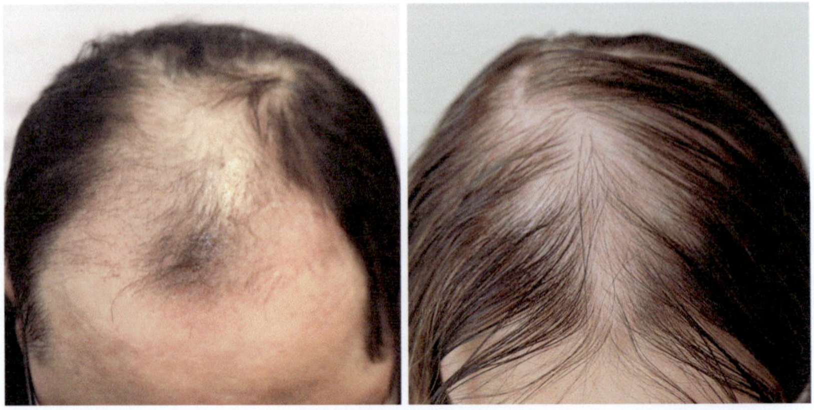

Fig. 12.2 Patterns of androgenetic alopecia in men and women

anagen (growth) phase, ultimately resulting in hair shaft thinning [1].

- In men, the process most prominently affects the frontal hairline (M-shaped recession) and the vertex (crown area), whereas in women, it typically presents as diffuse thinning along the central parting and the crown (Fig. 12.2) [1, 4].
- The rate and extent of progression vary widely among individuals.

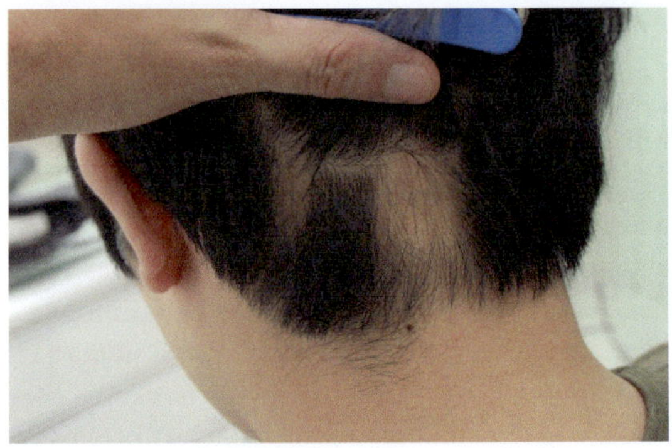

Fig. 12.3 Alopecia areata

12.2.2 Alopecia Areata

- Alopecia areata is characterized by a rapid inflammatory cell infiltration around hair follicles due to an autoimmune mechanism, resulting in well-circumscribed, round patches of hair loss (Fig. 12.3) [5].
- Mild cases may exhibit spontaneous hair regrowth within weeks to months, whereas severe forms can progress to alopecia totalis or alopecia universalis, often requiring immunosuppressive therapy [5].

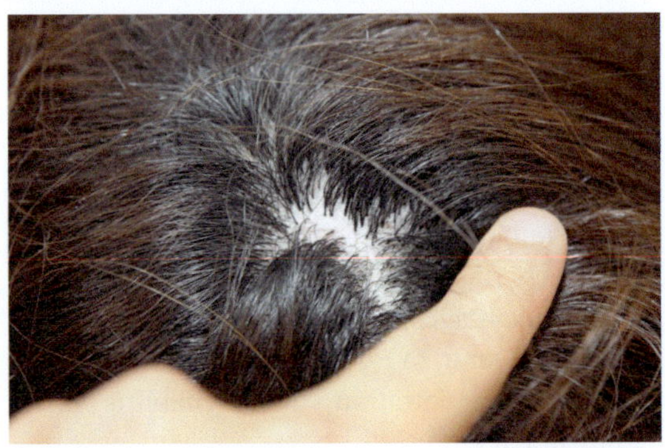

Fig. 12.4 Clinical presentation of scarring alopecia

12.2.3 Other Forms of Scarring and Inflammatory Alopecia

Scarring and inflammatory alopecia can arise from various causes, including burns, lupus erythematosus, seborrheic dermatitis, and trauma [6]. In cases where the scalp tissue sustains severe damage, permanent destruction of hair follicles occurs, leading to scarring and irreversible hair loss with a permanent reduction in hair density (Fig. 12.4) [6].

12.3 Mechanisms of Action of Injectable Therapies

Injectable therapies for hair loss aim to achieve relatively rapid and targeted effects by directly delivering regenerative agents, immunomodulators, and growth factors into the scalp [3]. The specific mechanisms are as follows:

- *Inflammation and immune modulation*: Agents such as corticosteroids and PDRN/PN suppress perifollicular inflammation and alleviate immune-mediated hair loss, including alopecia areata.
- *Improvement of blood circulation*: Agents such as botulinum toxin and adenosine relax scalp muscles and dilate the microvasculature, enhancing oxygen and nutrient delivery.
- *Growth factor stimulation and tissue regeneration*: Injections of PRP, growth factor cocktails, and PDRN/PN activate follicular cells, promote extracellular matrix (ECM) remodeling, and stimulate collagen production, fundamentally improving the scalp environment.
- *Normalization of the hair cycle*: Hair loss is characterized by a shortened anagen phase and a prolonged telogen phase. Injectable therapies work to extend the anagen phase or shorten the telogen phase, enhancing follicular activity.

12.4 Major Types of Injectable Therapies for Hair Loss

The table below categorizes major injectable therapies based on their mechanisms of action and clinical applications (Table 12.1).

Table 12.1 Key injectable therapies for hair loss

Agent	Mechanisms and key features
PRP (platelet-rich plasma)	Autologous blood-derived; delivers growth factors (PDGF, VEGF, EGF) to activate hair follicles and promote angiogenesis
PDRN (polydeoxyribonucleotide)	Enhances tissue regeneration, suppresses inflammation, and remodels the ECM to improve scalp health
PN (polynucleotide)	Exhibits anti-inflammatory effects, stimulates angiogenesis and ECM regeneration; known for rapid penetration and responsiveness based on molecular composition
PDLLA (poly-DL-lactic acid)	Improves scalp elasticity through collagen production and ECM remodeling; requires management of initial inflammation and potential adverse effects
PDO (polydioxanone)	Gradually degrades to induce localized collagen production, contributing to improved scalp structure and resilience
Botulinum toxin	Relaxes scalp muscles, enhances microcirculation, and inhibits TGF-beta expression, thereby preventing follicular miniaturization and optimizing the hair growth environment
Corticosteroids	Suppress inflammatory and immune responses to protect and regenerate hair follicles; effective short-term but long-term use requires caution due to potential side effects
HA (hyaluronic acid)	Provides potent moisturization and ECM stabilization, indirectly supporting hair growth by preventing scalp dryness
Adenosine	Enhances cellular metabolism and microvascular dilation, stimulating hair follicle activity and increasing growth factor expression
Placental extract	Supplies a variety of bioactive substances (peptides, vitamins, minerals) that promote follicular proliferation and hair growth
Autologous micrograft	Involves injecting crushed scalp tissue from the patient to regenerate follicles and activate growth factors, with long-term effects and no risk of immune rejection
Dutasteride mesotherapy	Delivers potent DHT inhibition locally via injection, minimizing systemic side effects while preventing follicular miniaturization and hair loss progression

12.4.1 PRP (Platelet-Rich Plasma)

PRP involves collecting a small volume of the patient's blood, centrifuging it to concentrate the platelets, and directly injecting the resulting plasma into areas affected by hair loss. Platelet-derived growth factors such as PDGF, VEGF, and EGF promote follicular cell proliferation and angiogenesis, thereby inducing hair growth [7].

Because the patient's own blood is used, allergy risk remains low, and aside from transient pain and swelling immediately after the procedure, significant adverse effects are rare (Fig. 12.5) [8].

Typically, 10–20 mL of the patient's blood is collected, placed into a commercial kit, and subjected to centrifugation to isolate PRP, which is then injected into the areas affected by hair loss (Fig. 12.6).

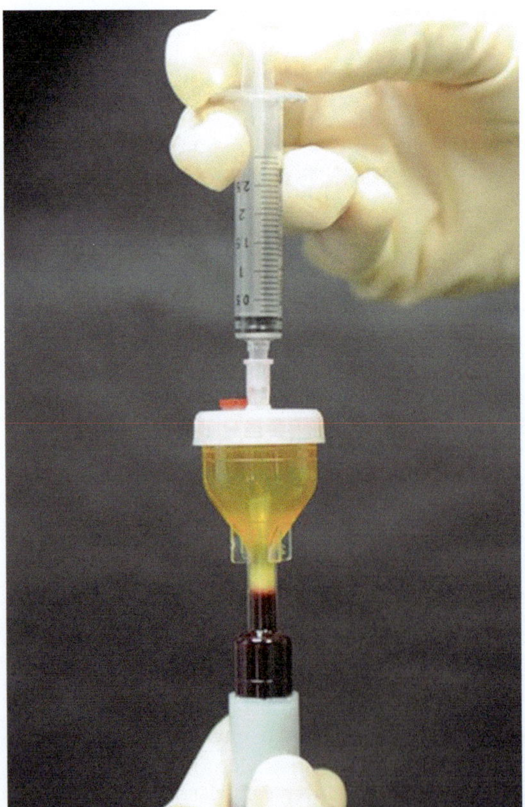

Fig. 12.5 Separation of PRP using a commercial kit

Recent studies have demonstrated that PRP treatment can lead to significant improvements in hair shaft thickness and density among patients with androgenetic alopecia. Gkini et al. reported notable enhancements in both parameters following PRP injections [9]. Furthermore, Kaiser et al. observed that the combination of PRP with oral or topical therapies produced a synergistic effect, yielding better outcomes than monotherapy alone [10].

12.4.2 Polynucleotides and Polymer-Based Agents (PDRN, PN, PDLLA, PDO)

This category of substances primarily acts by promoting tissue regeneration, collagen synthesis, and anti-inflammatory effects, ultimately improving the scalp environment and supporting follicular function.

1. PDRN (Polydeoxyribonucleotide)
Polydeoxyribonucleotide (PDRN), originally derived from sources such as salmon sperm or human placenta, was first utilized for applications in skin regeneration and wound healing [11].

More recently, research has demonstrated that these regenerative properties are also effective within the scalp, drawing increasing interest in PDRN as an adjunctive therapy for hair loss due to its dual role in inflammation modulation and cellular activation [12].

Chronic inflammation in the scalp can damage the perifollicular environment, disrupting the normal hair growth cycle [13]. PDRN binds to A2A

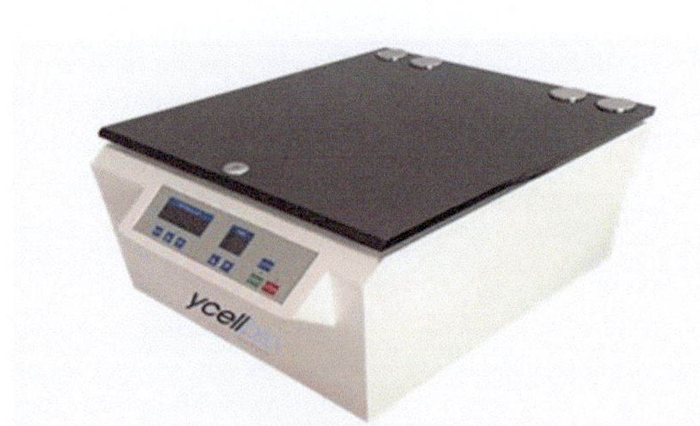

Fig. 12.6 PRP centrifuge

adenosine receptors, suppressing the excessive release of inflammatory cytokines [14]. This interaction stabilizes the scalp microenvironment and promotes fibroblast activation. Fibroblasts are critical for maintaining tissue health as they produce structural proteins such as collagen and elastin, thereby enhancing scalp elasticity and improving the conditions around hair follicles [15].

Additionally, PDRN stimulates collagen production and remodeling of the extracellular matrix (ECM), further contributing to improved scalp elasticity and microcirculation. Enhanced blood flow supplies oxygen and nutrients to hair follicles more effectively, encouraging dormant hairs in the telogen phase to re-enter the anagen (growth) phase.

When used in combination with standard treatments such as minoxidil or finasteride, PDRN appears to exert complementary effects, potentially improving overall therapeutic outcomes.

Moreover, its anti-inflammatory and tissue repair properties suggest potential applications in inflammatory types of hair loss, such as alopecia areata, where it may help prevent disease progression and recurrence.

PDRN treatment is generally administered via direct scalp injections or combined with microneedling techniques to enhance absorption (Fig. 12.7). Topical application following laser therapy has also been explored.

Clinical reports to date indicate that serious adverse effects are rare, although larger studies are needed to better define its long-term efficacy and safety profile.

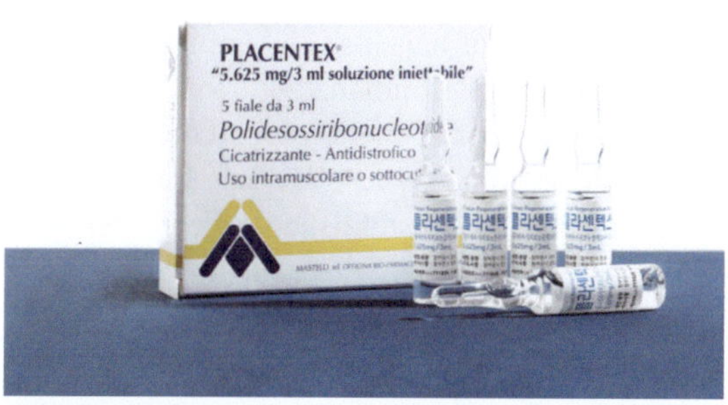

Fig. 12.7 PDRN

In summary, PDRN offers a multi-faceted mechanism of action in hair loss treatment through inflammation reduction, cellular activation, and ECM remodeling. It may enhance the efficacy of conventional therapies and holds promise across a range of hair loss conditions.

Future large-scale clinical trials are necessary to fully establish its long-term benefits and expand its role in the field of hair restoration.

2. PN (Polynucleotide)

Polynucleotides (PNs) are emerging candidates for hair loss treatment and have recently attracted attention in clinical research. While PDRN is typically extracted from sources such as salmon sperm or placenta and is widely used for its anti-inflammatory and tissue regenerative properties, PN differs in molecular weight and source, suggesting the potential for broader biological activity.

Similar to PDRN, PN has been reported to improve the scalp environment by exerting anti-inflammatory effects, promoting angiogenesis, and facilitating extracellular matrix (ECM) remodeling. However, PN is characterized by a different molecular profile, particularly a higher proportion of low-molecular-weight components, which may allow for more rapid tissue penetration and faster biological responses [16]. These differences suggest that the therapeutic effects and duration of action within the scalp may differ between PN and PDRN.

Currently, PN is not yet widely adopted as a standard agent for hair loss treatment (Fig. 12.8). Nonetheless, early clinical studies have shown promising results. In one study involving patients with androgenetic alopecia (AGA), four sessions of PN injections administered at 4-week intervals led to increased hair shaft diameter and density, along with an 82.1% improvement in patient-reported satisfaction [17]. These outcomes imply that PN may support follicular health by simultaneously promoting anti-inflammatory effects, angiogenesis, and ECM regeneration.

Although PN and PDRN share fundamental mechanisms related to tissue regeneration, differences in molecular structure and composition

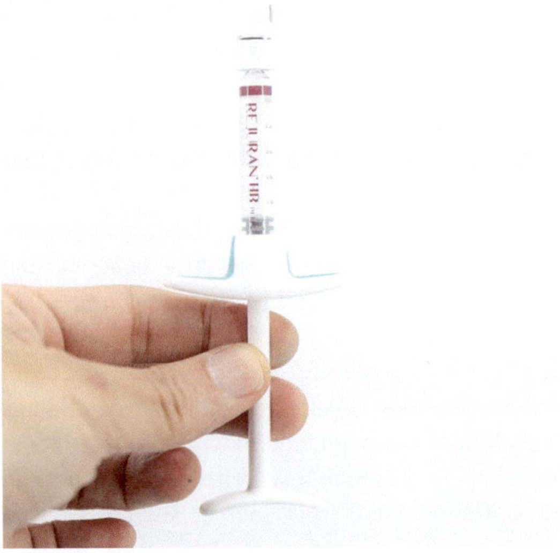

Fig. 12.8 Polynucleotide

may influence their penetration depth, onset of action, and treatment longevity within the scalp.

To clearly define the therapeutic role of PN in hair restoration, larger-scale clinical trials and long-term safety assessments are needed. As evidence accumulates, PN may emerge as a complementary agent to PDRN or as an independent modality, potentially offering a new therapeutic option in the evolving field of hair loss management.

3. PDLLA (Poly-DL-Lactic Acid)

Poly-DL-lactic acid (PDLLA) is a biodegradable synthetic polymer that has been widely used as a dermal filler for facial wrinkle correction and volume restoration. One of its key features is the gradual degradation at the injection site, which induces neocollagenesis over time (Fig. 12.9) [18].

Studies in skin regeneration have shown that PDLLA injections stimulate collagen and extracellular matrix (ECM) remodeling, enhancing tissue elasticity and structural integrity. These effects are now being explored in the context of the scalp, where they are expected to improve the supporting environment around hair follicles and enhance blood circulation, thereby optimizing the conditions for hair growth [19].

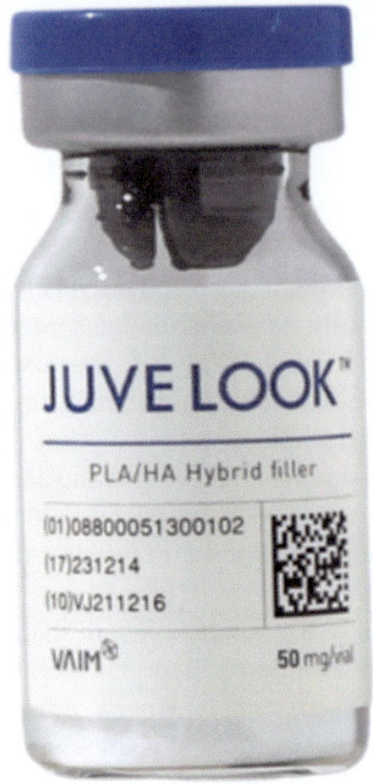

Fig. 12.9 PDLLA

In dermatologic applications, the effects of PDLLA appear gradually but have been reported to persist for several months to up to a year [20]. However, early adverse events—such as local inflammation or nodule formation due to product clumping—may occur, underscoring the importance of meticulous technique and practitioner expertise during administration [18].

When properly managed, PDLLA injected into the scalp can gradually stimulate collagen production, improving the structural resilience and elasticity of scalp tissue. In turn, enhanced microcirculation may increase oxygen and nutrient delivery to the follicles, potentially slowing the progression of hair loss and contributing to a healthier scalp environment.

Although clinical studies specifically investigating the use of PDLLA for hair loss are currently limited, its established effects on skin regeneration suggest a theoretical basis for its application in scalp therapy. The underlying mechanism—tissue remodeling through neocollagenesis—may offer a novel therapeutic avenue in the treatment of alopecia.

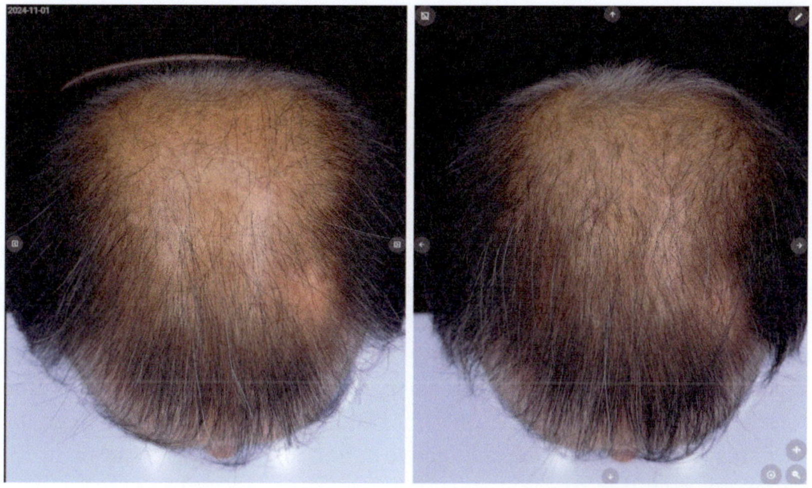

Fig. 12.10 Before and after three PDLLA sessions at monthly intervals

In a small number of test cases conducted by the author, an increase in hair density was observed following PDLLA injection into the scalp (Fig. 12.10). The formation of new collagen within the scalp may strengthen the structural support surrounding hair follicles, while improved microcirculation enhances nutrient delivery. Together, these effects may contribute to normalization of the hair growth cycle and potentially delay the progression of hair loss.

To clearly establish the therapeutic potential of PDLLA in hair loss treatment, dedicated studies focusing on scalp application are required, building upon existing preclinical and clinical research in skin regeneration.

Future investigations should systematically evaluate parameters such as injection dosage, treatment intervals, extent of collagen synthesis within scalp tissue, changes in vascular perfusion, and hair growth rate. These metrics will be essential for assessing both the safety and long-term efficacy of PDLLA-based scalp therapy.

4. PDO (Polydioxanone)

Polydioxanone (PDO) is a synthetic, bioabsorbable suture material widely used in aesthetic procedures such as thread lifting for facial rejuvenation and wrinkle correction [21]. When inserted or injected into tissue, PDO gradually degrades and stimulates localized collagen production, thereby enhancing tissue elasticity and structural stability [22].

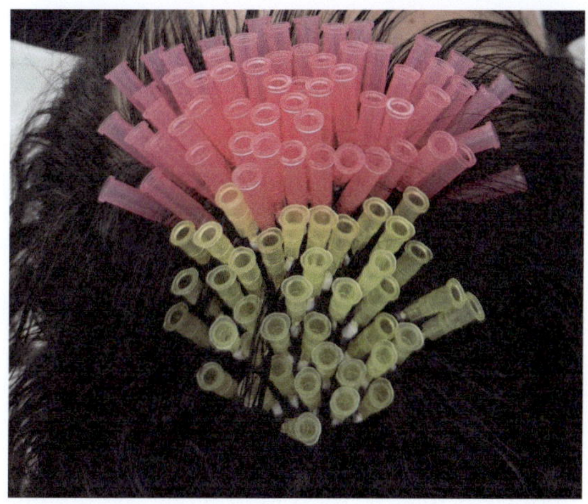

Fig. 12.11 Scalp application of PDO threads for hair loss treatment

Recently, efforts have been made to apply these properties to the scalp (Fig. 12.11). When administered in the form of fine particles or short-cut threads via injection or implantation, the degradation process of PDO triggers collagen synthesis, which may promote scalp tissue regeneration. This could lead to improved scalp elasticity and enhanced microcirculation, allowing for better oxygen and nutrient delivery to hair follicles and thereby optimizing the environment for hair growth [23].

Preliminary trials involving scalp application of PDO have shown a modest increase in hair shaft thickness. However, these findings are from early-stage studies, and further large-scale clinical research is needed to validate both the efficacy and safety of this approach.

An additional advantage of PDO lies in its slow degradation and sustained action, which may contribute to long-term scalp remodeling and potentially delay the progression of hair loss.

To further clarify the role of PDO in the treatment of hair loss, comprehensive preclinical and clinical studies are needed. These should systematically investigate optimal dosing strategies, injection intervals, and long-term safety specific to scalp applications. Based on such findings, PDO may emerge as a viable adjunctive option in hair restoration therapy.

12.4.3 Botulinum Toxin

Botulinum toxin, originally developed for aesthetic procedures such as wrinkle reduction and facial lifting, functions by blocking neuromuscular transmission, leading to localized muscle relaxation [24]. When applied to the scalp, this action can relieve tension in the scalp musculature and promote vasodilation in the microvasculature, thereby increasing blood flow to the scalp and enhancing the delivery of oxygen and nutrients to hair follicles [25].

Beyond muscle relaxation alone, botulinum toxin may exert additional hair growth-relevant physiological effects. It has been shown to reduce the expression of transforming growth factor-beta (TGF-β), a key molecule known to inhibit hair growth and induce follicular miniaturization [26]. This mechanism may contribute to a more favorable environment for follicular regeneration and help slow the progression of alopecia.

Clinically, botulinum toxin is typically administered via multiple small injections into the frontal and vertex scalp areas, with treatments repeated every 3–6 months. A typical total dose per session ranges from 50 to 150 units. Careful attention to dosage and frequency is critical, as excessive use or overly frequent injections may increase the risk of antibody formation or lead to adverse cosmetic effects such as eyelid ptosis or forehead asymmetry due to unintended diffusion into adjacent muscles.

Some patients may experience visible improvement as early as 1 month post-treatment, although clinical effects generally begin to emerge around 3 months following the procedure (Figs. 12.12, 12.13, 12.14, and 12.15).

To date, evidence suggests that botulinum toxin does not directly promote hair growth but may act as an effective adjunctive treatment by improving scalp vascularization and reducing TGF-β levels. As larger clinical studies continue to validate its efficacy and safety, botulinum toxin may become an important therapeutic tool in the management of androgenetic alopecia (AGA) and potentially other forms of hair loss.

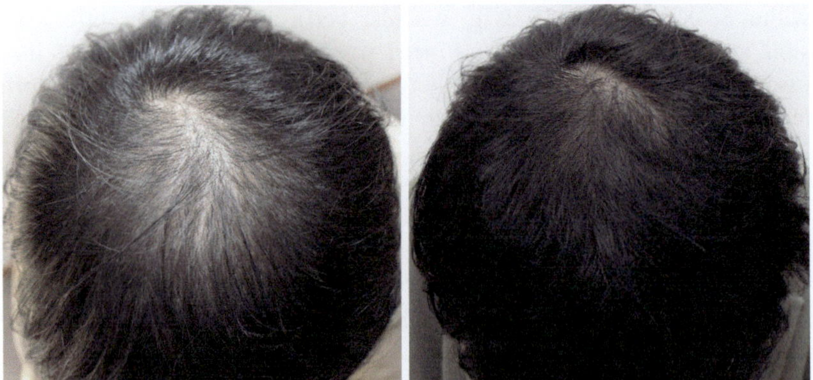

Fig. 12.12 Male androgenetic alopecia before (left) and 3 months after (right) botulinum toxin treatment

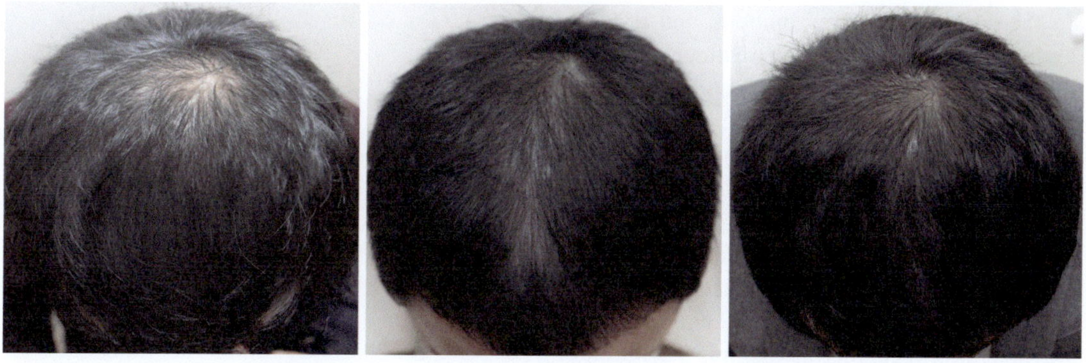

Fig. 12.13 Serial comparison of hair growth in male AGA treated with botulinum toxin

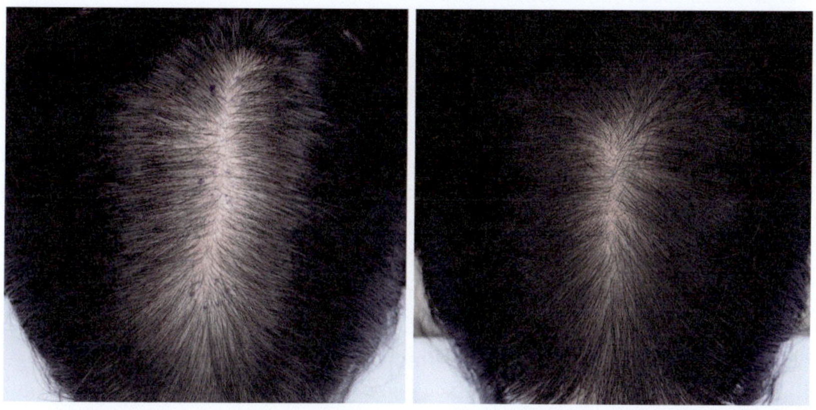

Fig. 12.14 Improvement in female pattern hair loss 5 months after botulinum toxin therapy

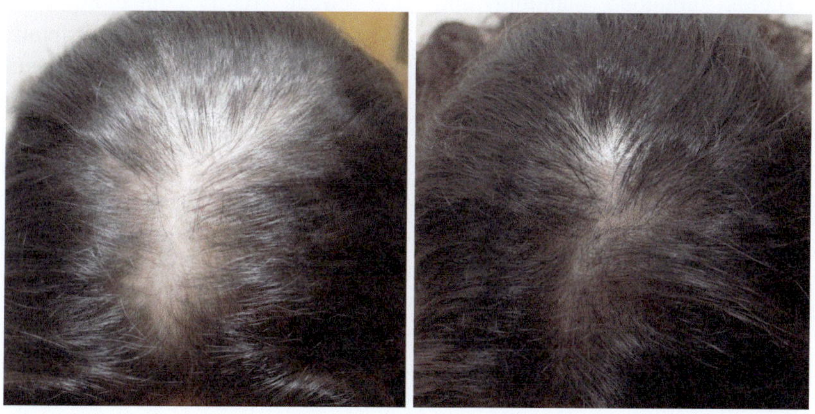

Fig. 12.15 Female hair loss before and 5 months after botulinum toxin treatment

12.4.4 Steroids

Alopecia areata is an autoimmune disorder wherein immune cells attack hair follicles, resulting in rapid hair loss and significant psychological distress [27]. Intralesional corticosteroid injections are commonly used to suppress local inflammation and immune activity, thereby protecting hair follicles and providing rapid symptomatic relief [28].

Triamcinolone acetonide is the most widely used agent for intralesional steroid therapy. It acts by quickly reducing inflammation, improving the perifollicular environment, and promoting hair regrowth. A typical treatment protocol involves injecting affected areas at 4-week intervals for two to three sessions. This approach is particularly effective in resolving acute inflammatory phases and providing prompt clinical improvement [29].

However, long-term and repeated steroid use poses a risk of adverse effects. Potential complications include skin atrophy, pigmentary changes, and systemic effects such as Cushing's syndrome. For this reason, corticosteroids should be administered in limited doses and localized strictly to the affected areas to minimize risk.

These considerations emphasize that while corticosteroid therapy is highly effective in the short term, long-term treatment strategies must be approached with caution [30].

Recent reviews have confirmed that intralesional corticosteroids play an important role in the acute management of alopecia areata by promoting rapid symptom resolution and supporting follicular regeneration. However, further studies are needed to better evaluate the risk of side effects and long-term safety. These findings highlight the dual nature of corticosteroids—as a potent short-term solution and a treatment that requires judicious planning and side effect monitoring.

12.4.5 Hyaluronic Acid (HA)

Hyaluronic acid (HA) is a naturally occurring glycosaminoglycan known for its exceptional hydrating properties. In the context of scalp health, HA contributes to extracellular matrix (ECM) stabilization and plays a crucial role in maintaining skin and follicular hydration (Fig. 12.16) [31].

When applied to the scalp, HA binds and retains water, preventing dryness and helping to maintain an optimal microenvironment around hair follicles [32].

Beyond simple moisturization, HA supports ECM integrity, enhances tissue elasticity, and facilitates effective delivery of oxygen and nutrients to the follicular unit [33]. These effects indirectly contribute to improved scalp circulation and overall hair maintenance.

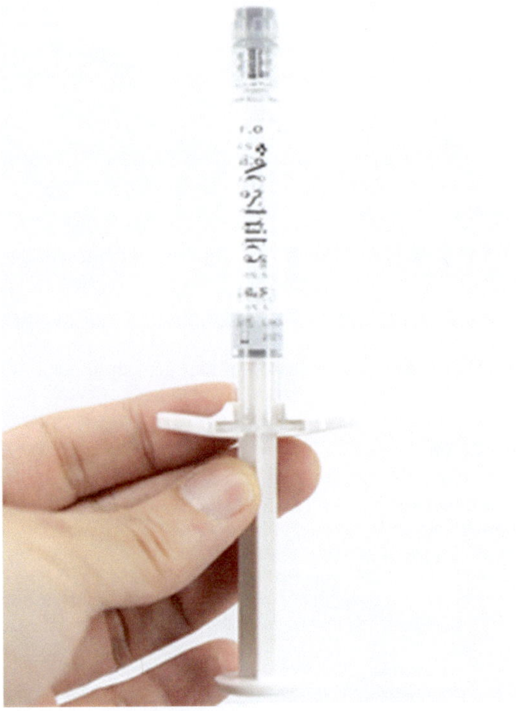

Fig. 12.16 Non-cross-linked hyaluronic acid

However, HA alone has limited hair growth-stimulating potential and does not directly induce anagen phase transition [34]. For this reason, it is often included in mesotherapy cocktails to support the action and penetration of other bioactive ingredients. It also helps reduce post-injection discomfort and irritation, making it a valuable adjunctive agent [35].

In summary, HA contributes to hair restoration not as a direct growth promoter but as a supportive agent that improves scalp hydration and ECM stability. When combined with other active ingredients in mesotherapy formulations, its synergistic effects may be maximized. Further research on optimal concentrations and formulation ratios may expand its use as an effective adjunct in hair loss therapy.

12.4.6 Adenosine

Adenosine is a naturally occurring nucleoside derivative known to enhance cellular metabolism and promote microvascular dilation, thereby improving oxygen and nutrient delivery to hair follicles [36]. This mechanism may contribute to follicular activation and modulation of the hair growth cycle, supporting its use as an adjunctive treatment for hair loss.

Early studies examined topical formulations such as adenosine-based scalp tonics, which showed efficacy in improving the perifollicular environment and stimulating the regeneration of telogen-phase hair. These topical products offered ease of use and a low risk of side effects but were limited by insufficient drug concentration reaching the follicular target [37].

To overcome these limitations, recent approaches have incorporated adenosine into injectable formulations. Delivered via mesotherapy, adenosine can reach the follicular unit in higher concentrations, thereby enhancing the expression of growth factors essential for hair development and maximizing microvascular expansion. This technique may be particularly effective in areas of advanced hair thinning; however, further studies are necessary to establish optimal dosing and safety [38].

In summary, adenosine contributes to hair loss management by promoting cellular metabolism and vascular perfusion around hair follicles [39]. Its use has evolved from simple topical applications to more targeted intradermal injections, with future clinical trials expected to clarify the ideal protocol, long-term efficacy, and safety.

12.4.7 Placental Extract

Placental extract contains a complex mixture of bioactive peptides, vitamins, and minerals derived from animal placenta and has demonstrated regenerative and anti-inflammatory effects. These properties have been investigated not only for skin rejuvenation but also for their potential role in promoting hair growth [40].

Several clinical and preclinical studies have reported that placental extract stimulates dermal papilla cell proliferation and enhances follicular development [41, 42]. Notably, its efficacy has been shown to be comparable to minoxidil in female pattern hair loss, indicating its value as a non-hormonal therapeutic option [43]. The proposed mechanisms include prolongation of the anagen phase and upregulation of follicular growth factor expression, leading to improvements in both hair thickness and density [44].

In chemotherapy-induced alopecia, human-derived placental extract has demonstrated regenerative effects by suppressing apoptosis and enhancing follicular proliferation [45]. When used in combination with minoxidil, studies suggest a synergistic effect, allowing for effective hair regrowth even at lower drug concentrations [44].

Despite its therapeutic promise, robust clinical evidence remains limited. Additional randomized controlled trials are required to confirm its efficacy and define standardized protocols for long-term use [46]. With further validation, placental extract may become a reliable adjunct or alternative in the development of hair loss treatments.

12.4.8 Autologous Micrograft Technique

The autologous micrograft technique is a regenerative therapy that involves harvesting a small amount of healthy scalp tissue—typically from the occipital region—followed by mechanical disaggregation to produce a cellular suspension rich in stem cells, fibroblasts, and extracellular matrix (ECM) components. This biologically active solution is then injected into areas of hair thinning (Figs. 12.17 and 12.18) [47].

The micrograft suspension stimulates endogenous regenerative mechanisms by activating growth factors and signaling pathways associated with follicular repair. It also promotes anagen phase induction and facilitates cell–cell interaction in damaged follicular environments, improving both hair density and shaft thickness. Because the treatment utilizes autologous

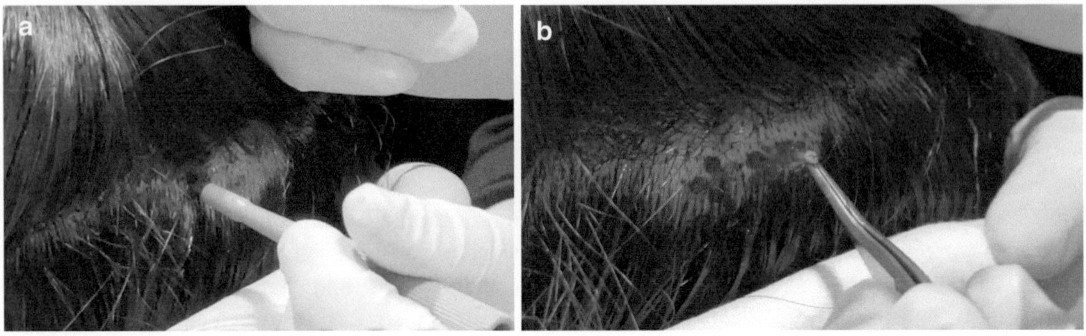

Fig. 12.17 Follicular tissue harvest during autologous micrograft procedure. (**a**) The hair follicle is harvested using a kit similar to a punch biopsy. (**b**) It is carefully extracted with forceps

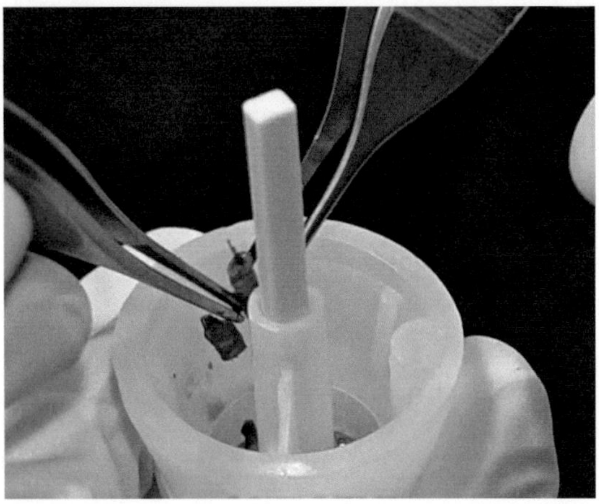

Fig. 12.18 Preparing harvested scalp tissue in micrograft kit

tissue, it carries minimal risk of immune rejection or allergic response and has been reported to yield results lasting 6–12 months after a single session [48].

However, the effectiveness of this technique can vary depending on the donor tissue quality and cell extraction efficiency. Concerns include possible cell viability reduction during the disaggregation process, minor downtime due to scalp injury, and the need for long-term efficacy data [47]. While the technique can be synergistically combined with medical therapies or hair transplantation, its consistency and standalone efficacy are yet to be fully established. Further randomized controlled trials are needed to optimize variables such as cell concentration, solution composition, and injection frequency [47].

12.4.9 Dutasteride Mesotherapy

Dutasteride mesotherapy is an emerging treatment that involves the intradermal injection of dutasteride—a potent 5α-reductase inhibitor—into the scalp using mesotherapy or microneedling techniques [49]. This approach aims to harness the drug's powerful dihydrotestosterone (DHT) suppression effects locally while minimizing systemic adverse effects commonly associated with oral administration [50].

Dutasteride differs from its first-generation counterpart, finasteride, in that it inhibits both type I and type II isoenzymes of 5α-reductase, resulting in over 90% suppression of serum DHT levels [49, 50]. While oral administration has demonstrated strong efficacy, it carries the risk of sexual side effects and long drug half-life. Mesotherapy offers a localized delivery alternative, reducing systemic absorption and improving the safety profile [51].

Retrospective studies involving large patient cohorts have shown that dutasteride mesotherapy is safe and effective over a 6-month treatment course, with only minor adverse effects such as transient pain or mild edema at injection sites [51]. However, the efficacy of this technique is highly dependent on injection parameters such as site accuracy, drug concentration, and frequency. The absence of standardized protocols remains a limitation [49].

Some cases have reported adverse events, including localized scarring alopecia at injection sites, potentially linked to cytotoxic effects of solvents (e.g., ethanol) used in the formulation

[52]. Recent studies have also explored the synergistic use of microneedling with dutasteride and low-dose minoxidil, reporting superior improvements in hair density and thickness compared to dutasteride alone—likely due to enhanced drug penetration and tissue regeneration [53].

In conclusion, dutasteride mesotherapy provides a targeted and effective means of inhibiting follicular miniaturization and promoting regrowth while minimizing systemic exposure. Further clinical trials are required to establish long-term efficacy, optimal dosing, and standardized treatment protocols.

12.4.10 Summary of Injectable Agents

Each injectable treatment option should be selected based on the degree of hair loss, scalp condition, and individual therapeutic goals. In early-stage hair loss, agents such as PRP or hyaluronic acid can improve scalp health and promote hair growth. Inflammatory or autoimmune-mediated alopecia, such as alopecia areata, may benefit more from corticosteroids or nucleotides like PDRN/PN.

In more advanced cases with hair shaft miniaturization, botulinum toxin or collagen-inducing polymers (e.g., PDO, PDLLA) may be employed to enhance follicular support and microcirculation. For patients who seek potent DHT inhibition without systemic side effects, dutasteride mesotherapy is a promising alternative.

Ultimately, treatment must be personalized. A comprehensive consultation and evaluation are essential prior to initiating therapy, and combination approaches are often necessary to achieve optimal outcomes.

12.5 Injection Techniques for Hair Loss Treatment

Injectable therapy for scalp alopecia can be broadly classified into three primary delivery methods:

1. *Manual injections*
2. *Mesogun-assisted delivery* (single or multi-needle systems)
3. *Microjet devices*

Additionally, microneedling-assisted topical application—either pre- or post-needle insertion—can be used to enhance transdermal drug absorption [54].

Manual Injections

The manual injection technique involves direct administration of therapeutic agents using a fine needle. It allows the practitioner to precisely control the depth and angle of penetration, facilitating targeted drug distribution across specific areas of the scalp (Fig. 12.19). This method is advantageous in tailoring treatment based on individual scalp characteristics and lesion distribution [55].

Mesogun-Assisted Injection Technique

The mesogun technique utilizes a mechanized injector equipped with either single- or multi-needle arrays to deliver therapeutic agents at a consistent depth, pressure, and speed. Single-needle systems allow for focused drug delivery in specific areas, while multi-needle configurations enable broader coverage in less time, enhancing procedural efficiency.

This device-assisted technique offers uniform drug distribution, and its controlled needle arrangement and injection pressure have been shown to contribute positively to treatment outcomes [56].

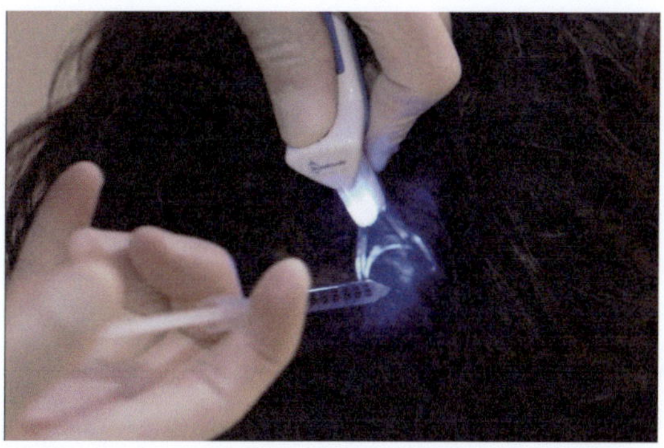

Fig. 12.19 Direct injection technique using a syringe

Microjet Technique

The microjet method employs an ultra-fine jet injection system to administer drugs at low pressure with high precision (Fig. 12.20). This technique minimizes tissue trauma and injection-site discomfort while ensuring even drug dispersion throughout the scalp.

Due to its minimally invasive nature, the microjet approach is particularly beneficial for sensitive scalp areas or when extremely localized drug delivery is required [57].

Microneedling-Assisted Topical Drug Application

Microneedling can be used in conjunction with injectable therapy as an adjunctive technique, wherein topical agents are applied to the scalp before or after microneedling (Fig. 12.21). This approach creates microchannels in the stratum corneum, significantly enhancing transdermal drug absorption.

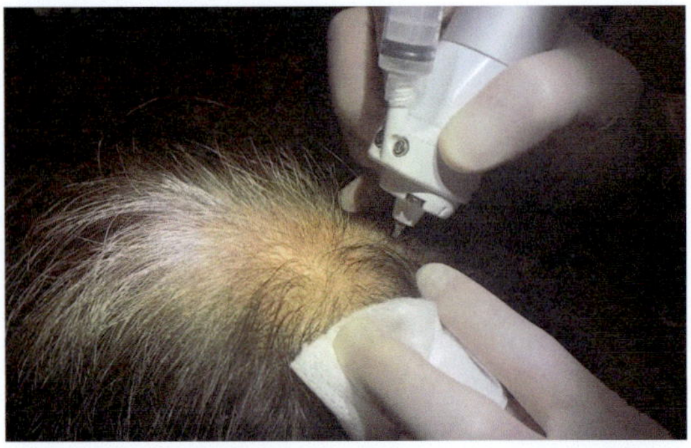

Fig. 12.20 Microjet delivery method

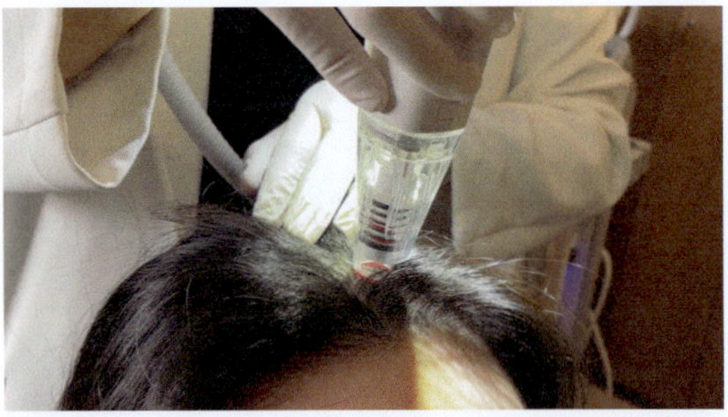

Fig. 12.21 Microneedling technique for scalp drug delivery

Additionally, microneedling has been shown to improve local blood circulation and stimulate tissue regeneration, further potentiating the therapeutic effects of hair loss treatments [58–60]. As such, microneedling-assisted delivery is increasingly recognized as a valuable complementary method to enhance the efficacy of conventional injection techniques.

12.6 Adverse Effects

With the wider adoption of injectable therapies for alopecia, growing attention is also being paid to potential adverse effects. Common side effects at the injection site include pain, bruising, edema, infection, and hypersensitivity reactions, with the incidence and severity varying based on the type of substance used and the delivery method.

Mild bleeding and bruising at needle entry points are common and may be accompanied by localized pain lasting 1–3 days post-procedure. These symptoms are usually self-limiting and resolve spontaneously without specific treatment.

Post-injection edema typically results from localized tissue irritation and transient changes in scalp microcirculation. Although usually mild and short-lived, persistent swelling in some patients may necessitate supportive management.

Given the invasive nature of injection therapy, infection risk remains an inherent concern. Strict aseptic technique and proper disinfection of instruments and the scalp are imperative to prevent microbial contamination, as infections can impair follicular regeneration and scalp integrity.

Hypersensitivity reactions are rare but more likely to occur with non-autologous agents such as polynucleotides or placental extracts. In contrast, autologous products (e.g., PRP, micrografts) carry minimal risk due to immunologic compatibility [61]. Thorough screening for allergy history is recommended prior to treatment.

12.7 Conclusion and Future Directions

Injectable treatments for alopecia represent an innovative modality that addresses limitations of traditional oral and topical therapies by delivering regenerative agents directly to the scalp and hair follicles. A variety of injectables—including PRP, PDRN/PN, botulinum toxin, corticosteroids, and autologous micrografts—have demonstrated efficacy in enhancing hair density, increasing hair thickness, and slowing the progression of hair loss across multiple clinical studies.

Looking ahead, personalized and combinatorial approaches are poised to drive the next evolution in hair loss management. Tailored protocols based on an individual's genetic profile, scalp condition, and alopecia type may include synergistic combinations such as PRP with botulinum toxin, PDRN with corticosteroids, or PRP with autologous micrografts.

Additionally, emerging technologies such as stem cell-derived exosomes, next-generation growth factors, and advanced biodegradable polymers are being explored as novel agents in injectable formats. These innovations may enhance drug bioavailability, prolong therapeutic duration, and reduce adverse effects.

Despite its promise, injectable therapy remains a relatively new frontier in alopecia management. Large-scale, prospective studies are needed to establish evidence-based protocols and clinical guidelines. Such research will refine safety and efficacy benchmarks and help optimize integration with other modalities such as oral medication, topical treatments, surgical hair restoration, and lifestyle interventions.

Alopecia is a multifactorial and chronic disorder, and while injectables cannot serve as a universal solution, they offer a powerful therapeutic option. As protocols are refined, injectable therapies are likely to become a central pillar of future hair loss care.

References

1. Hamilton JB. Patterned loss of hair in man. Types and incidence. Ann N Y Acad Sci. 1951;53(3):708–28.
2. Rogers NE, Avram MR. Medical treatments for male and female pattern hair loss. J Am Acad Dermatol. 2008;59(4):547–66.
3. Gentile P, Garcovich S. Systematic review of platelet-rich plasma use in androgenetic alopecia compared with Minoxidil®, Finasteride®, and adult stem cell-based therapy. Int J Mol Sci. 2020;21:2702.
4. Gupta M, Mysore V. Classifications of patterned hair loss: a review. J Cutan Aesthet Surg. 2016;9(1):3–12.
5. Shapiro J. Current treatment of alopecia areata. J Investig Dermatol Symp Proc. 2013;16(1):S42–4. https://doi.org/10.1038/jidsymp.2013.14.
6. Asati DP, Singh S, Sharma VK. Dermatoses misdiagnosed as deliberate injuries. Med Sci Law. 2012;52(4):245–51.
7. Rodrigues BL, Montalvão SAL, Cancela RBB, et al. Treatment of male pattern alopecia with platelet-rich plasma: a double-blind controlled study with analysis of platelet number and growth factor levels. J Am Acad Dermatol. 2019;81(3):694–702.
8. Roohaninasab M, Goodarzi A, Ghassemi M. Systematic review of platelet-rich plasma in treating alopecia: focusing on efficacy, safety, and therapeutic durability. Dermatol Ther. 2021;34(6):e14768.
9. Gkini MA, Kouskoukis AE, Tripsianis G, Rigopoulos D, Stravrakakis P. Study of platelet-rich plasma injections in the treatment of androgenetic alopecia through an one-year period. J Cutan Aesthet Surg. 2014;7(4):213–9.
10. Kaiser MA, Ferrari LM, Gaumond SI, et al. Platelet rich plasma combination therapies for treatment of androgenetic alopecia: a systematic review. J Cutan Aesthet Surg. 2023;16(3):45–53.
11. Nguyen TH, Wang SL. Recent advances on polydeoxyribonucleotide extraction and its novel application in cosmeceuticals. Int J Biol Macromol. 2024;230:780–90.
12. Cho SB, Zheng Z, Kang JS, Kim H. Therapeutic efficacy of 1,927-nm fractionated thulium laser energy and polydeoxyribonucleotide on pattern hair loss. Med Lasers. 2016;5(3):20–7.
13. Sadgrove N, Batra S, Barreto D, Rapaport J. An updated etiology of hair loss and the new cosmeceutical paradigm in therapy: clearing 'the big eight strikes'. Cosmetics. 2023;10:106.
14. Veronesi F, Dallari D, Sabbioni G, Fini M. Polydeoxyribonucleotides (PDRNs) from skin to musculoskeletal tissue regeneration via adenosine A2A receptor involvement. J Cell Physiol. 2017;232(9):2298–307.

15. Dan X, Li S, Chen H, Xue P, Liu B, Ju Y, Lei L, Li Y. Tailoring biomaterials for skin anti-aging. Mater Today Bio. 2024;20:45–53.
16. Marques C, Porcello A, Cerrano M, Hadjab F, Chemali M, Lourenço K, Hadjab B, Raffoul W, Applegate LA, Laurent AE. From polydeoxyribonucleotides (PDRNs) to polynucleotides (PNs): bridging the gap between scientific definitions, molecular insights, and clinical applications of multifunctional biomolecules. Biomolecules. 2025;15:148.
17. Thanasarnaksorn W, Limsuchaiwat N, Sirithanabadeekul P, Charoensuksira S, Suwanchinda A, Meephansan J. Polynucleotides as a novel therapeutic approach in androgenetic alopecia: an analysis of effectiveness and safety. Arch Dermatol Res. 2025;317(1):399.
18. Lee KWA, Chan LKW, Lee AWK, Lee CH, Wong STH, Yi K-H. Poly-D,L-lactic acid (PDLLA) application in dermatology: a literature review. Polymers. 2024;16:2583.
19. Oh S, Seo SB, Kim G, Batsukh S, Son KH, Byun K. Poly-D,L-lactic acid stimulates angiogenesis and collagen synthesis in aged animal skin. Int J Mol Sci. 2023;24:7986.
20. Lin CY, Lin JY, Yang DY, Lee SH, Kim JY, Kang M. Efficacy and safety of poly-D,L-lactic acid microspheres as subdermal fillers in animals. Plast Aesthet Res. 2019;6:16.
21. Velazco de Maldonado GJ, Suarez-Vega DV, Miller-Kobisher B, Víctor GG. Smart PDOs™ and the Cartesian Technique™: a milestone in facial rejuvenation with bioactive scaffolds. J Cutan Aesthet Surg. 2024;17(4):292–306.
22. Yue H, Zhou L, Zou R, et al. Promotion of skin fibroblasts collagen synthesis by polydioxanone mats combined with concentrated growth factor extracts. J Biomater Appl. 2019;34(4):487–97.
23. Sherif MESA, Ibrahim MK, Abd-Elkareem IMAE. Evaluation of efficacy and safety of scalp threading with polydioxanone (PDO) monofilament threads in the treatment of male androgenetic alopecia. Al-Azhar Int Med J. 2024;4:65–75.
24. Meretsky CR, Umali JP, Schiuma AT. A systematic review and comparative analysis of Botox treatment in aesthetic and therapeutic applications: advantages, disadvantages, and patient outcomes. Cureus. 2024;16(8):1–10.
25. Freund BJ, Schwartz M. Treatment of male pattern baldness with botulinum toxin: a pilot study. Plast Reconstr Surg. 2010;126(5):79–85.
26. Shon U, Kim MH, Lee DY, Kim SH, Park BC. The effect of intradermal botulinum toxin on androgenetic alopecia and its possible mechanism. J Am Acad Dermatol. 2020;83(5):1231–8.
27. Abarca YA, Scott-Emuakpor R, Tirth J, Moroz O, Others. Alopecia areata: understanding the pathophysiology and advancements in treatment modalities. Cureus. 2025;2025:15–22.
28. Kumaresan M. Intralesional steroids for alopecia areata. Int J Trichology. 2010;2(1):63–5.
29. Yee BE, Tong Y, Goldenberg A, Hata T. Efficacy of different concentrations of intralesional triamcinolone acetonide for alopecia areata: a systematic review and meta-analysis. J Am Acad Dermatol. 2020;82(4):1018–21.
30. Shaath T, Liu DY, Rajpara AN, Hanson C. Safe and efficacious use of intralesional steroids for the treatment of focally resistant mycosis fungoides. J Drugs Dermatol. 2015;14:466–71.
31. Bukhari SNA, Roswandi NL, Waqas M, Habib H. Hyaluronic acid, a promising skin rejuvenating biomedicine: a review of recent updates and pre-clinical and clinical investigations on cosmetic and nutricosmetic effects. Int J Biol Macromol. 2018;120:1682–95.
32. Fernández-Martos S, Calvo-Sánchez M. Sustained human hair follicle growth ex vivo in a glycosaminoglycan hydrogel matrix. Int J Mol Sci. 2019;20(7):1741.
33. Luttrell T, Rosenberry S, Estacado N. Novel use of a biologically active-prefabricated-random-three-dimensional-polymer scaffold of hyaluronic acid (HYAFF) to facilitate complicated wound closure. In: Burns, infections and wound care. Cham: Springer; 2018. p. 75–86.
34. Ding YW, Li Y, Zhang ZW, Dao JW, Wei DX. Hydrogel forming microneedles loaded with VEGF and Ritlecitinib/polyhydroxyalkanoates nanoparticles for mini-invasive androgenetic alopecia treatment. Bioact Mater. 2024;38:85–96.
35. Sommatis S, Capillo MC, Liga E, Maccario C, Rauso R. Biological efficacy evaluation of a non-cross-linked hyaluronic acid dermal filler for biomedical application in inflammatory scalp conditions. Life. 2021;12(1):Article 2.
36. Hartmann DA, Coelho-Santos V. Pericyte control of blood flow across microvascular zones in the central nervous system. Annu Rev Physiol. 2022;84:85–96.
37. Tsuboi R, Itami S, Inui S, Ueki R, Katsuoka K. Guidelines for the management of androgenetic alopecia (2010). J Dermatol. 2012;39:113–20.
38. Guo H, Gao W, Endo H, McElwee K. Experimental and early investigational drugs for androgenetic alopecia. Expert Opin Investig Drugs. 2017;26:917–32. https://doi.org/10.1080/13543784.2017.1353598.
39. Kim J, Shin JY, Choi Y-H, Kang NG, Lee S. Anti-hair loss effect of adenosine is exerted by cAMP mediated Wnt/β-catenin pathway stimulation via modulation of Gsk3β activity in cultured human dermal papilla cells. Molecules. 2022;27:2184.
40. Ngawhirunpat T, Rangsimawong W, Tansathien K, Suriyaamporn P. In vitro biological activity and in vivo human study of porcine-placenta-extract-loaded nanovesicle formulations for skin and hair rejuvenation. Pharmaceutics. 2022;14(9):1846.
41. Rangsimawong W, Duangjit S, Sritananuwat P. Potential of deer placenta extract in hair cell regeneration and its nanoniosome-microspicule gel as a transfollicular delivery system. Cosmetics. 2024;11(6):204.

42. Sanguanboonyaphong P, Sritananuwat P, Duangjit S. Evaluating the efficacy of goat placenta extract in PEGylated liposomes and microspicules for chemotherapy-induced hair loss. Pharmaceuticals. 2024;17(8):1084.
43. Barat T, Abdollahimajd F, Dadkhahfar S, Moravvej H. Evaluation of the efficacy and safety of cow placenta extract lotion versus minoxidil 2% in the treatment of female pattern androgenetic alopecia. Int J Womens Dermatol. 2020;6(4):318–21.
44. Kwon TR, Oh CT, Park HM, Han HJ, Ji HJ, Kim BJ. Potential synergistic effects of human placental extract and minoxidil on hair growth-promoting activity in C57BL/6J mice. Clin Exp Dermatol. 2015;40(6):672–81.
45. Kim MH, Kim K, Lee H, et al. Human placenta induces hair regrowth in chemotherapy-induced alopecia via inhibition of apoptotic factors and proliferation of hair follicles. BMC Complement Med Ther. 2020;20:230.
46. Szendzielorz E, Spiewak R. Placental extracts, proteins, and hydrolyzed proteins as active ingredients in cosmetic preparations for hair loss: a systematic review of available clinical evidence. Appl Sci. 2024;14:10301.
47. Gasteratos K, Kouzounis K, Goverman J. Autologous stem cell-derived therapies for androgenetic alopecia: a systematic review of randomized control trials on efficacy, safety, and outcomes. Plast Reconstr Surg Glob Open. 2024;12(2):e5606.
48. Chunmei W, Xian H, Yang B, Alkouz Z. Clinical trial efficacy of autologous cellular micrografts in androgenic alopecia. Res Sq. 2023. https://doi.org/10.21203/rs.3.rs-2613149/v1.
49. Herz-Ruelas ME, Álvarez-Villalobos NA, Millán-Alanís JM, de León-Gutiérrez H, Ocampo-Garza SS, Gómez-Flores M, Grimalt R. Efficacy of intralesional and oral dutasteride in the treatment of androgenetic alopecia: a systematic review. Skin Appendage Disord. 2020;6(6):338–45.
50. Sobhy N, Aly H, El Shafee A, El Deeb M. Evaluation of the effect of injection of dutasteride as mesotherapeutic tool in treatment of androgenetic alopecia in males. Our Dermatol Online. 2013;4(1):40–5.
51. Saceda-Corralo D, Moustafa F, Moreno-Arrones Ó, Jaén-Olasolo P, Vañó-Galván S, Camacho F. Mesotherapy with dutasteride for androgenetic alopecia: a retrospective study in real clinical practice. J Drugs Dermatol. 2022;21(7):742–7.
52. Reguero Del Cura L, De Quintana Sancho A, Rubio Lombraña M, López Sundh AE, González López MA. Two cases of paradoxical nonscarring alopecia after mesotherapy with dutasteride. Skin Appendage Disord. 2022;8(1):46–8.
53. Essam R, Selim H, Ehab R. The boosting effect of minoxidil 0.1% when combined with dutasteride 0.01% and microneedling in the treatment of female pattern hair loss. J Egypt Womens Dermatol Soc. 2024;21(1):29–35.
54. Panda A, Matadh VA, Suresh S, et al. Non-dermal applications of microneedle drug delivery systems. Drug Deliv Transl Res. 2022;12:67–78.
55. Li J, Zhang S, Zhao W, Yang F, Liu M, Li X, Jiang X. Intradermal injection in balding region versus intramuscular injection in surrounding muscles: a split-scalp, randomized trial on BoNT for androgenetic alopecia. Dermatol Ther (Heidelb). 2024;14(6):1671–82. https://doi.org/10.1007/s13555-024-01189-x. Epub 2024 Jun 2. PMID: 38824483; PMCID: PMC11169350.
56. Kim S, Kye J, Lee M, Park B. Evaluation of mesotherapy as a transdermal drug delivery tool. Skin Res Technol. 2016;22(2):158–63.
57. Hong JY, Lee YH, Kim HJ, Park KY. Therapeutic performance of needle injection versus needle-free jet injector system for polynucleotide filler in skin rejuvenation. J Cosmet Dermatol. 2025;24(1):e16595.
58. Jia L, Xiong J, Guo R, Li Y, Jiang H. A comprehensive review of microneedling as a potential treatment option for androgenetic alopecia. Aesth Plast Surg. 2022;46(6):2979–94.
59. Pei D, Zeng L, Huang X, Wang B, Liu L, Zhang G. Efficacy and safety of combined microneedling therapy for androgenic alopecia: a systematic review and meta-analysis of randomized clinical trials. J Cosmet Dermatol. 2024;23(5):1560–72.
60. Fertig RM, Gamret AC, Cervantes J, Tosti A. Microneedling for the treatment of hair loss? J Eur Acad Dermatol Venereol. 2018;32(4):564–9.
61. Fitzgerald R, Bertucci V, Sykes JM, Duplechain JK. Adverse reactions to injectable fillers. Facial Plast Surg. 2016;32(5):532–55.

13 Advanced Techniques in Botulinum Toxin Injection

Jeongmok Cho and Won Lee

13.1 Introduction

13.1.1 Mechanism of Action and Types of Botulinum Toxin

Botulinum toxin is a neurotoxin produced by the anaerobic, Gram-positive bacterium *Clostridium botulinum*. To date, eight serotypes (A, B, C_1, C_2, D, E, F, G) have been identified [1]. Clinically, type A and type B toxins are primarily used, with type A exhibiting the most potent effect, followed by type B [1]. Botulinum toxin disrupts nerve transmission by blocking acetylcholine release at the neuromuscular junction, inducing paralysis in the target muscle [2].

This action occurs through a process where the toxin's heavy chain binds to nerve terminal receptors, allowing entry into the cell. Subsequently, the light chain cleaves SNARE proteins (such as SNAP-25, VAMP, and Syntaxin) necessary for synaptic vesicle fusion, thereby blocking acetylcholine release [2] (Fig. 13.1).

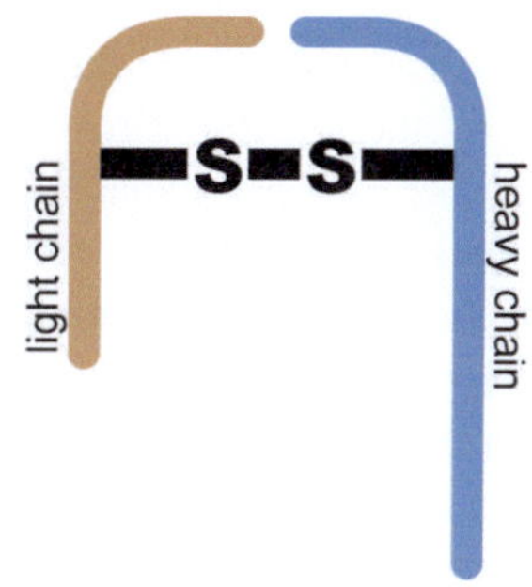

Fig. 13.1 Structure of botulinum toxin

13.1.2 Muscle Relaxation Mechanism and Nerve Transmission Process

While the blockade of acetylcholine release at the neuromuscular junction by botulinum toxin, leading to temporary relaxation (paralysis) of skeletal muscle, is irreversible, it is not permanent [2]. Over time, nerve sprouting occurs around the intact nerve terminals, initiating the

J. Cho
Etonne Plastic Surgery Clinic,
Seoul, Republic of Korea

W. Lee (✉)
Yonsei E1 Plastic Surgery Clinic,
Anyang, Kyonggi-do, Korea (Republic of)

W. Lee (ed.), *Innovative Injectable Techniques in Minimally Invasive Aesthetics*,
https://doi.org/10.1007/978-981-95-2161-6_13

recovery of muscle function. Typically, the effects gradually diminish about 3–4 months after the procedure [3]. Although some patients may experience sustained effects for 4–6 months, it remains a temporary treatment requiring periodic re-injection for maintenance [2].

13.1.3 Historical Changes in Botulinum Toxin Use

Botulinum toxin was first used by Dr. Alan B. Scott in 1977 for the correction of strabismus. It received its initial US FDA approval in 1989 for strabismus treatment. Since then, it has been used for various therapeutic purposes in neurology (dystonia), cerebral palsy spasticity, migraine prevention, and hyperhidrosis treatment [1]. Subsequently, its application expanded widely in the field of cosmetic surgery, including forehead, glabellar, periorbital, and perioral wrinkles, masseter (square jaw) reduction, and neck wrinkle improvement [4].

13.1.4 Potency and Clinical Effects of Botulinum Toxin

The molecular potency of botulinum toxin is measured by the total amount of active neurotoxin in the drug. Since this molecular potency can vary between manufacturers, standardized methods are necessary for clinical use. Manufacturers typically standardize this potency based on LD50 (lethal dose 50—the amount of a substance that kills 50% of test animals under specific conditions). Theoretically, 100 U of botulinum toxin should possess the same amount of toxicity, but errors can occur during the manufacturing process. Clinically approved botulinum toxin preparations must have minimal variability within the specified dosage range. The preparation process before injection is crucial, as active neurotoxin can be inactivated due to various factors, including the reconstitution process and storage conditions.

The use of botulinum toxin for cosmetic purposes can be broadly divided into two main objectives. The first is to block the movement of facial expression muscles to prevent wrinkle formation. The second utilizes the atrophy phenomenon that occurs when muscles or salivary glands remain inactivated after injection, leading to a reduction in size. For safe clinical procedures, a consistent response to a given dose is essential for both objectives. However, the size and location of facial expression muscles and salivary glands vary among individuals, necessitating adjustments in the botulinum toxin dosage. Furthermore, clinical effects can differ based on patient factors such as gender, facial structure, and age. The injection method can also influence clinical outcomes, with variations in injection site, needle angle, and botulinum toxin dilution potentially altering results.

13.1.5 Botulinum Toxin Resistance

1. Mechanisms of Botulinum Toxin Resistance
Botulinum toxin resistance is categorized into immunological and biological mechanisms. Immunological resistance occurs when the body's immune system recognizes the toxin as an antigen due to repeated administration, leading to the production of neutralizing antibodies (NAbs). Botulinum toxin formulations consist of the core neurotoxin and complexing proteins. Among these, complexing proteins play a crucial role in inducing an immune response. These complexing proteins and other contaminating proteins (like bacterial flagellin) can act as adjuvants, activating innate immunity and triggering an adaptive immune response against the toxin [5].

In this process, dendritic cells engulf and process the toxin, activating T cells and B cells to produce large amounts of toxin-specific antibodies (especially IgG type). With repeated administration, this immune response becomes faster and stronger, leading to secondary nonresponse, where the clinical effect of botulinum toxin diminishes or disappears. On the other hand, biological resistance (non-immunological factors) includes nerve regeneration and changes at the neuromuscular junction at the injection site or alterations in neurotransmission components.

However, the primary cause of clinically significant resistance is currently considered to be the immunological mechanism. Ultimately, the formation of neutralizing antibodies interferes with the action of botulinum toxin, leading to treatment failure, known as secondary resistance. Conversely, cases where the effect is minimal from the beginning (congenital lack of efficacy) are classified as primary resistance [6].

2. Incidence

The actual incidence of botulinum toxin resistance varies among studies but is generally reported to be low. According to large-scale meta-analyses, the rate of neutralizing antibody formation for botulinum toxin type A is approximately less than 0.5%, with clinically significant resistance (secondary nonresponse) occurring in less than 0.1% of cases. For example, one meta-analysis of 33 clinical trials (involving about 5876 participants) found the NAb incidence rate to be 0.5%, with only 0.08% leading to loss of treatment effect. However, the incidence of resistance varies depending on the indication and treatment setting. Cases involving repeated high-dose injections for neurological disorders (e.g., cervical dystonia, strabismus) showed higher antibody incidence rates compared to cosmetic procedures (e.g., wrinkle improvement). Meta-analysis results indicated that while the NAb incidence rate in cervical dystonia was low at around 2.1%, studies on blepharospasm or spasmodic torticollis reported rates exceeding 20%. Furthermore, the number of treatments and total administered dose influence the risk of resistance. The NAb incidence rate was 23 times higher in patients with repeated injections compared to inexperienced individuals, and the risk increased with higher doses (a 5% increase in resistance risk for every 100 U increase in dose) [7].

One study found that about 54% of cosmetic clinicians had encountered patients with botulinum toxin resistance, with most estimating the incidence rate to be less than 1%. Internationally, the frequency of resistance is generally low, but reports vary widely from 0.3% to 27.6%. This variation is attributed to differences in target diseases and study methodologies. There are concerns that the increasing trend of cosmetic procedures involving repeated injections from a young age may make immune resistance a more significant issue in the future [S2]. In summary, while botulinum toxin resistance is rare overall, the risk increases with factors like dose and frequency, necessitating preventive management in clinical practice.

3. Treatment and Solutions

When botulinum toxin resistance is confirmed, several treatment strategies can be considered. First, switching toxin products and serotypes is common. This involves changing to a different botulinum toxin type A formulation or, in some cases, switching to botulinum toxin type B. Type B toxin has low cross-reactivity with type A, and it has been reported to be effective in patients who have developed antibodies against type A. Specifically, incobotulinumtoxin A, a highly purified formulation free of complexing proteins, has lower immunogenicity and has shown clinical efficacy in patients resistant to type A. In a study involving 33 cervical dystonia patients resistant to other toxin preparations, treatment with incobotulinumtoxin A for 1 year resulted in significant improvement in symptom scores, with 75% of patients showing clinical improvement (symptom reduction of 30% or more) [8]. Additionally, neutralizing antibody titers tended to decrease or stabilize during treatment, suggesting that switching agents can help overcome resistance [9]. Second, optimizing the administration strategy is important. Using the minimum effective dose, maintaining sufficient intervals between injections (at least 3 months), and avoiding unnecessary booster injections are recommended [10]. Third, immunosuppressive therapy or desensitization is not yet standardized but is being discussed at the research level. For instance, laboratory-level development of monoclonal antibodies that neutralize anti-botulinum antibodies or desensitization therapy using genetic recombination techniques are being explored. However, these approaches require further research before clinical application. Lastly, alternative treatments should be considered when resistance occurs. The desired effects of botulinum toxin (e.g., improvement of dystonia, wrinkle reduction) can be supplemented with other drugs or procedures. For example, oral anticonvulsants or physical therapy can be combined for dystonia, while cosmetic wrinkle improvement can be addressed with device-based treatments (radiofrequency, HIFU, etc.) or fillers. In conclusion, prevention is the best treatment for botulinum toxin resistance. Clinicians should carefully control the number of injections and dosage and educate patients to avoid unnecessary procedures. If resistance develops, switching serotypes or using highly purified formulations may be effective, and other treatment methods can be combined as needed to manage the patient's clinical condition. These latest research findings contribute to establishing strategies for preserving the long-term safety and efficacy of botulinum toxin treatment and hold significant clinical importance.

13.2 Procedure Preparation

13.2.1 Reconstitution of Botulinum Toxin

With the exception of some products, most botulinum toxins are supplied as lyophilized powder in vials. The powder is hydrated by injecting physiological saline into the vial, typically using 2–4 mL. Precise dosage injection is crucial for achieving consistent and stable clinical effects without side effects. To reduce the inconvenience of calculating the required volume in mL based on the diluted concentration each time, using 2 mL of saline for 100 U of botulinum toxin is a very useful method. After reconstitution, 0.1 mL contains 5 U of botulinum toxin, and injecting 1 U requires a volume of 0.02 mL (Table 13.1).

Table 13.1 Conversion table when 100 U of botulinum toxin is hydrated with 2 mL of saline

Botulinum toxin dose (U)	Total injection volume (mL)
100	2
5	0.1
1	0.02

Using insulin syringes for botulinum toxin procedures is very advantageous (Fig. 13.2). Insulin syringes are designed to minimize dead space and deliver small, precise doses of insulin, making them highly suitable for accurately injecting small amounts of botulinum toxin.

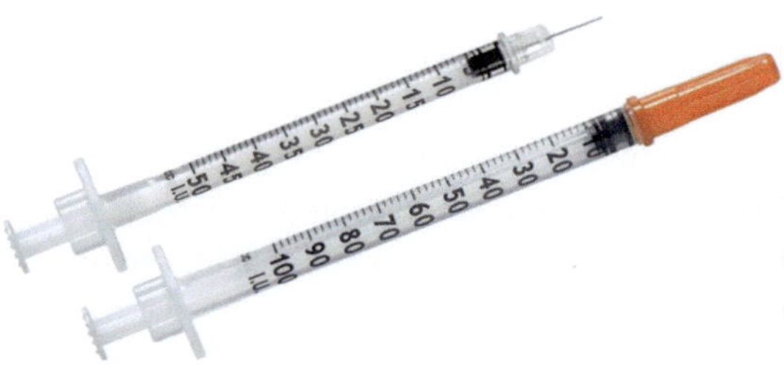

Fig. 13.2 Insulin syringes (0.5, 1 mL)

Generally, using a 1 mL insulin syringe is convenient, and a syringe equipped with a 31G, 8 mm needle is sufficient for injecting into facial areas at the desired depth. Insulin syringes have different scale markings compared to standard syringes. A 1 mL insulin syringe is marked such that 1 scale unit corresponds to 2 U (international units of insulin), which is equivalent to 0.02 mL. When 100 U of botulinum toxin is hydrated with 2 mL of saline, 0.02 mL contains 1 U of botulinum toxin. Therefore, when using an insulin syringe, 1 scale mark intuitively represents the injection of 1 U of botulinum toxin, allowing the practitioner to quickly and accurately inject the desired dose.

13.2.2 Storage of Reconstituted Botulinum Toxin

Botulinum toxin is manufactured in various dosages depending on the manufacturer, with 50, 100, and 200 U being commonly used. Since it is rare to use an entire vial of botulinum toxin in a single procedure, the hydrated toxin is often stored in a refrigerator. Manufacturer recommendations typically advise using the hydrated toxin within 24 h. However, in actual clinical practice, it is often stored in the refrigerator and used over a slightly longer period. Some studies report that botulinum toxin stored refrigerated for up to 4–6 weeks after reconstitution does not show a significant decrease in wrinkle improvement effects, suggesting that storage for up to 1 month is acceptable, after which it should be discarded [11]. Exposure to room temperature (approx. 20–25 °C) can easily denature the protein structure, accelerating the loss of activity. One study reported that the activity of reconstituted toxin could decrease by more than half if left at room temperature for several hours [12]. Therefore, it is recommended to maintain refrigeration as much as possible even during use in the injection or procedure room or to minimize temperature changes using ice packs.

13.2.3 Botulinum Toxin Injection Method

When injecting reconsituted botulinum toxin, it is necessary to administer the precise dose at the correct site. Adjusting the amount of solution drawn into the insulin syringe according to the practitioner's hand size is useful. If the practitioner has small hands, injecting with a fully filled 1 mL insulin syringe can be uncomfortable, so using multiple insulin syringes divided by area may be more practical. If a large amount of solution is drawn into a single syringe and used for multiple sites, the needle can become dull, making penetration difficult and causing pain during the procedure. Especially for sites where the injection involves touching the bone, repeated use can dull the needle tip, increasing resistance when piercing the skin. Approximately, it is useful to draw enough solution into one insulin syringe to inject one area on both the left and right sides of the face, typically around 12–30 U.

Since botulinum injections are generally not very painful, local anesthesia is usually unnecessary. However, applying ice packs before the procedure is very beneficial [13]. Lowering the skin temperature reduces pain and constricts nearby blood vessels, decreasing the likelihood of bruising [14]. Applying ice for a short time immediately before the procedure can reduce patient discomfort and increase post-procedure satisfaction, making it a useful method.

13.2.4 Botulinum Toxin in Combination Treatments

Recently, to maximize treatment effects, botulinum toxin injections are often performed concurrently with other procedures like fillers or energy-based devices (EBDs). Since botulinum toxin is a drug-based treatment, careful consideration of the procedure order is necessary when combining it with EBD treatments. EBDs can potentially have negative effects on the toxin, so it is generally advisable to perform the EBD treatment before the injection [15]. When considering combination treatments, the treatment plan should account for the intended effects and target tissue layers of each procedure. The potential side effects of each treatment must also be considered to ensure that the combination yields synergistic effects without increasing adverse events.

Combining botulinum toxin and filler injections is also very common [16]. Since both involve injecting substances via needles, there can be various opinions regarding the order of procedures. If both are performed on the same day, it is recommended to inject the botulinum toxin first, followed by the filler. Botulinum toxin injections involve administering very small amounts of the drug into the muscle or dermis, whereas fillers are injected into the dermis or subdermal layer to add volume. Therefore, injecting botulinum toxin after filler placement could potentially alter the shape, and if the toxin flows into the layer containing the filler, it could spread throughout the filler space, leading to unintended results. If the procedures are not performed on the same day, injecting botulinum toxin first to induce muscle relaxation can make subsequent filler injection easier and yield better results [17].

13.3 Botulinum Toxin Injection Methods for Facial Wrinkle Improvement

13.3.1 Overview

Facial wrinkles arise from various causes. Wrinkles amenable to improvement with botulinum toxin are dynamic wrinkles caused by the repetitive action of facial expression muscles. It is useful to consider the anatomical location of these muscles to eliminate expressions that make one look older or convey negative emotions. Using excessive doses of botulinum toxin when treating facial expression muscles can result in a "masked" appearance due to lack of facial expression. Injecting botulinum toxin near the eyebrows can, if done incorrectly, lead to ptosis (drooping eyelid) if the toxin affects the levator palpebrae superioris muscle. Although the action of botulinum toxin is irreversible at the molecular level, muscle function recovers as new motor nerve sprouts grow. Therefore, most side effects resolve spontaneously over time. However, to achieve aesthetically stable results, a thorough understanding of anatomy and injection of effective doses at precise locations are crucial.

13.3.2 Horizontal Forehead Lines

Forehead wrinkles are a significant factor contributing to the perception of aging. The causes of excessive frontalis muscle use leading to horizontal forehead lines are varied. However, with age, the eyebrows often descend compared to their youthful position, frequently causing the upper eyelid skin to droop significantly. Coupled with weakened eyelid-opening strength, individuals may compensate by using eyebrow elevation to open their eyes. This habit can lead to pronounced horizontal wrinkles in the central forehead due to frequent frontalis muscle contraction.

Inhibiting the action of the frontalis muscle with botulinum toxin can improve horizontal forehead lines. Typically, 12–18 U of botulinum toxin is used, divided into six injection points (Fig. 13.3). As the arrangement of the frontalis muscle varies among individuals, it is best to directly observe the horizontal wrinkles that appear when the patient raises their eyebrows and determine the injection sites accordingly. The frontalis muscle extends slightly lateral to the temporal crest, so insufficient treatment in the lateral areas can cause the lateral eyebrows to arch upward ("Spock brow"), requiring caution [18].

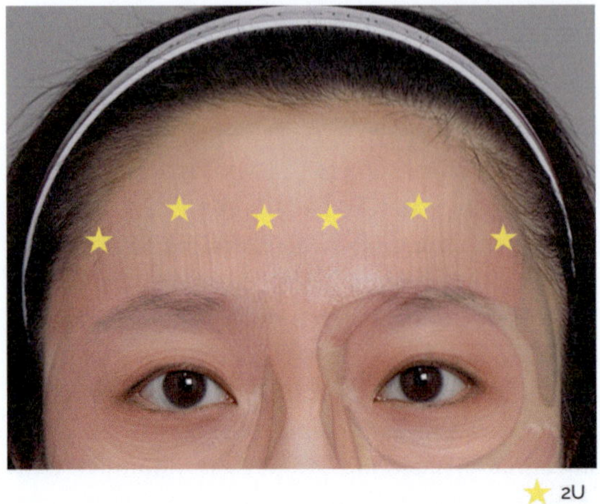

Fig. 13.3 Botulinum toxin injection sites for horizontal forehead lines

Patients who habitually use eyebrow elevation to open their eyelids may complain of discomfort opening their eyes or that their eyes appear smaller after frontalis botulinum toxin treatment. Before treating horizontal forehead lines with botulinum toxin, it is advisable to check if the patient experiences significant difficulty opening their eyes while manually preventing eyebrow elevation.

13.3.3 Glabellar Lines

Glabellar lines, often formed when frowning, can create deep vertical wrinkles in the area between the eyebrows. The corrugator supercilii muscle, which pulls the eyebrows downward, consists of oblique and transverse bellies. It originates from the superomedial orbital rim and extends superolaterally at an approximate 30-degree angle, inserting into the dermis of the medial eyebrow [19]. Patients often seek treatment for glabellar lines when vertical wrinkles have already started to form, frequently inquiring about filler injections rather than botulinum toxin. Filler injections in the glabellar region carry a risk of blindness, necessitating cautious procedures [20]. In cases of glabellar wrinkles, the corrugator supercilii muscle is often hypertrophied and frequently used, increasing the likelihood of filler migration after injection. Therefore, weakening the muscle with botulinum toxin before treating any remaining wrinkles with filler is a safer approach. In cases of significant muscle hypertrophy, the area medial to the eyebrow may appear bulky, creating an illusion of hollowness in the forehead above the brow. When consulting patients desiring forehead fillers, it is important to assess whether the glabellar muscles are thick. If the glabellar muscles are hypertrophied, filler migration is more likely after forehead filler injection, making prior botulinum toxin treatment advisable.

To determine the injection sites for glabellar lines, it is important to have the patient frown and identify the location of the vertical wrinkles and any skin depressions above the medial eyebrow. The corrugator supercilii muscle attaches to the bone medial to the vertical wrinkles, so injection in this area should involve feeling the needle touch the bone before injecting. The skin depression superior to the medial eyebrow corresponds to the muscle's dermal insertion; injection here should not touch the bone and should only penetrate just below the dermis. Typically, 3–4 U of botulinum toxin is used per site, with 3 U generally sufficient for women and 4 U recommended for men with thicker muscles (Fig. 13.4). If the muscle is thick, causing bulging above the eyebrow, shortening the treatment interval (e.g., every 4 months instead of 6) can help reduce muscle volume.

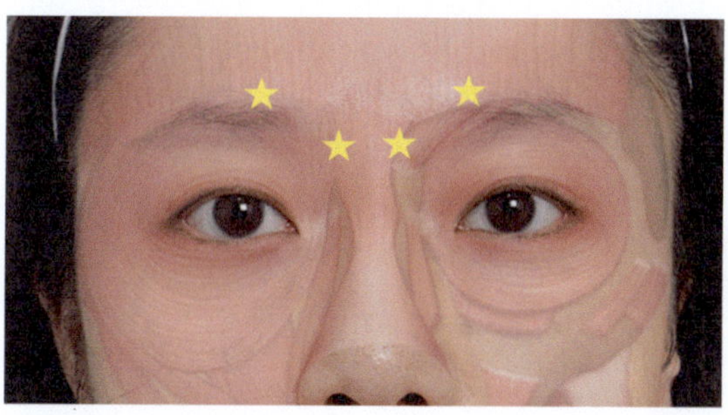

Fig. 13.4 Botulinum toxin injection sites for glabellar lines

13.3.4 Crow's Feet (Periorbital Lines)

Crow's feet are a major reason patients perceive themselves as aging and seek anti-aging treatments. Various factors contribute to severe crow's feet, including thin skin and frequent smiling. Injecting botulinum toxin into the lateral portion of the orbicularis oculi muscle can partially weaken the wrinkles around the eyes. Some patients are hesitant about botulinum toxin treatment due to concerns about unnatural eye expressions. However, avoiding excessive doses can improve crow's feet without significantly impairing expression.

Treatment for crow's feet typically involves injecting three sites per side, totaling six points. Instead of relying on fixed measurements like "a certain number of centimeters from the lateral canthus," it is better to determine the injection sites based on the individual patient's muscle location and wrinkles. Immediately before the procedure, ask the patient to squeeze their eyes shut tightly and note the location of the deep wrinkles. Generally, target three areas: lateral to the eye corner, just below the lateral eyebrow, and below the eye corner. Depending on the wrinkle pattern, injecting slightly more toxin into deeper wrinkles can be considered. Use 2–3 U of botulinum toxin per site (Fig. 13.5). The orbicularis oculi muscle has an average thickness of about 1.56 mm and is located 0.88–2.8 mm below the skin surface [21]. Therefore, injections should preferably be intradermal or just below the dermis to avoid unnatural expressions. Especially in the area below the eye corner, injecting too

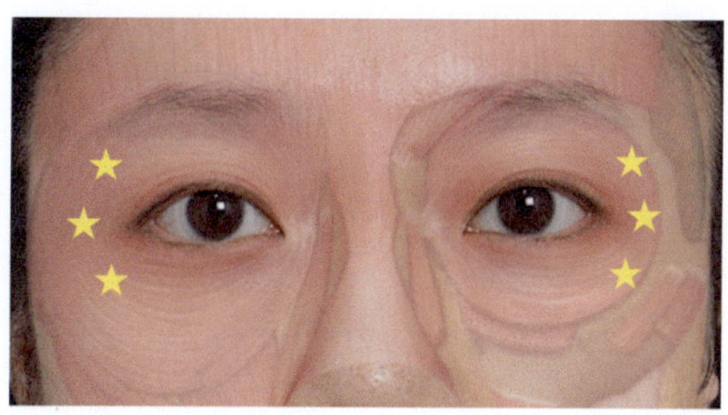

Fig. 13.5 Botulinum toxin injection sites for crow's feet

deeply in patients with lean faces can inadvertently affect the zygomaticus major muscle. This can lead to an unnatural smile, so injections in the periorbital area should generally be superficial. Periorbital veins are often easily visible; avoiding these vessels during injection helps prevent bruising. A superficial, intradermal injection technique is preferable to deep injection, as it minimizes the risk of venous injury and bruising, and also prevents a "frozen" or expressionless appearance.

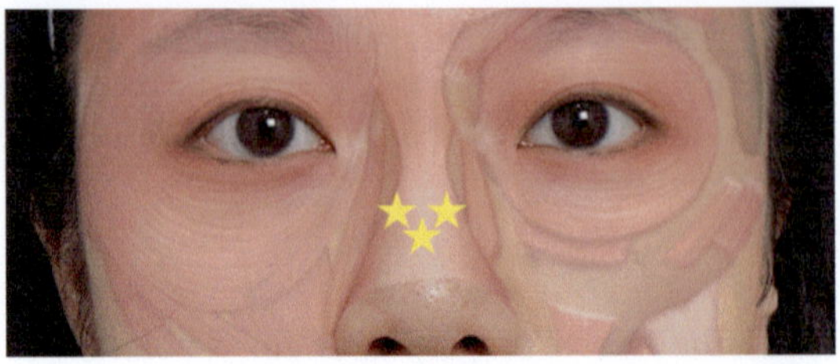

Fig. 13.6 Botulinum toxin injection sites for bunny lines

13.3.5 Bunny Lines (Nasal Wrinkles)

Bunny lines are wrinkles on the bridge of the nose caused by the nasalis muscle. They become very prominent when scrunching the face and rarely leave permanent wrinkles like glabellar lines. However, because they are highly emphasized during facial scrunching, relaxing the muscle with botulinum toxin can soften the expression. Patients rarely notice their own bunny lines as they seldom look in the mirror while making this expression. Nevertheless, these lines can significantly impact the impression given to others when frowning. Therefore, it's advisable to check for bunny lines during consultations for periorbital botulinum toxin and recommend treatment if appropriate. When treating glabellar and crow's feet, checking for bunny lines and suggesting treatment can help create a more favorable impression.

The injection sites are three points along the area where bunny lines form, using 2–3 U of botulinum toxin per site (Fig. 13.6). The injection targets the nasalis muscle located just beneath the dermis. The skin in this area is relatively thin, so injecting 2–3 U will spread thinly and sufficiently cover the wrinkled area.

13.3.6 Gummy Smile

The muscles responsible for lifting the upper lip are the levator labii superioris alaeque nasi (LLSAN), levator labii superioris (LLS), and zygomaticus minor (Zmi). Botulinum toxin treatment can improve the appearance for patients bothered by excessive gingival display when smiling. Particularly in patients with strong LLSAN contraction, smiling can create a depression medial to the nasolabial fold, resulting in an unnatural facial expression. Botulinum toxin can be useful in creating a better impression in these cases [22].

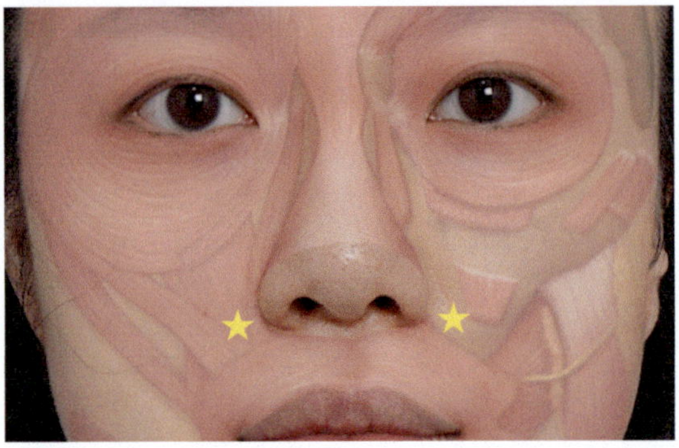

Fig. 13.7 Botulinum toxin injection sites for gummy smile (LLSAN)

The injection site is lateral to the nasal ala, where the nasolabial fold begins. Ask the patient to smile and inject into the area where skin depression is visible, typically one point on each side (total two points). Inject 2–3 U of botulinum toxin per side, ensuring the injection is not too deep (Fig. 13.7).

13.3.7 Depressor Anguli Oris (DAO) Muscle

The depressor anguli oris (DAO) muscle pulls the corners of the mouth downward and can contribute to a negative appearance when the mouth is tightly closed. For patients seeking anti-aging treatments or surgery due to jawline sagging, the DAO muscle is an important target. Habitual use of the DAO muscle due to incorrect muscle habits can lead to fine lines below the marionette lines and a downturned appearance of the mouth corners, worsening the overall impression.

The optimal injection site is where a wrinkle forms in the center of the marionette line when the patient makes an "ee" sound (Fig. 13.8). In patients who frequently use the DAO, identifying this wrinkle is usually straightforward. However, if the muscle is used subconsciously, finding the exact wrinkle can be difficult. In such cases, the injection site can be determined as the midpoint on the marionette line between the corner of the mouth and the jawline [23]. Inject 3–4 U of botulinum toxin at this site. Injecting too superiorly may affect the risorius muscle, leading to an unnatural smile. Injecting too inferiorly and medially could affect the depressor labii inferioris (DLI) muscle, causing asymmetry or distortion of the lip shape during smiling, so caution is needed.

13.3.8 Chin (Mentalis Muscle)

The mentalis muscle can cause a "cobblestone" or "orange peel" appearance on the chin when the lips are pursed tightly. In individuals with a short chin, strong activation of the mentalis muscle can make the chin appear even shorter. Patients with a habit of tightly closing their mouths often overuse both the DAO and mentalis muscles. The shortened chin can make the jawline appear less defined, contributing to an aged appearance, especially if the jawline is already sagging. The mentalis muscle is also important during chin filler procedures. In patients with hypertrophied mentalis muscles, filler migration is more likely, and the augmented chin length may shorten more quickly.

The mentalis muscle originates near the alveolar bone and descends inferolaterally, inserting into the chin dermis [24]. While the dermal insertions cause wrinkling, the overall muscle contraction shortens the chin. Therefore, botulinum toxin should ideally be injected into the center of the mentalis muscle. Ask the patient to purse their lips to create chin wrinkles, and inject into the points on the left and right sides of the chin where wrinkling is most severe. The needle should be directed slightly superomedially, injecting 4–5 U per site (Fig. 13.9).

13.3.9 Jawline (Nefertiti Lift)

Loss of jawline definition is one of the most common complaints among patients distressed by an aging appearance. As soft tissues lose elasticity, the jawline sags downward, contributing to an older look, prompting many to seek various treatments to prevent this. The platysma muscle, continuous with the facial SMAS layer, extends from

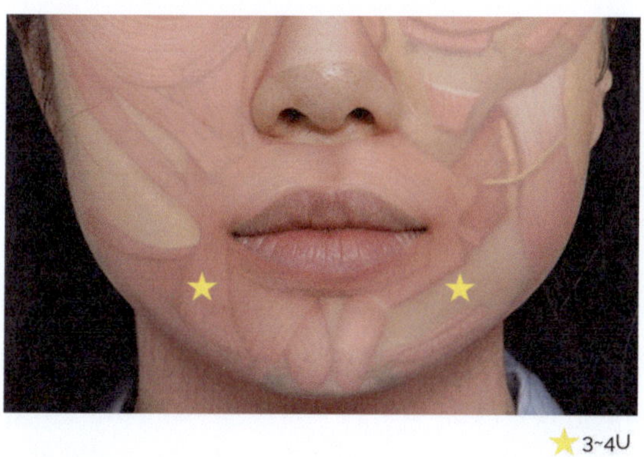

Fig. 13.8 Botulinum toxin injection sites for depressor anguli oris (DAO)

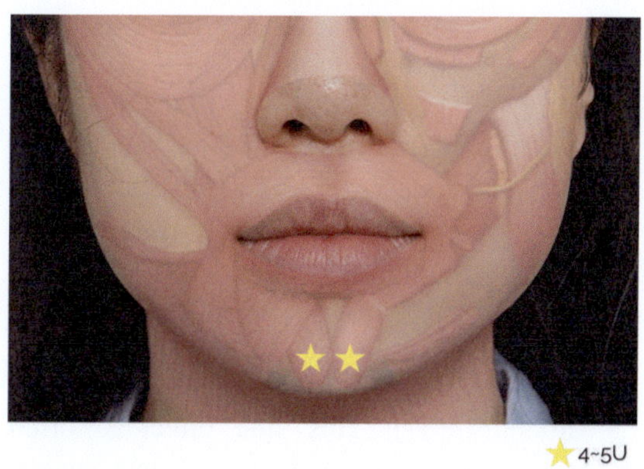

Fig. 13.9 Botulinum toxin injection sites for the chin (mentalis muscle)

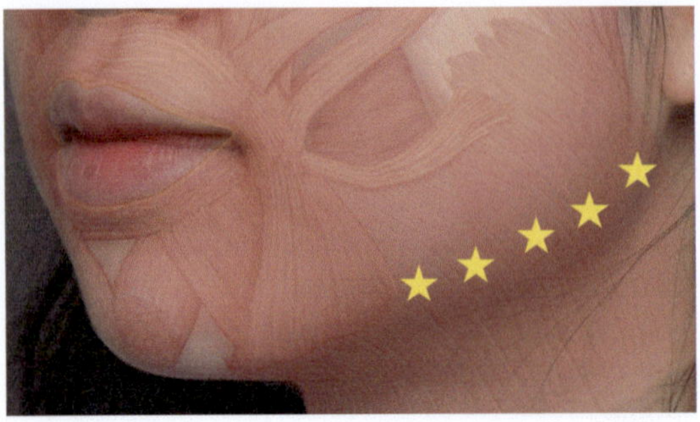

Fig. 13.10 Botulinum toxin injection sites along the jawline

the jawline down the neck. Platysma contraction can make the jawline appear obtuse and, in severe cases, cause visible vertical bands in the neck. Relaxing the platysma with botulinum toxin can not only reduce vertical neck bands but also help sharpen the jawline contour [25].

Inject a total of 15–20 U of botulinum toxin per side, distributed along the jawline in five to six points (Fig. 13.10). The platysma is a very thin muscle, so injections should be placed just below the dermis or intradermally. Injecting too medially can affect perioral muscles, so caution is advised.

13.4 Ptosis Following Botulinum Toxin Injection

13.4.1 Mechanism of Ptosis

Ptosis (upper eyelid drooping), a rare complication following facial botulinum toxin injections, primarily occurs due to local diffusion of the toxin, inhibiting the function of the levator palpebrae superioris muscle [26]. For instance, when botulinum toxin is injected into the forehead/glabellar region to eliminate frown lines, the toxin can potentially pass through the orbital septum or spread into the orbit, reaching the levator muscle and causing temporary paralysis, leading to eyelid drooping [27]. This side effect is often reported to result from an insufficient understanding of the anatomical structures of the injection site and toxin diffusion pathways. Injection points that are too low (near the orbital rim) or too deep increase the risk of unintended toxin leakage into the levator muscle, causing ptosis. Ultimately, botulinum toxin-induced ptosis is understood as an extension of its local muscle-paralyzing action, occurring specifically when the toxin reaches the levator palpebrae superioris and its accessory muscle, Müller's muscle, weakening the nerve stimulation required to lift the upper eyelid [26].

13.4.2 Incidence of Ptosis

The incidence of ptosis following botulinum toxin use for cosmetic purposes, such as forehead or glabellar wrinkle improvement, is relatively low, reported to be around 1–5% depending on the study [26, 28]. For example, a clinical trial involving 264 subjects reported transient eyelid drooping in 5.4% of cases, typically resolving within a month. A meta-analysis combining several studies estimated the average incidence rate to be around 1.8% [26]. Ptosis symptoms usually begin 2–10 days post-procedure. Mild cases often resolve spontaneously within a few weeks without specific treatment, with full recovery typically occurring within 2–3 months [28]. While ptosis is rare in cosmetic indications (approx. 1–5%), recent literature consistently indicates that the incidence may be higher in therapeutic indications, particularly when treating conditions like blepharospasm.

13.4.3 Treatment and Prevention

Management of botulinum toxin-induced ptosis focuses on alleviating symptoms and minimizing patient discomfort until the toxin's effects wear off. For mild ptosis (eyelid droop <2 mm), alpha-adrenergic agonist eye drops can improve symptoms. Apraclonidine 0.5% eye drops (Iopidine) are commonly used; they stimulate the sympathetic nerves of Müller's muscle (superior tarsal muscle), providing about 1–2 mm of eyelid elevation. These drops are typically administered two to three times daily for temporary eyelid lift, with effects lasting several hours (6–8 h), helping to improve patient satisfaction [26, 28]. More recently, oxymetazoline HCl 0.1% ophthalmic solution has become the only FDA-approved drug for acquired blepharoptosis. This alpha-agonist also contracts Müller's muscle, temporarily lifting the eyelid, and has shown significant improvement in clinical studies [29]. If the ptosis is severe (e.g., ≥3–4 mm) or the patient desires faster improvement, additional botulinum toxin injection might be considered. Somewhat paradoxically, injecting a small amount of toxin into the pretarsal portion of the orbicularis oculi muscle of the affected eyelid can reduce the tension of the eyelid-closing muscle, thereby enhancing the relative action of the levator muscle [28]. Small case series have confirmed that injecting 1–2 units of toxin into the upper eyelid orbicularis muscle resulted in approximately 1–2 mm elevation of the droopy eyelid, with patients regaining normal eyelid function within weeks [28, 29]. Notably, a 2023 case study involving eight cases of severe ptosis (≥3 mm) post-botulinum toxin injection reported significant recovery in all patients treated with a combination of pretarsal toxin reinjection and oxymetazoline eye drops [29]. Thus, non-invasive treatment with eye drops and localized botulinum toxin reinjection, used alone or in combination, can shorten the duration of ptosis and improve the patient's functional and aesthetic discomfort. Prevention strategies for ptosis are also emphasized in recent literature. Practitioners are advised to have precise knowledge of facial anatomy and inject the toxin superficially above the orbital rim to minimize diffusion into surrounding muscles [26]. For example, during glabellar wrinkle treatment, injection points should be placed above the superior orbital rim, and injections at the medial end of the eyebrow should avoid being too medial or deep [26]. Techniques such as using the minimum effective dose, avoiding unnecessary injections into the lateral tails of the corrugator muscles, or reducing the number of injections are suggested. Applying gentle upward pressure for about 30 s after injection to prevent downward diffusion toward the orbit has also been described. Instructing patients to avoid rubbing or massaging the treated area is crucial to prevent the toxin from spreading beyond the intended site [28]. These preventive measures can further reduce the risk of ptosis, which can occur even with experienced injectors, thereby enhancing patient satisfaction and safety. In conclusion, although botulinum toxin-induced ptosis is a rare side effect, its psychological and functional impact on patients can be significant. Therefore, it is clinically important to actively manage it using treatments suggested by recent research (e.g., alpha-agonist eye drops, additional toxin injections) and adhere to safe injection techniques and preventive strategies from the outset. Recent reports emphasize that these approaches effectively resolve most temporary issues, and normal function is restored as the toxin's effects diminish over time. Consequently, practitioners who are knowledgeable about the mechanism and risk factors of ptosis, provide realistic explanations about its incidence, and fully inform patients about treatment options and prognosis in case of side effects can offer safer and more satisfactory botulinum toxin treatments.

13.5 Botulinum Toxin Injection Methods for Facial Contouring

13.5.1 Overview

Patients desiring a smaller facial size often seek various procedures and surgeries to achieve their desired facial shape. While facial bone surgery is a definitive method for altering facial shape, many patients prefer non-surgical options, leading to high demand for procedures that make the face appear smaller. Although EBDs are often used to reduce the fat layer and achieve facial slimming, botulinum toxin-induced nerve blockade inhibits muscle contraction, leading to gradual atrophy and size reduction of unused muscles. Clinically, injecting botulinum toxin into hypertrophied masseter muscles results in a reduction in muscle thickness and volume after several weeks, narrowing the lower face [30]. Studies have observed structural changes in muscle tissue post-injection, including increased expression of atrophy-related genes and decreased muscle fiber diameter. Repeated injections have also been reported to cause cumulative muscle atrophy leading to fibrosis [30]. Notably, single injections of low-frequency, low-dose toxin primarily cause temporary muscle weakness, whereas high-dose or repeated injections can induce more pronounced and sustained muscle volume reduction [31].

Botulinum toxin also inhibits acetylcholine release at autonomic nerve endings. Therefore, injecting it into salivary glands blocks nerve stimulation for saliva secretion. Blocking the cholinergic secretomotor nerves of glands like the parotid and submandibular glands reduces saliva production and puts the gland tissue into a functional resting state, ultimately decreasing gland volume and activity [32]. This demonstrates that the nerve blockade mechanism applies similarly to salivary glands as it does to muscles. Quantitative studies on salivary gland size changes post-toxin injection have shown significant volume reduction in injected parotid glands, with only minor recovery (5–8%) observed after 3 months [33]. This indicates that toxin can be used to temporarily shrink salivary glands, improving lower facial contours. The effects of botulinum toxin typically begin within 2–3 days post-injection, peak at 1–2 weeks and last for about 3–4 months in both muscles and salivary glands, after which nerve function gradually recovers, returning them to their original state [34]. The duration of effect can be cumulative with repeated treatments; some studies report muscle reduction effects lasting beyond 6 months, even up to 1–2 years, with repeated treatments [35]. In conclusion, botulinum toxin inhibits the function and reduces the size of target muscles and salivary glands through nerve transmission blockade, with the intensity and duration of effects varying depending on the dose and number of treatments.

13.5.2 Square Jaw Reduction (Masseter Reduction)

The masseter is a masticatory muscle located at the angle of the mandible. Especially in Asians, congenital factors or chronic habits like bruxism can lead to hypertrophy, resulting in a square jaw appearance. Injecting botulinum toxin into this area causes muscle atrophy, leading to a slimmer jawline contour [30, 36]. Clinically, many patients in their 20s and 30s with a wide-appearing jaw undergo toxin injections for masseter reduction. Significant reduction in the maximum width of the lower face has been reported approximately 4–8 weeks post-procedure [34].

The injection sites should be determined based on the location of the masseter bulge when the patient clenches their teeth firmly. It is best to inject 1–2 cm above the mandibular angle at the most prominent point, dividing the dose into three to four points spaced about 1 cm apart (Fig. 13.11). Injecting too superficially can cause the toxin to enter facial expression muscles, leading to side effects. It is recommended to insert the needle until it touches the bone, then withdraw slightly before injecting. Typically, 25–30 U of botulinum toxin is used per side. For men with very thick muscles, up to 50 U per side may be used. Research on cost-effectiveness suggests that using 24 U per side (total 48 U) was most efficient [37]. Therefore, it is reasonable to start with a total of 50 U for the first treatment, potentially increasing to 60 U for patients with relatively large masseters.

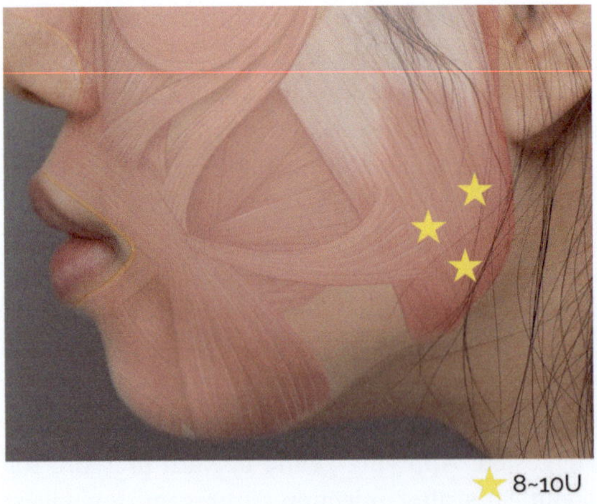

Fig. 13.11 Botulinum toxin injection sites in the masseter muscle

Occasionally, a localized bulge may appear in the masseter muscle after the procedure. Anatomically, the masseter is divided into superficial and deep layers by the deep inferior tendon (DIT). If the toxin is injected only into the deep layer, the superficial layer may contract compensatorily, causing the bulge [38]. This can be easily resolved by injecting an additional 10–15 U of botulinum toxin into the protruding area. Since this phenomenon is not common, it is not necessary to routinely inject both deep and superficial layers. Injecting too superficially can cause problems with facial expression muscles. Therefore, the standard approach is to inject into the deepest part initially and perform additional injections only if a localized bulge occurs.

13.5.3 Temporal Region Reduction (Temporalis Muscle Treatment)

The temporalis muscle is a broad masticatory muscle attached to the temple area, working with the masseter to close the jaw. While the lower masseter is typically the main determinant of facial width aesthetically, a bulging appearance on the side of the head may indicate temporalis muscle hypertrophy [39]. This can be particularly noticeable in patients with chronic bruxism. If palpation reveals a bulging muscle in the temporal crest area when the patient clenches their teeth, botulinum toxin injection into the temporalis muscle can reduce its volume. Such temporal hypertrophy can be found even in patients without significant masseter enlargement. Temporal reduction can be a useful method to decrease overall facial size and create a softer, more curved facial contour.

The injection sites for the temporalis muscle are typically three to four points in the area of maximum bulge when the muscle is contracted (Fig. 13.12). Generally, a dose similar to that used for the masseter is employed, with 25–30 U of botulinum toxin per side being useful. Unlike the masseter, the temporalis muscle is spread over a wider area, so dividing the dose into more points may be beneficial in some cases.

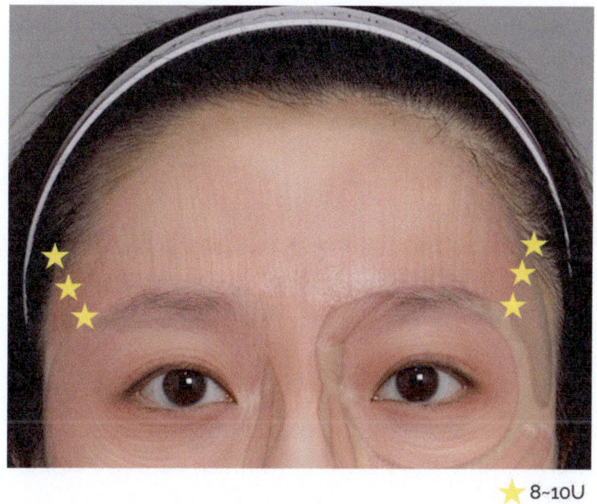

Fig. 13.12 Botulinum toxin injection sites for the temporal muscle

Injection into the temporalis muscle can lead to a slight reduction in temple muscle thickness and head circumference. One study reported an approximate 55% reduction in temporalis muscle thickness and a 1.1 cm decrease in head circumference post-procedure, although the latter change was statistically minimal [39]. While the change in temporal contour may not be as dramatic as with masseter reduction, it can help relax muscle tension and provide subtle contour improvement.

13.5.4 Parotid Gland Reduction

The parotid gland is a major salivary gland in the face. Enlargement due to obesity, systemic diseases, or chronic irritation can cause bulging in the lower face area. Parotid gland hypertrophy can make the area just above the jawline and below the ear appear widened laterally, contributing to a larger facial appearance [40]. Injecting botulinum toxin into the salivary gland blocks cholinergic secretomotor nerves, reducing saliva production. This principle has long been used therapeutically to treat sialorrhea (excessive drooling) [32]. Cosmetically, reducing salivary gland function can decrease gland size and volume, softening the bulge in the lower face. Studies have confirmed a reduction in parotid gland thickness on ultrasound after botulinum toxin injection, along with improved facial contours [40]. Therefore, toxin injection can be considered for patients with parotid gland hypertrophy or facial swelling due to excessive saliva production.

Accurate anatomical knowledge of the parotid gland is crucial for toxin injection. The toxin is injected into the palpable gland area located just above the jawline and below the ear. Typically, 20–30 U of botulinum toxin is used per side (Fig. 13.13). In men with larger faces, up to 50 U may be used. Unlike muscle, botulinum toxin does not diffuse easily within the salivary gland, so dividing the dose into multiple points is beneficial. Depending on the size, injecting 5 U into four to six separate locations is effective. The parotid gland is often better palpated with the patient lying down rather than sitting. Asking the patient to clench their masseter muscle helps identify its location by observing the volume change, making it easier to palpate the parotid gland volume separate from the masseter. If necessary, ultrasound guidance can be considered for precise injection [41].

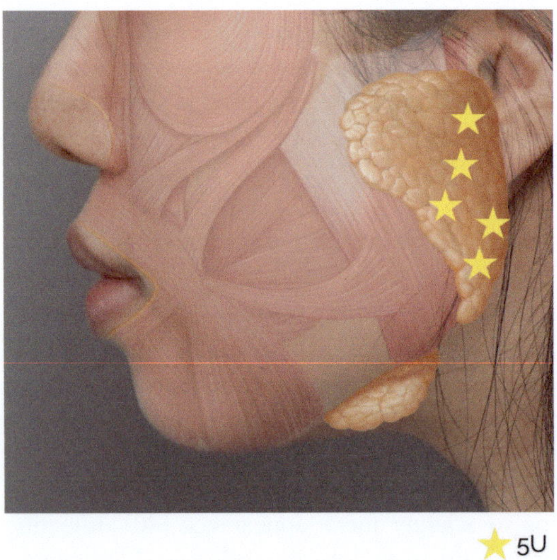

Fig. 13.13 Botulinum toxin injection sites for parotid gland

Following toxin injection into the salivary gland, saliva reduction typically begins within about a week, peaking at 2–4 weeks. Dry mouth due to reduced saliva production may occur, although it is generally less frequent than with submandibular gland injections. A noticeable reduction in parotid gland volume can occur within weeks, improving the bulge below the jawline. A 6-month follow-up study showed a significant decrease in gland thickness, resulting in a slimmer facial shape with reduced facial contour curvature on photographic analysis [41]. The duration of effect is generally around 3–4 months, after which nerve function recovers, and the gland size often returns to baseline as salivary function normalizes [30].

13.5.5 Submandibular Gland Reduction

Submandibular gland hypertrophy can cause bilateral bulging under the chin, mimicking a double chin appearance. Similar to parotid gland treatment, botulinum toxin can induce atrophy of the submandibular gland. The injection site is best identified by palpating the protruding gland under the chin. Asking the patient to swallow helps identify the firm, mobile gland. Generally, the submandibular gland is located posterior to the facial vein, so locating the facial artery and palpating the gland behind it can be useful. Due to its proximity to the facial artery, it is important to avoid injecting too anteriorly [42]. When the needle enters the correct location, a firm resistance is typically felt. Usually, 20 U of botulinum toxin is injected per side. Since the gland is not as wide as the parotid, dividing the dose into two points and injecting 10 U into each is useful (Fig. 13.14).

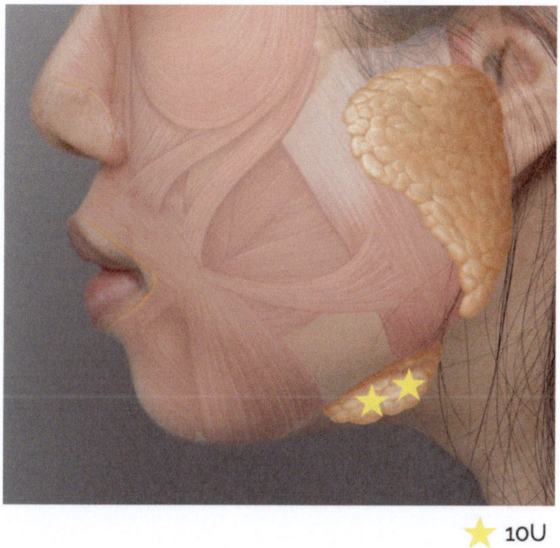

Fig. 13.14 Botulinum toxin injection sites for submandibular gland

13.6 Other Botulinum Toxin Injection Techniques (Microbotox/Mesobotox)

Fundamentally, botulinum toxin works by blocking acetylcholine release at the neuromuscular junction, thereby inhibiting muscle function. For salivary glands, inhibiting acetylcholine release suppresses saliva secretion, allowing for cosmetic applications. However, studies have shown that injecting small amounts of botulinum toxin into the dermal layer can positively affect pore size, skin elasticity, sebum production, and scars [43]. This technique, often termed "Mesobotox" or "Microbotox," involves injecting highly diluted toxin solution into the superficial layers of the skin (dermis) using multiple microinjections. It aims to improve fine lines, pores, sebum production, and redness. Reports suggest benefits for facial flushing and mild acne as well [44]. Rather than causing deep muscle paralysis like traditional injections, Microbotox focuses on improving overall skin quality by acting on superficial structures (sebaceous glands, capillaries, etc.). The key aspect of Microbotox is the use of very dilute toxin (e.g., diluted two to four times more than standard dilutions or even higher) injected into the dermis or superficial subcutaneous layer, creating small blebs. These micro-doses reaching the superficial skin layers act on the non-neuronal cholinergic system in the epidermis/dermis, leading to skin improvements. Acetylcholine is known to stimulate secretion from exocrine glands like sweat and sebaceous glands, and it influences the function of skin cells (keratinocytes, melanocytes—affecting proliferation, pigmentation), microcirculation in capillaries, and immune/inflammatory responses. By blocking these acetylcholine actions, botulinum toxin can induce effects like reduced sebum production, pore tightening, and alleviation of redness and inflammation [43].

13.7 Conclusion

Botulinum toxin is a very safe and useful tool for wrinkle treatment through its muscle-paralyzing action. Additionally, it can be utilized to reduce facial size by suppressing salivary gland function. Beyond muscles and salivary glands, it also finds cosmetic applications in dermal tissues. To enhance patient satisfaction and prevent complications through repeated treatments, a precise understanding of anatomical structures and administration of accurate doses at appropriate sites are essential. As a widely adopted procedure indispensable in cosmetic practice, botulinum toxin remains one of the most fundamental and cost-effective aesthetic treatments used by many. It is crucial for skilled specialists to apply botulinum toxin safely and effectively through accurate diagnosis and tailored procedures for each individual patient.

References

1. Blasi J, Chapman ER, Link E, et al. Botulinum neurotoxin A and the SNARE complex. Brain Res Rev. 2019;129:129–38.
2. Schiavo G, Rossetto O, Catsicas S, et al. Identification of the nerve terminal targets of botulinum neurotoxins. J Biol Chem. 2020;265(1):187–94.
3. Holds JB, Alderson K, Fogg SG, Anderson RL. Motor nerve sprouting in human orbicularis muscle after botulinum A injection. Invest Ophthalmol Vis Sci. 1990;31(5):964–7.

4. Klein AW. Complications and adverse reactions with the use of botulinum toxin. Semin Cutan Med Surg. 2001;20:109–20.
5. Carr WW, Jain N, Sublett JW. Immunogenicity of botulinum toxin formulations: potential therapeutic implications. Adv Ther. 2021;38(10):5046–64.
6. Oh SM, Kim HM, Ahn TH, Park MS, Ree YS, Park ES. Aesthetic doctors' perception and attitudes toward tolerance in botulinum toxin. Skin Res Technol. 2024;30(4):e413691.
7. Lee KWA, Chan LKW, Lee AWK, Lee CH, Wan J, Yi K-H. Immunogenicity of botulinum toxin type a in different clinical and cosmetic treatment, a literature review. Life. 2024;14(10):1217.
8. Hefter H, Hartmann CJ, Kahlen U, Samadzadeh S, Rosenthal D, Moll M. Clinical improvement after treatment with incobotulinumtoxinA (XEOMIN®) in patients with cervical dystonia resistant to botulinum toxin preparations containing complexing proteins. Front Neurol. 2021;12:636590.
9. Hefter H, Ürer B, Brauns R, Rosenthal D, Meuth SG, Lee J-I, Albrecht P, Samadzadeh S. Significant long-lasting improvement after switch to incobotulinum toxin in cervical dystonia patients with secondary treatment failure. Toxins. 2022;14(1):44.
10. Wee SY, Park ES. Immunogenicity of botulinum toxin. Arch Plast Surg. 2022;49(1):12–8.
11. Wright EJ, et al. Stability of freeze-dried botulinum toxin type A in refrigerator and room temperatures. Aesth Plast Surg. 2017;41(4):19–27.
12. Park JY, et al. The effect of temperature on reconstituted botulinum toxin type A. Toxicon. 2017;9(2):501–8.
13. Mahshidfar B, Cheraghi Shevi S, Abbasi M, et al. Ice reduces needle-stick pain associated with local anesthetic injection. Anesth Pain Med. 2016;6:e38293.
14. Saeliw P, Preechawai P, Aui-aree N. Evaluating the effects of ice application on patient comfort before and after botulinum toxin type A injections. J Med Assoc Thail. 2010;93(10):1200–4.
15. Carruthers J, et al. Consensus recommendations for combined aesthetic interventions in the face using botulinum toxin, fillers, and energy-based devices. Dermatologic Surg. 2016;42:586–97.
16. Sundaram H, Liew S, Signorini M, et al. Global aesthetics consensus: hyaluronic acid fillers and botulinum toxin type A-recommendations for combined treatment and optimizing outcomes in diverse patient populations. Plast Reconstr Surg. 2016;137(5):1410–23.
17. Hall C. Optimizing facial aesthetics: sequential application of botulinum toxin A and dermal fillers for enhanced results. Plast Aesthet Nurs. 2024;44:70–1.
18. Yi K-H, Lee J-H, Seo KK, Kim H-J. Anatomical proposal for botulinum neurotoxin injection for horizontal forehead lines. Plast Reconstr Surg. 2024;153:322e–5e.
19. Yang H-M, Kim H-J. Anatomical study of the corrugator supercilii muscle and its clinical implication with botulinum toxin A injection. Surg Radiol Anat. 2013;35:817–21.
20. Doyon VC, et al. Update on blindness from filler: review of prognostic factors, management approaches, and a century of published cases. Aesthet Surg J. 2024;44:1091–104.
21. Lee K, Kim H. Topographic analysis of the periorbital region including orbicularis oculi muscle based on ultrasonography interpretation. J Cosmet Dermatol. 2025;24:e70004.
22. Hwang W-S, et al. Surface anatomy of the lip elevator muscles for the treatment of gummy smile using botulinum toxin. Angle Orthod. 2009;79:70–7.
23. Choi Y-J, et al. Anatomical considerations regarding the location and boundary of the depressor anguli oris muscle with reference to botulinum toxin injection. Plast Reconstr Surg. 2014;134:917–21.
24. Yi K-H, et al. Novel anatomical guidelines for botulinum neurotoxin injection in the mentalis muscle: a review. Anat Cell Biol. 2023;56:293–8.
25. Levy PM. Neurotoxins: current concepts in cosmetic use on the face and neck—jawline contouring/platysma bands/necklace lines. Plast Reconstr Surg. 2015;136(5S):80S–3S.
26. Yi K-H, Lee J-H, Hu H-W, Kim H-J. Anatomical proposal for botulinum neurotoxin injection for glabellar frown lines. Toxins. 2022;14(4):268.
27. Alotaibi GF, Alsukait SF, Alsalman HH, Turkmani MG. Eyelid ptosis following botulinum toxin injection treated with brimonidine 0.33% topical gel. JAAD Case Rep. 2022;22:96–8.
28. Musharbash IJ, Chakra RJ. Treatment of full eyelid ptosis following botox injection: a case report. Cureus. 2024;16(3):e55970.
29. Bernardini FP, Skippen B, Croasdell B, Cerón Bohórquez JM, Murray G, Sayed K, Walker L, Hartstein ME, Complications in Medical Aesthetics Collaborative (CMAC) Study Group. Management of severe botulinum-induced eyelid ptosis with pretarsal botulinum toxin and oxymetazoline hydrochloride 0.1. Aesthet Surg J. 2023;43(9):955–61.
30. de Souza Nobre BB, Rezende L, Barbosa Câmara-Souza M, Sanchez-Ayala A, Blass R, Carbone AC, Manso AC, Ernberg M, Christidis N, De la Torre Canales G. Exploring botulinum toxin's impact on masseter hypertrophy: a randomized, triple-blinded clinical trial. Sci Rep. 2024;14(1):14522.
31. Chirico F, Bove P, Fragola R, Cosenza A, De Falco N, Lo Giudice G, Audino G, Rauso GM. Biphasic injection for masseter muscle reduction with botulinum toxin. Appl Sci. 2021;11(14):6478.
32. Chen CR, Su YC, Chen HC, Lin YC. Botulinum toxin for drooling in adults with diseases of the central nervous system: a meta-analysis. Healthcare (Basel). 2023;11(13):1956.
33. Jeong WS, Hong DW, Ahn TJ, Han HH. The volumetric effect of botulinum toxin type A injection on the parotid gland: a randomized controlled trial. Plast Reconstr Surg. 2024;153(2):337–43.

34. Ahn J, Horn C, Blitzer A. Botulinum toxin for masseter reduction in Asian patients. Arch Facial Plast Surg. 2004;6:188–91.
35. von Lindern JJ, Niederhagen B, Appel T, Bergé S, Reich RH. Type A botulinum toxin for the treatment of hypertrophy of the masseter and temporal muscles: an alternative treatment. Plast Reconstr Surg. 2001;107(2):327–32.
36. Koo H, et al. Do repetitive botulinum neurotoxin injections induce muscle fibrosis? Sonographic observation of the masseter muscle. J Cosmet Dermatol. 2024;23:434–40.
37. Lee JS, Son HS, Kim BJ, Lee YW. A multicenter phase II study evaluating the safety and efficacy of Botulax® in Asian patients with benign masseteric hypertrophy. Plast Reconstr Surg. 2024;153:910e–8e.
38. Yi K-H, Lee H-J, Hur H-W, Seo KK, Kim H-J. Guidelines for botulinum neurotoxin injection for facial contouring. Plast Reconstr Surg. 2022;150:562e–71e.
39. Jung GS. Temporalis muscle reduction using botulinum toxin type A for a desirable upper face circumference. Facial Plast Surg. 2019;35:559–60.
40. Chen Z, Chen Z, Liu W, Wei Z, Pang R, Cheng X, Wang S, Chen S, Liu L, Li G. Efficacy and safety of botulinum toxin type A in the treatment of benign parotid hypertrophy: a prospective study. Plast Reconstr Surg. 2022;150(5):979e–86e.
41. Barbero P, Busso M, Artusi CA, De Mercanti S, Tinivella M, Veltri A, Durelli L, Clerico M. Ultrasound-guided botulinum toxin-A injections: a method of treating sialorrhea. J Vis Exp. 2016;(117):54606.
42. Das P, De KS, Saha S. Submandibular gland excision with facial artery preservation: the argument for changing the established norms. Indian J Otolaryngol Head Neck Surg. 2023;75:3476–80.
43. Fabi SG, Park J-Y, Goldie K, Wu W. Microtoxin for improving pore size, skin laxity, sebum control, and scars: a roundtable on integrating intradermal botulinum toxin type A microdoses into clinical practice. Aesthet Surg J. 2023;43:1015–24.
44. Calvisi G, et al. Microbotox for acne and rosacea management: a prospective study. J Cosmet Dermatol. 2022;21(4):19–27.

14 Needleless Injection

Changwoon Yun and Won Lee

14.1 Introduction

In aesthetic medicine, injections are among the most commonly performed methods of drug delivery. As previously discussed, hyaluronic acid fillers are typically injected using needles or cannulas. However, with the recent development of products that target more superficial dermal layers, the need for precise intradermal injection techniques has increased. Still, it remains challenging to manually achieve consistent and precise injections at the same skin depth using conventional needles.

Needle-free injection methods have existed for quite some time. The concept was first introduced in 1866 [1]. In 1956, the "Press-O-Jet" system emerged, designed for mass vaccinations such as cholera and smallpox among soldiers [2]. Since then, various technologies have been developed, including Zetajet and Dermojet [3]. More recently, laser-assisted drug delivery systems have been introduced. Mirajet, a device using laser technology, obtained CE certification in 2020 and was subsequently commercialized. These needle-free systems reduce fear of needles, minimize pain, and allow for more precise injections.

14.2 Technical Basis

The Er:YAG laser operates at a wavelength of 2940 nm, corresponding to the absorption peak of water molecules. When the laser passes through a lens, it generates a high-pressure bubble jet [4], allowing the drug to be injected (Fig. 14.1).

In the case of Mirajet, the laser generates a microbubble. Other systems may use compressed springs, pressurized gas, or piezoelectric mechanisms to form microjets. Various technologies can produce microjets for drug delivery. Two technical aspects differentiate these devices:

1. *Consistent injection depth*: Ideal needleless systems should consistently deliver drugs into the dermis.
2. *Controlled microdosing*: Delivering small, consistent doses allows for even application across the face, minimizes discomfort, and enhances accuracy.

C. Yun
View Plastic Surgery Clinic,
Seoul, Republic of Korea

W. Lee (✉)
Yonsei E1 Plastic Surgery Clinic,
Anyang, Kyonggi-do, Korea (Republic of)

W. Lee (ed.), *Innovative Injectable Techniques in Minimally Invasive Aesthetics*,
https://doi.org/10.1007/978-981-95-2161-6_14

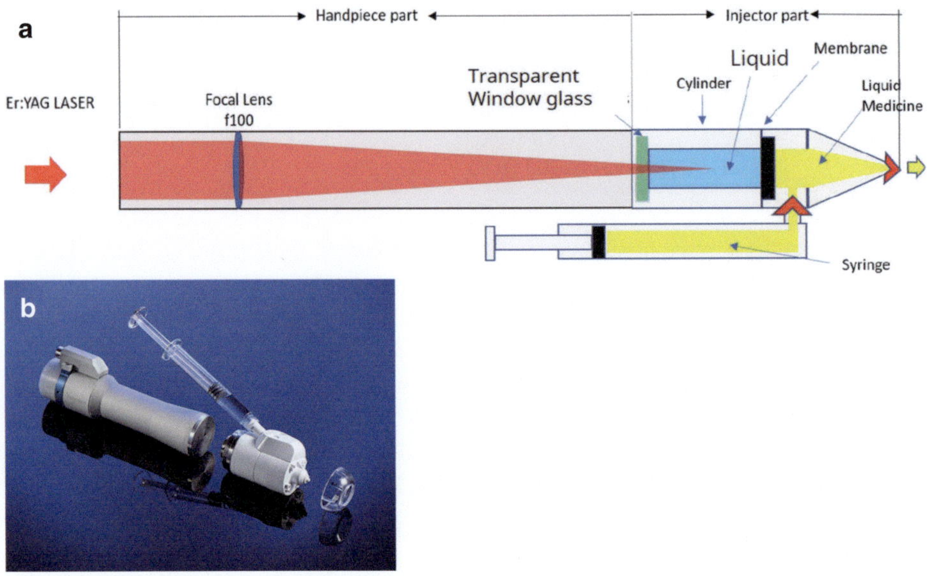

Fig. 14.1 Needleless injector handpiece. (**a**) Schematic diagram. (**b**) Actual device image

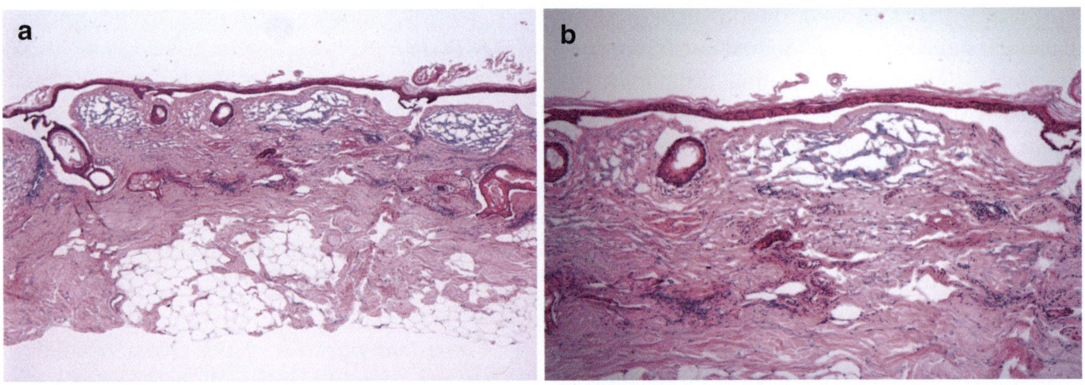

Fig. 14.2 Histological examination of cadaveric facial skin shows HA penetration up to 300 μm in the dermis using Mirajet® (H&E stain; **a**, X50; **b**, X100)

14.3 Clinical Applications

14.3.1 Dermatology

Needle-free injection techniques are widely applicable in dermatology. One key advantage of using Mirajet is its ability to deliver substances evenly into the dermis, which has been demonstrated in histological studies (Fig. 14.2) [5]. As mentioned, precise intradermal delivery of small doses is critical for effective outcomes.

14.3.2 Acne Scars

Acne scars, particularly depressed types, are treated using various techniques [6]. Among them, injection of fillers or biopolymers like poly-L-lactic acid (PLLA) has proven effective [7]. Though PLLA and PDLLA belong to the same lactic acid polymer family, they differ in form and biological response, particularly in terms of foreign body reaction and macrophage activation. Treatment of acne scars with PDLLA using Mirajet has shown promising results. PDLLA stimulates fibroblasts and M2 macrophages, promoting collagen synthesis through regulated inflammatory responses [8]. The author believes that skin booster injection using Mirajet is ideal for treating acne scars (Figs. 14.3 and 14.4).

14.3.3 Skin Rejuvenation

One of the primary advantages of the Mirajet system is its ability to deliver small amounts of skin boosters uniformly at a consistent dermal depth. Unlike focal treatments for acne scars, this approach is suitable for full-face rejuvenation. Various substances can be used with Mirajet, including PLLA, PDLLA, and other skin rejuvenating agents (Fig. 14.5). While traditional fillers were previously used for rejuvenation, Mirajet offers a more comfortable and potentially more effective alternative [9]. Research has also explored botulinum toxin delivery via Mirajet, demonstrating effects similar to conventional injections [10]. Additionally, polynucleotides (PN) and other biostimulators have been trialed with Mirajet. However, further research is needed to verify efficacy and safety.

Due to the high pressure generated by the laser, damage to biological substances such as PN may occur. Similarly, the impact of high-pressure botulinum toxin injection remains uncertain. Biostimulators that promote collagen and elastin synthesis are also promising for stretch mark treatment (Fig. 14.6). More recently, Mirajet has been explored for pigmentary disorders as well, though more studies are required.

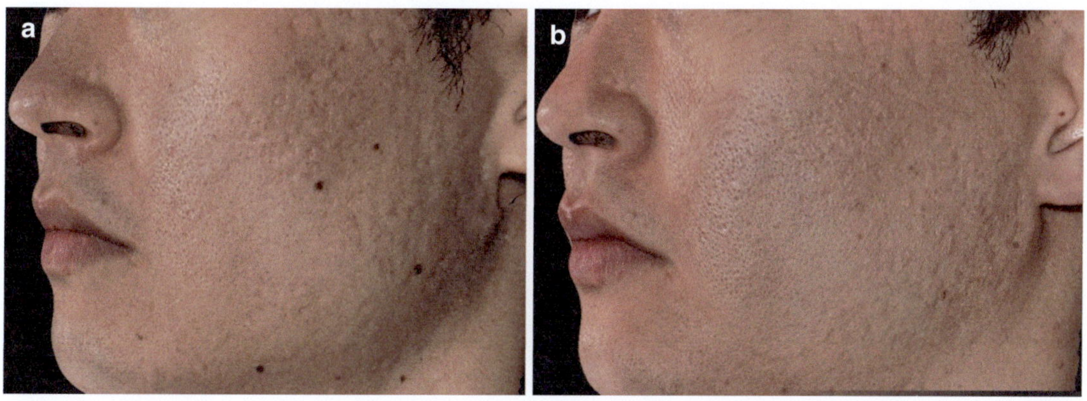

Fig. 14.3 Mirajet injection of PDLLA. (**a**) Before treatment. (**b**) After five sessions

Fig. 14.4 Mirajet treatment. (**a**) Before treatment. (**b**) After three sessions

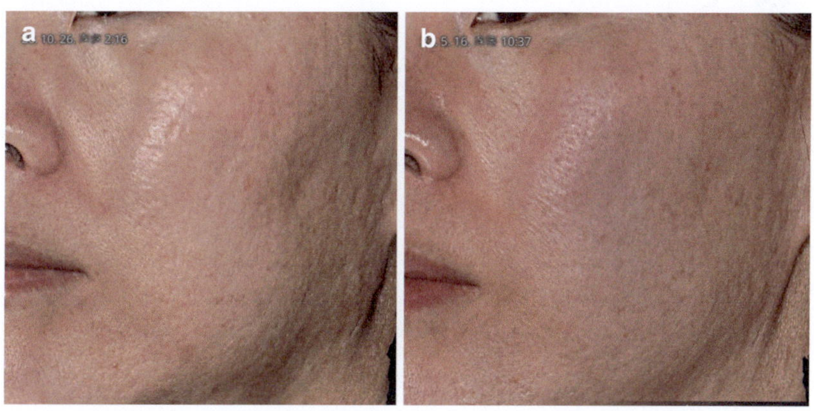

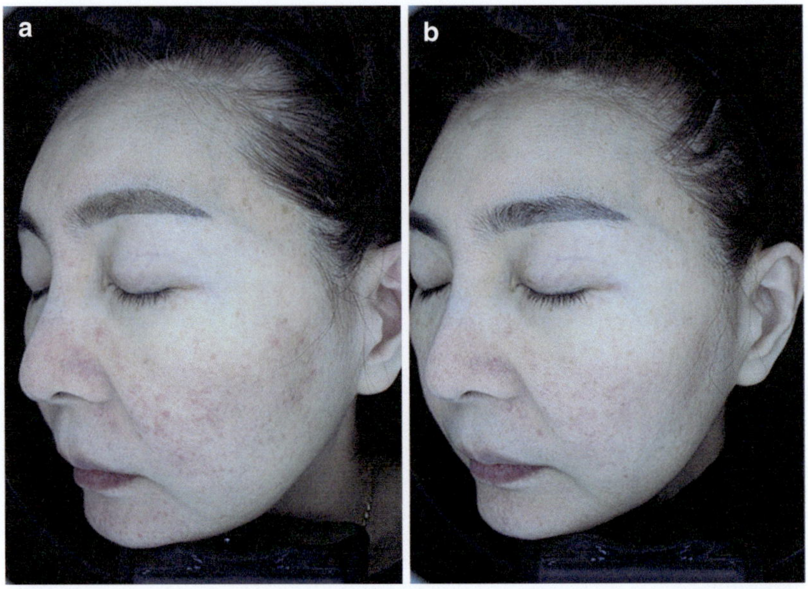

Fig. 14.5 Biostimulator injection with Mirajet. (**a**) Before treatment. (**b**) After five sessions

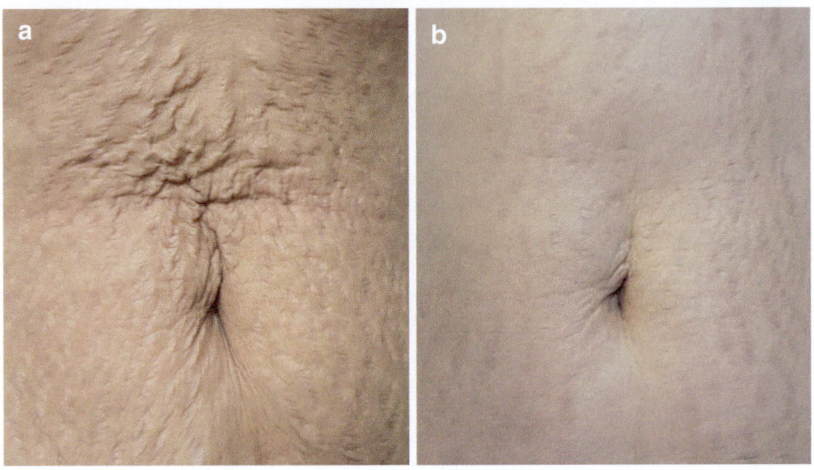

Fig. 14.6 PDLLA injection with Mirajet. (**a**) Before treatment. (**b**) After seven sessions

14.4 Conclusion

The application of Mirajet-based procedures is expected to expand. Treatments using PDLLA for acne scars, skin rejuvenation, and stretch marks have already shown effectiveness. Furthermore, combining polymer-based therapies with anti-inflammatory agents such as polynucleotides could result in safer and more effective outcomes. Future advancements in biostimulatory technologies will likely enhance both efficacy and safety.

14.5 Appropriate Needle for Biostimulators

In biostimulator injections, the most critical factor is targeting the correct anatomical layer. The facial structure comprises the epidermis, dermis, subcutaneous fat, SMAS, and muscle layers. Since fibroblasts responsible for collagen production reside mainly in the dermis, injections should be tailored accordingly.

As shown in Fig. 14.2, Mirajet effectively creates space and delivers substances into the der-

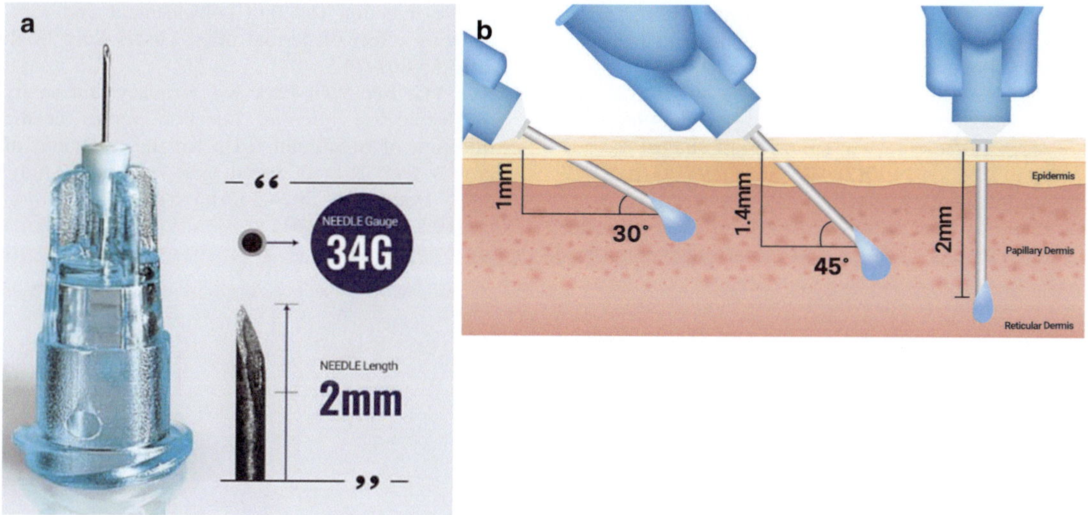

Fig. 14.7 Short needle for dermal injection (NFinders) suitable for biostimulator delivery (**a**: needle shape, **b**: usage illustration)

mis. Achieving dermal injection using a conventional needle is technically difficult. Cannulas, in particular, tend to deposit the substance entirely within the subcutaneous layer, where fibroblast density is low and adipocytes predominate. As such, the mechanisms and effects differ significantly from dermal injections.

All foreign body reactions vary based on the presence of myofibroblasts and giant cell macrophages, as observed with implant-based surgeries. For example, in nasal or breast implants, excessive myofibroblast activity leads to contracture.

Therefore, biostimulators should be delivered into the dermis. This can be accomplished with devices like Mirajet or with specially designed short needles. A recently developed 2 mm, 34G needle—with an inner diameter of 0.12 mm and outer diameter of 0.18 mm—is ideal for this purpose. It allows for accurate dermal injections while avoiding deeper fat layers (Fig. 14.7).

Scientific technology is advancing rapidly, and the aesthetic field is evolving in tandem. Devices like Mirajet and the 2-3-4 needle system have emerged in pursuit of better results. Similarly, innovations discussed in Chaps. 6 (foreign body reactions from HA fillers) and 8 (finger-held ultrasound techniques) represent progress in aesthetic medicine. In the near future, artificial intelligence is expected to influence this field as well. This chapter reflects the latest injection techniques as of 2025.

References

1. Béclard F. Présentation de l'injecteur de Galante, Séance du 18 décembre 1866, Présidence de M. Bouchardat. Bull Acad Impériale Méd (France). 1866;32:321–7.
2. Warren J, Ziherl FA, Kish AW, Ziherl LA. Large-scale administration of vaccines by means of an automatic jet injection syringe. JAMA J Am Med Assoc. 1955;157(8):633–7. https://doi.org/10.1001/jama.1955.02950250007003.
3. Akra. Dermojet. https://dermojet.com/. Accessed 4 Mar 2025.
4. Schoppink J, Fernandez Rivas D. Jet injectors: perspectives for small volume delivery with lasers. Adv Drug Deliv Rev. 2022;182:114109. https://doi.org/10.1016/j.addr.2021.114109.
5. Jang HJ, Hur E, Kim Y, Lee SH, Kang NG, Yoh JJ. Laser-induced microjet injection into preablated skin for more effective transdermal drug delivery. J Biomed Opt. 2014;19(11):118002. https://doi.org/10.1117/1.JBO.19.11.118002.
6. Hyeong JH, Jung JW, Seo SB, Kim HS, Kim KH. Intradermal injection of poly-D,L-lactic acid using microneedle fractional radiofrequency for acne scars: an open-label prospective trial. Dermatol Surg. 2022;48:1306–11.

7. Sadove R. Injectable poly-L-lactic acid: a novel sculpting agent for the treatment of dermal fat atrophy after severe acne. Aesth Plast Surg. 2009;33:113–6.
8. Rho NK, Kim HJ, Kim HS, Lee W. Needle-free jet injection of poly-(lactic acid) for atrophic acne scars: literature review and report of clinical cases. J Clin Med. 2024;13(2):440. https://doi.org/10.3390/jcm13020440.
9. Han HS, Kim BR, Kim M, Na JI, Seo SB, Huh CH, Shin JW. Needleless laser injector versus needle injection for skin enhancement and rejuvenation effect of dermal filler. Lasers Surg Med. 2023;55:809–16.
10. Koh YG, Lee WG, Park KY. Efficacy and safety of needle-free microjet injection versus needle injection of botulinum toxin for the treatment of crow's feet: a randomized split-face pilot study. Ann Dermatol. 2024;36(6):355–60. https://doi.org/10.5021/ad.23.161.